HANDBOOK OF COGNITIVE-BEHAVIORAL THERAPIES

Handbook of Cognitive-Behavioral Therapies

SECOND EDITION

Edited by
Keith S. Dobson

THE GUILFORD PRESS
New York   London

© 2001 The Guilford Press
A Division of Guilford Publications, Inc.
72 Spring Street, New York, NY 10012
www.guilford.com

Printed in the United States of America

This book is printed on acid-free paper.

Last digit is print number: 9 8 7 6 5 4 3 2 1

Library of Congress Cataloging-in-Publication Data

Handbook of cognitive-behavioral therapies / edited by Keith S.
  Dobson.—2nd ed.
      p. cm.
   Includes bibliographical references and index.
   ISBN 1-57230-601-7
      1. Cognitive therapy—Handbooks, manuals, etc.   2. Behavior
therapy—Handbooks, manuals, etc.   I. Dobson, Keith S.

  RC489.C63 H36 2000
  616.89'142—dc21

                                                      00-064027

About the Editor

Keith S. Dobson, PhD, is a full professor and director of clinical psychology in the Department of Psychology at the University of Calgary, Calgary, Alberta, Canada. His research interests are in the domain of mental health, and he conducts active research in the two primary areas of clinical depression and psychotherapy research. Dr. Dobson has over 120 publications, 7 books, and numerous conference presentations and clinical workshops to his credit, as well as active grants from the Alberta Heritage Foundation for Medical Research and the National Institute of Mental Health. In addition to his research interests, Dr. Dobson is actively involved in professional psychology, and has served on provincial and national organizations of social science, health, and psychology, including a former post as president of the Canadian Psychological Association. He maintains an active clinical practice in the area of cognitive therapy.

Contributors

Aaron T. Beck, MD, Department of Psychiatry, University of Pennsylvania, Philadelphia, Pennsylvania

Larry E. Beutler, PhD, Graduate School of Education, University of California at Santa Barbara, Santa Barbara, California

Kirk R. Blankstein, PhD, Department of Psychology, University of Toronto at Mississauga, Mississauga, Ontario, Canada

Lauren Braswell, PhD, Department of Psychology, University of St. Thomas, St. Paul, Minnesota

Roslyn Caldwell, PhD, Graduate School of Education, University of California at Santa Barbara, Santa Barbara, California

Joan Davidson, PhD, San Francisco Bay Area Center for Cognitive Therapy and Department of Psychology, University of California at Berkeley, Berkeley, California

Keith S. Dobson, PhD, Department of Psychology, University of Calgary, Calgary, Alberta, Canada

Robert J. DeRubeis, PhD, Department of Psychology, University of Pennsylvania, Philadelphia, Pennsylvania

David J. A. Dozois, PhD, Department of Psychology, University of Western Ontario, London, Ontario, Canada

Windy Dryden, PhD, PACE, Goldsmiths' College, University of London, New Cross, London, England

Thomas J. D'Zurilla, PhD, Department of Psychology, State University of New York at Stony Brook, Stony Brook, New York

Albert Ellis, PhD, Albert Ellis Institute for Rational Emotive Behavior Therapy, New York, New York

T. Mark Harwood, PhD, Graduate School of Education, University of California at Santa Barbara, Santa Barbara, California

Rick E. Ingram, PhD, Department of Psychology, Southern Methodist University, Dallas, Texas

Philip C. Kendall, PhD, ABPP, Department of Psychology, Temple University, Philadelphia, Pennsylvania

Robert A. Neimeyer, PhD, Department of Psychology, University of Memphis, Memphis, Tennessee

Arthur M. Nezu, PhD, Department of Clinical and Health Psychology, MCP Hahnemann University, Philadelphia, Pennsylvania

Jacqueline B. Persons, PhD, San Francisco Bay Area Center for Cognitive Therapy and Department of Psychiatry, University of California at San Francisco, San Francisco, California

Jonathan D. Raskin, PhD, Department of Psychology, State University of New York at New Paltz, New Paltz, New York

Lynn P. Rehm, PhD, Department of Psychology, University of Houston, Houston, Texas

Paul D. Rokke, PhD, Department of Psychology, North Dakota State University, Fargo, North Dakota

Zindel V. Segal, PhD, Center for Addiction and Mental Health—Clarke Division, Departments of Psychiatry and Psychology, University of Toronto, Toronto, Ontario, Canada

Greg J. Siegle, PhD, Department of Psychiatry, Western Psychiatric Institute, University of Pittsburgh School of Medicine, Pittsburgh, Pennsylvania

Tony Z. Tang, PhD, Department of Psychology, Northwestern University, Evanston, Illinois

Acknowledgments

A large number of individuals have contributed to the development of the field of cognitive-behavioral therapies; I have had the opportunity to talk to and work with many of these over the approximately two decades that I have worked as a researcher and clinician. My original mentor in this endeavor was Brian Shaw, with whom I still meet from time to time, and I always appreciate his perspective. Other key figures in my own development, and to whom I owe a great debt of gratitude, include the late Neil Jacobson, Steve Hollon, Tim Beck, Jack Rachman, Jeff Young, and Leslie Sokol. I have been involved in the field of cognitive-behavioral therapies during their nascence and ascendancy to what is arguably the dominant position in the field of psychotherapy. I have had the luxury of witnessing the growth in the clinical richness of the field, as well as the incredible advances in the evaluation of the efficacy of these models. The field has now grown to the point where it is almost impossible to keep abreast of the development, manualization, and evaluation of the cognitive-behavioral therapies. To those who participate in this overall endeavor, and with whom I have had the opportunity to talk, I give my acknowledgment.

When the first edition of this volume was published in 1988, I noted that a key impetus for the book was a graduate seminar in psychotherapy that I was teaching. I have been gratified over the years since the original publication to hear from many people whom I respect, who have told me that they used the book in their own universities. One of the most enjoyable aspects of my own career is the opportunity to work with graduate students—the intelligent, enthusiastic group of people who become the next generation of psychotherapists and researchers. I deeply appreciate my interactions with these individuals, and their energy is part of why a second edition of this book was completed.

A second clear factor behind the development of this second edition has been the ongoing support and enthusiasm of Seymour Weingarten, as editor-in-chief of The Guilford Press. His steady hand has been an important factor in bringing this book to the reader. I also want to acknowledge his editorial assistant Carolyn Graham, copy editor Marie Sprayberry, and senior production editor Jeannie Tang, all of The Guilford Press. The authors of this work obviously also deserve a round of applause for their extremely thoughtful and positive contributions to this book. Edna Haatainen and Karen McClure provided secretarial support for this book.

Finally, I want to acknowledge here the ongoing emotional support and encouragement I receive from my family: my wife, Debbie, my son, Chris, and my daughter, Beth. My children have largely grown up in the intervening time between the publication of the first edition and the current one, and it has been my particular pleasure to watch their development from children to young adults. Although I still have a number of years before even considering retirement, I hope to grow old and contented watching both my children and the field of cognitive-behavioral therapy emerge into full adulthood.

Preface

This book, like any second edition, reflects a continuing belief in the importance of the topic. What is perhaps somewhat unusual about this second edition is the fact that in the 13 years since the publication of the first edition, there has been a veritable explosion of innovative developments within the field of cognitive-behavioral therapies. This book is an effort to reflect that growth, while being sensitive to the fact that there remains much to do. As I noted in the preface to the first edition, at that time there really was no comprehensive book, written by the best experts in the field, that covered the broad domain of cognitive-behavioral therapy. Since then, a number of authored and edited books have undertaken this task, with varying degrees of success. The completion of this book obviously reflects the publisher's and my own belief that it fills an important place in the books on the topic.

An attempt is made in this volume to approach the cognitive-behavioral therapies from a theoretical perspective. The chapter topics were specifically chosen to sample the different approaches to cognitive-behavioral therapy, rather than to provide a technological or practice-oriented text. The intended audience is one that is learning about the field of psychotherapy and wishes to explore the growth of the various cognitive-behavioral models. In our adoption of this approach to the field, several issues have emerged that warrant some discussion here.

Many of the works that deal with cognitive-behavioral therapy use various disorders or clinical problems as the organizing framework for the exposition of the treatment. Such an approach is particularly useful for readers who want to learn how to deal with various clinical syndromes. In principle, it is potentially possible even to derive the theoretical substrate to these interventions by reading them in detail. My belief (based on my own clinical training, plus what is now considerable experience in training others) leads me to a somewhat different starting point, which is that what beginning therapists need most is a conceptual framework to help them understand what they are doing. My assumption is that acquiring this framework will make the more technical aspects of choosing and applying specific interventions to individual clients *relatively* simpler tasks. (On this point I do not want to be misunderstood; I do not believe that learning how to conduct competent psychotherapy is easy. Even if one knows or is told exactly what to do, considerable training and supervision are still required to do that work well.)

One of the basic questions raised in the first edition of this volume was that of what constitutes a "cognitive-behavioral therapy." This question is still valid today, and when I speak with others, it is not at all unusual to have someone ask about the difference among behavior therapy, cognitive therapy, and cognitive-behavioral therapy. Indeed, with the development of approaches such as schema-focused cognitive therapy and constructivist therapy, I continue to question myself on the conceptual limits to the field. Broadly speaking, my perception is that in order for a treatment to be accurately labeled a cognitive-behavioral therapy, it must be based on the mediational model. A therapist using this model is presumed to make the assumption that cognitive change will mediate or lead to behavioral change. Furthermore, cognitive-behavioral therapy rests on a pragmatic concern on the therapist's part about the client's adaptive (i.e., behavioral) functioning. Cognitive-behavioral therapists therefore use treatment methods to effect cognitive change in the service of behavioral change; furthermore, in order to assess their outcomes, both cognitive and behavioral (and in most instances emotional) assessment is required.

As I noted in the preface to the first edition, an important distinction can be made between those cognitive-behavioral therapies that focus on the process of therapy, and those that focus on cognitive content or on the hypothesized structure of cognitions. Thus some of the approaches are general in nature, and potentially could be applied to a number of content areas. In this regard, problem-solving therapy is an excellent example: It explicitly focuses on a process of approaching real-world problems, but is considerably less focused on the content of those problems. In contrast, approaches such as rational emotive behavior therapy or cognitive therapy make theory-based assumptions about the content of clients' cognitions, and therefore seeks changes in the content (and perhaps even structure) of these cognitions as therapeutic goals. Whether process changes, content changes, or both are the critical features of cognitive-behavioral therapies remains to be fully understood, however.

A phenomenon has recently begun that will have important consequences in psychotherapy. I am referring to the movement toward empirically supported treatments. This approach has taken the bold step of specifying the criteria by which treatments can be judged to have accumulated sufficient empirical evidence to warrant a decision that they are either well established or probably efficacious, and it has actually started to name treatments meeting those criteria. Although clinical psychology has espoused the perspective that science should inform practice, just as practice should inform science, there has been considerable resistance to implementing practice guidelines or standards based on empirical evidence about which treatments actually have documented positive outcomes. The establishment of criteria for empirically supported treatments therefore has the potential to advance this agenda considerably. Although the field must be sensitive to the quality of the evidence base, as well as to conceptual and practical limitations in the accumulation of evidence, it is nonetheless increasingly my view that the field of psychotherapy must move to a transparent, common-sense, evidence-based set of practices as soon as possible, in order to fulfill the mission of providing a human service worthy of the public's investment of trust, confidence, time, energy, and money. In this regard, I strongly endorse the movement toward empirically supported treatments. I also take some measure of satisfaction in the strong representation of cognitive-behavioral therapies amongst those therapies that have been recognized as empirically supported. One of my fervent hopes is that the field of cognitive-behavioral therapy continues its strong tradition of gathering outcome markers related to treatment efficacy.

One last theme that I want to touch upon briefly here is that of mechanisms of action in the cognitive-behavioral therapies. As readers of this volume are aware, the vast majority of the cognitive-behavioral therapies actually involve multiple components, which are often staged in a sequential set of learning experiences. Furthermore, the treatment manuals for many of the cognitive-behavioral therapies make the assumption that a sound working alliance, or collaborative set, between a therapist and client is an important prerequisite for the treatment to be maximally effective. To date, there is scant evidence that speaks to the question of what the necessary and sufficient elements of cognitive-behavioral therapy are. As the field develops, I believe that an important issue will be whether or not research can isolate those aspects of these treatments that perhaps account for most of the benefits associated with them. If so, it may then be possible to develop purer, or more hybridized, models to maximize patient benefit. It may also be possible to analyze, in a way that is not possible now, which aspects of treatment best interact with particular client characteristics to optimize treatment outcome.

Although the field of cognitive-behavioral therapies has advanced a long distance in the period of time between the first edition of this book and the current one, there remains much to be done. There are questions about the models that underlie these treatments, their conceptual relations, the mechanisms of action, which treatments are efficacious, which treatments are most efficacious, which treatments are most efficacious for which client groups, the acceptability of these treatments to patients, the best ways to train and disseminate these treatments, the age specificity of these treatments, the transportability of these treatments among various cultural and language groups, and many other issues as well. There is little doubt in my mind that the next decade will see at least as many innovations as the one just past. I look forward to participating in that process.

KEITH S. DOBSON, PHD
Calgary, Alberta, Canada

Contents

PART ONE: CONCEPTUAL ISSUES

1 Historical and Philosophical Bases   3
   of the Cognitive-Behavioral Therapies
      Keith S. Dobson and David J. A. Dozois

2 Cognitive Assessment: Issues and Methods   40
      Kirk R. Blankstein and Zindel V. Segal

3 Cognitive-Behavioral Case Formulation   86
      Jacqueline B. Persons and Joan Davidson

4 Cognition and Clinical Science: 111
   From Revolution to Evolution
      Rick E. Ingram and Greg J. Siegle

5 Cognitive-Behavioral Therapy   138
   and Psychotherapy Integration
      *Larry E. Beutler, T. Mark Harwood,
      and Roslyn Caldwell*

PART TWO: THE THERAPIES

6 Self-Management Therapies   173
     Paul D. Rokke and Lynn P. Rehm

7 Problem-Solving Therapies   211
     Thomas J. D'Zurilla and Arthur M. Nezu

8 Cognitive-Behavioral Therapy with Youth   246
     Lauren Braswell and Philip C. Kendall

9 Rational Emotive Behavior Therapy   295
     Windy Dryden and Albert Ellis

10 Cognitive Therapy   349
     Robert J. DeRubeis, Tony Z. Tang,
     and Aaron T. Beck

11 Varieties of Constructivism in Psychotherapy   393
     Robert A. Neimeyer and Jonathan D. Raskin

Index   431

PART ONE

CONCEPTUAL ISSUES

1

Historical and Philosophical Bases of the Cognitive-Behavioral Therapies

KEITH S. DOBSON
DAVID J. A. DOZOIS

One of the difficulties that has persisted through the development of cognitive-behavioral therapies has been the definition of their scope. Although the earliest of the cognitive-behavioral therapies emerged in the early 1960s (Ellis, 1962), it wasn't until the 1970s that the first major texts on "cognitive-behavior modification" appeared (Kendall & Hollon, 1979; Mahoney, 1974; Meichenbaum, 1977). The intervening period was one of considerable interest in cognition and in the application of cognitive theory to behavior change. Mahoney (1977), for example, noted that while psychology had generally undergone a "cognitive revolution," the same theoretical focus was being brought to bear upon clinical psychology. In creating a cognitive revolution in clinical psychology, different theorists and practitioners brought their own interests and perspectives to the problems at hand. As a result, a large number of models for cognitive and behavior change have been advanced, and a veritable armamentarium of clinical techniques has been added to the clinician's repertory.

This chapter reviews the major developments in the history of cognitive-behavioral therapies, with a focus on the period from the early 1960s to the mid-1970s. After briefly defining the current scope of cognitive-behavioral therapies and the essential nature of the general model for cognitive-behavioral therapy, we review the historical bases of this therapy. Six major reasons for the development of cognitive-behavioral therapy are proposed and discussed. The chapter then presents a formal chronology of the major cognitive-behavioral therapy approaches and summarizes their major philosophical underpinnings. The last section of the chapter emphasizes both the principles that all of these therapies share and those that vary from approach to approach.

DEFINING COGNITIVE-BEHAVIORAL THERAPY

At their core, all cognitive-behavioral therapies share three fundamental propositions:

1. Cognitive activity affects behavior.
2. Cognitive activity may be monitored and altered.
3. Desired behavior change may be affected through cognitive change.

Although using a slightly different title, Kazdin (1978) has argued a similar implicit set of propositions in his definition of cognitive-behavior modification: "The term 'cognitive-behavior modification' encompasses treatments that attempt to change overt behavior by altering thoughts, interpretations, assumptions, and strategies of responding" (p. 337). Cognitive-behavior modification and cognitive-behavioral therapy can thus be seen as nearly identical in their basic assumptions, and highly similar in treatment methods. Perhaps the one area where the two labels identify divergent therapies is with respect to treatment outcomes. Whereas cognitive-behavior modification seeks overt behavior change as an end result (Kazdin, 1978; Mahoney, 1974), some contemporary forms of cognitive-behavioral therapy focus their treatment effects on cognitions per se, in the belief that behavior change will follow. Ellis's (1962, 1979a; Dryden & Ellis, Chapter 9, this volume) efforts on belief change, for example, constitute a type of therapy that Kazdin's (1978) definition would not incorporate as a form of cognitive-behavior modification. The term "cognitive-behavioral therapy," therefore, is a broader term than "cognitive-behavior modification," subsuming cognitive-behavior modification within it (see also Dobson, Backs-Dermott, & Dozois, 2000).

The first of the three fundamental propositions of cognitive-behavioral therapy, that cognitive activity affects behavior, is a restatement of the basic mediational model (Mahoney, 1974). Although early theorists supporting cognitive-behavioral approaches had to document the theoretical and empirical legitimacy of this proposition (e.g., Mahoney, 1974), there is now overwhelming evidence that cognitive appraisals of events can affect the response to those events and that there is clinical value in modifying the content of these appraisals (e.g., Dobson et al., 2000; Granvold, 1994; Hollon & Beck, 1994). While debate certainly continues about the degree and exact nature of the appraisals an individual makes in different contexts (cf. Coyne, 1999; Held, 1995), the fact of mediation is no longer strongly contested.

The second fundamental proposition of cognitive-behavioral therapy is that cognitive activity may be monitored and altered. Implicit in this statement are a number of corollaries. For example, it is assumed that we may gain access to cognitive activity. As such, cognitions must be knowable and assessable. There is, however, reason to believe that access to cognitions is not perfect, and that people may report cognitive activities on the basis of their *likelihood* of occurrence rather than their *actual* occurrence (Nisbett & Wilson, 1977). Most researchers in the area of cognitive assessment, however, continue to attempt to document reliable and valid, cognitive assessment strategies, usually with behavior as the source of validational data (Merluzzi, Glass, & Genest, 1981; Segal & Shaw, 1988; Blankstein & Segal, Chapter 2, this volume). This area continues to be one where further research efforts are required (Clark, 1997).

Another corollary stemming from the second proposition is that assessment of cognitive activity is a prelude to the alteration of cognitive activity. This view, however, must be considered speculative. Although it makes conceptual sense that once we may measure a construct we may then begin to manipulate it, one does not *necessarily* follow from the other. In the arena of human change, the measurement of cognition may not necessarily assist change efforts. As has been written elsewhere (Mischel, 1981; Shaw & Dobson, 1981; Segal & Cloitre, 1993), most cognitive assessment strategies emphasize the content of cognitions and the assessment of cognitive results, rather than the cognitive process. Examining the process of cognition, as well as the interdependence among cognitive, behavioral, and affective systems, on the other hand, will most likely advance our understanding of change. This form of cognitive monitoring remains at a very rudimentary stage of development.

The third fundamental proposition of cognitive-behavioral therapy is a direct result of the adoption of the mediational model. It is that desired behavior change may be effected through cognitive change. Thus, while cognitive-behavioral theorists accept that overt reinforcement contingencies can alter behavior, they are likely to emphasize that there are alternative methods for behavior change, one in particular being cognitive change.

Due to the statement that cognitive change may influence behavior, many of the efforts of cognitive-behavioral researchers have been attempts to document a mediational influence. In one of the earliest demonstrations of this type, Nomikos, Opton, Averill, and Lazarus (1968) demonstrated that the same loud noise created different degrees of physiological disturbance, based upon the research participants' expectancy for the noise. In a similar vein, Bandura (1977) has employed the construct of self-efficacy to document that a subject's perceived ability to approach a fearful object is a strong predictor of actual behavior. Many studies have documented the role of cognitive appraisal processes in a variety of laboratory and clinical settings (Bandura, 1997).

Although the inference of cognitive activity has been generally accepted, it is still extremely difficult to document the further assumption that changes in cognition mediate behavior change. In order to do so, the assessment of cognitive change must occur independently of behavior. For example, if a phobic person approaches within 10 feet of a feared object, is treated through a standard type of systematic desensitization (including a graduated approach), and is then able to predict and demonstrate a closer approach to the feared object, making the inference that cognitive mediation of the behavior change has occurred is difficult at best and unnecessary at worst. On the other hand, if the same phobic person is treated with some form of cognitive intervention (e.g., imagined approach of the feared object), and then demonstrates the same behavior change, then cognitive mediation of that behavior change is much more plausible. Moreover, if that same phobic person demonstrates changes in his or her behavior toward objects previously feared but not specifically treated, then the cognitive mediation of that behavior change is essential, in that there must be some cognitive "matching" between the treated object and the other object of generalization.

WHAT CONSTITUTES COGNITIVE-BEHAVIORAL THERAPY?

A number of current approaches to therapy fall within the scope of cognitive-behavioral therapy as it is defined above. These approaches all share a theoretical perspective assuming that internal covert processes called "thinking" or "cognition" occur, and that cognitive events may mediate behavior change. Furthermore, these approaches all assume that behavioral change does not have to involve elaborate cognitive mechanisms. In some forms of cognitive-behavioral therapy, the interventions may have very little to do with cognitive appraisals and evaluations, but may be heavily dependent upon client action and behavior change. In fact, many cognitive-behavioral theorists explicitly state that because of the mediational hypothesis, not only is cognition *able* to alter behavior, but it *must* alter behavior, so that behavior change may thus be used as an indirect index of cognitive change. The actual outcomes of cognitive-behavioral therapy will naturally vary from client to client, but in general the two main indices used for change are cognition and behavior. To some extent emotional and physiological changes are also used as indicators of change, particularly where emotional or physiological disturbance is a major manifestation of the presenting problem in therapy (e.g., anxiety disorders, psychophysiological disorders).

There are three major classes of cognitive-behavioral therapies, each with a slightly different class of change goals (Mahoney & Arnkoff, 1978). The three classes of therapies are coping skills therapies, problem-solving therapies, and cognitive restructuring methods. Since a later section of this chapter details the specific therapies that fall within these categories of cognitive-behavioral therapies, this topic is not reviewed here. What is important to note, however, is that the different classes of therapy orient themselves toward different degrees of cognitive versus behavioral change. For example, coping skills therapies are of primary use in dealing with problems in which a person is largely reacting to events outside of him- or herself. In this case, therapy focuses on identifying and altering the ways in which the person may exacerbate the influence of negative events (e.g., engaging in anxiety-provoking thoughts and images) or employ strategies to lessen the impact of the negative events. Thus the primary markers of success within this form of therapy involve reductions in the consequences of negative events (e.g., less demonstrated anxiety) and behavioral signs of improved coping abilities. In the case of cognitive restructuring techniques, however, the desired change is more a result of disturbance created from within the person him- or herself.

Although cognitive-behavioral therapy targets both cognition and behavior as primary change areas, certain types of desired change would clearly fall outside the realm of cognitive-behavioral therapy. For example, a therapist who adopts a classical conditioning approach to the treatment of self-destructive behavior in an autistic child is not employing a cognitive-behavioral framework. In fact, any therapeutic regimen that adopts a stimulus–response model is not a cognitive-behavioral therapy. Only in instances where cognitive mediation can be demonstrated, and where cognitive mediation is an important component of the treatment plan, can the label "cognitive-behavioral" be applied.

Just as strictly behavioral therapies are not cognitive-behavioral, strictly cognitive therapies are also not cognitive-behavioral. For example, a therapeutic model that states that memories of a long-past traumatic event cause current disturbance, and that consequently targets those memories for change, is not a cognitive-behavioral therapy. It should be noted that this example carries the provision that no association between the current disturbance and past trauma is possible. In a case where a past trauma has occurred, but a recent event is highly similar to that past event and the client is experiencing distress as a function of both the past trauma and the current event, cognitive mediation is much more likely and the therapy may be cognitive-behavioral in nature.

Finally, therapies that base their theories in the expression of excessive emotions, as may be seen in cathartic models of therapy (Janov, 1970), are not cognitive-behavioral. Thus, although these therapies may posit that the emotions derived from extreme or negative mediational processes, the lack of a clear mediational model of change places them outside the field of cognitive-behavioral therapy.

HISTORICAL BASES
OF COGNITIVE-BEHAVIORAL THERAPY

As students of modern psychological history know, cognitive-behavioral therapies grew out of traditional behavior therapy, which in turn was an innovation from radical behavioral approaches to human problems. The major distinction between cognitive-behavioral and behavioral therapies, as previously stated, is the incorporation of the mediational perspective into the cognitive-behavioral approaches to problems. This incorporation phenomenon occurred at different times with different cognitive-behavioral approaches, but occurred mainly during the end of the 1960s and the early part of the 1970s (Kazdin, 1978). A number of specific factors conspired at this time to make the development of cognitive-behavioral theory possible, and cognitive-behavioral therapy a logical necessity:

1. Although the behavioral perspective had been a dominant force for some time, it was becoming apparent by the end of the 1960s that a nonmediational approach was not expansive enough to account for all of human behavior (Breger & McGaugh, 1965; Mahoney, 1974). Bandura's (1965, 1971) accounts of vicarious learning defied traditional behavioral explanation, as did the work on delay of gratification by Mischel (Mischel, Ebbesen, & Zeiss, 1972). Similarly, children were learning grammatical rules well out of the ability of most parents and educators to reinforce discriminatively (Vygotsky, 1962), and behavioral models of language learning were under serious attack. Yet another sign of dissatisfaction with behavioral models was the attempt to expand these models to incorporate "covert" behaviors (i.e., thought) (Homme, 1965). Although this approach met with some limited optimism, criticisms from behavioral quarters made it apparent that extensions of this sort were not consistent with the behavioral emphasis on overt phenomena.

2. Just as there was growing dissatisfaction with the strict stimulus–response nonmediational model of behavior, there continued to be a rejection of the strongest alternative perspective, the psychodynamic model of personality and therapy. Early writings in the area of cognitive-behavioral therapy (e.g., Beck, 1967, pp. 7–9; Ellis, 1973; Ellis, 1979a, p. 2) included statements that summarily rejected psychoanalytic emphases on unconscious processes, historical material, and the need for long-term therapy that relied heavily on the development of insight regarding the transference–countertransference relationship. Beyond philosophical disagreements with some of the basic tenets of psychodynamic models, reviews of the outcome literature suggested that the efficacy of traditional psychotherapy was not particularly impressive (Eysenck, 1969; Luborsky, Singer, & Luborsky, 1975; Rachman & Wilson, 1971, 1980). Perhaps the boldest evaluative comment about the demonstrated efficacy of psychodynamic therapies came from Rachman and Wilson (1980), who stated that "there still is no acceptable evidence to support the view that psychoanalysis is an effective treatment" (p. 76).

3. A third factor that facilitated the development of cognitive-behavioral therapy was the fact that the very nature of some problems, such as obsessional thinking, made noncognitive interventions irrelevant. As was appropriate, behavior therapy was applied to disorders that were primarily demarcated by their behavioral correlates. Also, where disorders were multifaceted, behavioral therapists targeted the behavioral symptoms for change (e.g., Ferster, 1974). This focus on behavior provided a significant increase in therapeutic potential over past efforts, but was not fully satisfying to therapists who recognized that entire problems or major components of problems were going untreated. The development of cognitive-behavioral treatment interventions helped to fill a void in clinicians' treatment techniques.

4. A number of mediational concepts were being developed, researched, and established within experimental psychology (Neisser, 1967; Paivio, 1971). These models, of which the most influential perhaps was the information-processing model of cognition, were explicitly mediational and were receiving considerable support from cognition laboratories. One of the developments that was perhaps natural was the extension of information-processing models to clinical constructs (e.g., Hamilton, 1979, 1980; Ingram & Kendall, 1986; Neufeld & Mothersill, 1980).

Even beyond the development of general cognitive models, a number of researchers in the 1960s and 1970s conducted basic research into the cognitive mediation of clinically relevant constructs. Lazarus and associates, for example, conducted a number of studies during this period in which they documented that anxiety involves cognitive mediation (Lazarus, 1966; Lazarus & Alfert, 1964; Lazarus & Averill, 1972; Lazarus, Opton,

Nomikos, & Rankin, 1965; Lazarus & Folkman, 1984; Monat, Averill, & Lazarus, 1972; Nomikos et al., 1968). Taken together, the two research areas of general cognitive psychology and what may be termed "applied cognitive psychology" challenged behavioral theorists to account for the data being accumulated. In essence, the challenge amounted to a need for behavioral models to redefine their limits and incorporate cognitive phenomena into the models of behavioral mechanisms. Perhaps one of the earliest signs of this attempt at incorporation can be seen in the self-regulation and self-control literature, which developed during the early part of the 1970s (Cautela, 1969; Goldfried & Merbaum, 1973; Mahoney & Thoresen, 1974; Rachlin, 1974; Stuart, 1972). All of these various attempts to delineate self-control perspectives on behavior modification shared the idea that the individual has some capacity to monitor his or her behavior, to set internally generated goals for behavior, and to orchestrate both environmental and personal variables to achieve some form of regulation in the behavior of interest. In order to develop these self-control models, several cognitive processes had to be hypothesized, including attempts to define self-control strategies largely in terms of internal "cybernetic" components of functioning (e.g., Jeffrey & Berger, 1982).

5. Another aspect of the early formation of the cognitive-behavioral therapies was the development and identification of a number of theorists and therapists who identified themselves as being cognitive-behavioral in orientation. Some of the people to begin this process explicitly were Beck (1967, 1970), Cautela (1967, 1969), Ellis (1962, 1970), Mahoney (1974), Mahoney and Thoresen (1974), and Meichenbaum (1973, 1977). The establishment of several key proponents of a cognitive-behavioral perspective clearly had the effect of creating a *Zeitgeist* that drew the attention of others in the field. In addition, the creation of a journal specifically tailored to the emerging cognitive-behavioral field helped to further this trend. Thus the establishment in 1977 of *Cognitive Therapy and Research*, with Michael Mahoney as editor, provided a forum "to stimulate and communicate research and theory on the role of cognitive processes in human adaptation and adjustment" (from the cover of the journal). The existence of a regular publication in the area of cognitive-behavioral theory and cognitive-behavior modification allowed researchers and therapists to present provocative ideas and research findings to a wide audience.

6. A final but not unimportant historical factor contributing to the continued interest in the cognitive-behavioral perspective has been the publication of research studies that have found cognitive-behavioral treatments to be as effective as, or more effective than, strictly behavioral approaches. In an early critical review of cognitive-behavior modification, Ledgewidge (1978) reviewed 13 studies that contrasted cognitive-behavior modification with behavioral therapies and found no demonstrated superiority for either.

He noted that the studies he reviewed were based upon analogue populations, and that clinical trials were required for a more summative judgment. His largely critical review prompted a reply that largely dismissed Ledgewidge's criticisms as "premature" (Mahoney & Kazdin, 1979). Since this early controversy about the efficacy of cognitive-behavioral therapies, a number of reviews have clearly demonstrated that cognitive-behavioral therapies have a positive clinical impact (Berman, Miller, & Massman, 1985; Dobson & Craig, 1996; Dush, Hirt, & Schroeder, 1983; Miller & Berman, 1983; Shapiro & Shapiro, 1982). Indeed, the cognitive-behavioral therapies are notable for their presence among the list of empirically supported therapies (Chambless et al., 1996; Chambless & Hollon, 1998). It is important to note, however, that meta-analyses of therapeutic effectiveness question the extent to which cognitive-behavioral treatments are superior to strictly behavioral treatments (Berman et al., 1985; Glogcuen, Cottraux, Cucherat, & Blackburn, 1998; Miller & Berman, 1983). As the data base is further enlarged, more definitive statements will be possible about the effectiveness of these types of therapy. Ideally, what will emerge from continued research will be not only specific conclusions about the overall efficacy of cognitive-behavioral therapies, but also specific statements about the relative efficacy of different types of cognitive-behavioral therapies with specific types of clinical problems.

It becomes apparent from the present review that a number of compelling reasons have existed and continue to exist for the development of cognitive-behavioral models of dysfunction and therapy. These reasons include dissatisfaction with previous models of therapy, clinical problems that emphasize the need for a cognitive-behavioral perspective, the research conducted into cognitive aspects of human functioning, the *Zeitgeist* phenomenon that has led to an identified group of cognitive-behavioral theorists and therapists, and the growing body of research that supports the clinical efficacy of cognitive-behavioral interventions. With this general trend in mind, this chapter now turns to providing more in-depth summaries of the historical developments behind the large number of specific cognitive-behavioral therapies that have evolved over the past 35 years.

CONTEMPORARY COGNITIVE-BEHAVIORAL THERAPIES: A CHRONOLOGY

Cognitive-behavioral therapies represent hybrids of behavioral strategies and cognitive processes, with the goal of achieving behavioral and cognitive change. However, even a brief overview of the major therapeutic procedures subsumed under the general heading of cognitive-behavioral therapy reveals a diversity of principles and procedures. The diversification in the development and implementation of the cognitive-behavioral approach may be explained, in part, by the differing theoretical orientations of those who generated intervention strategies based on this perspective. For example, Ellis and Beck, the founders of rational-emotive behavior therapy and cognitive therapy, respectively, came from psychoanalytic backgrounds. In contrast, Goldfried, Meichenbaum, and Mahoney were trained originally in the principles of behavior modification.

Mahoney and Arnkoff (1978) organized the cognitive-behavioral therapies into three major divisions: (1) cognitive restructuring, (2) coping skills therapies, and (3) problem-solving therapies. Therapies included under the heading of cognitive restructuring assume that emotional distress is the consequence of maladaptive thoughts. Thus the goal of these clinical interventions is to establish more adaptive thought patterns. In contrast, coping skills therapies focus on the development of a repertoire of skills designed to assist the client in coping with a variety of stressful situations. The problem-solving therapies may be characterized as a combination of cognitive restructuring techniques and coping skills training procedures. Problem-solving therapies emphasize the development of general strategies for dealing with a broad range of personal problems, and stress the importance of an active collaboration between client and therapist in the planning of the treatment program.

In the subsections that follow, the evolution of the major therapies associated with the cognitive-behavioral tradition is described. This review is not intended to be exhaustive, and therefore excludes a number of therapies that have not stimulated a significant amount of research or clinical application.

Rational Emotive Behavior Therapy

Rational emotive behavior therapy (REBT; formerly called rational–emotive therapy, or RET) is regarded by many as one of the premiere examples of the cognitive-behavioral approach. The basic theory and practice of REBT were formulated by Albert Ellis over 40 years ago. Following extensive training and experience in psychoanalysis, Ellis began to question the efficacy and efficiency of the classical analytic method. He observed that patients tended to remain in therapy for considerable periods of time and frequently resisted psychoanalytic techniques such as free association and dream analysis. Moreover, Ellis questioned whether the personal insight that was assumed to lead to therapeutic change according to psychoanalytic theory resulted in durable changes in behavior.

Still, however, I was not satisfied with the results I was getting. For, again, a great many patients improved considerably in a fairly short length of time, and felt much better after getting certain seemingly crucial insights. But few of them were really cured, in the sense of being minimally assailed with anxiety or hostility. And, as before, patient after patient would say to me: "Yes, I see exactly what bothers me now and why I am bothered by it; but I nevertheless still am bothered. Now what can I do about that?" (Ellis, 1962, p. 9)

Discouraged by the limitations of the analytic method, Ellis began to experiment with more active and directive treatment techniques. Through a process of clinical trial and error, he gradually formulated a theory of emotional disturbance and a set of treatment methods that emphasized a practical approach to dealing with life problems. Although advocates of analytic theory considered Ellis's methods heretical, the advent of behavior therapy in the 1960s and the growing acceptance of the role of cognitions in understanding human behavior eventually fostered the acceptance of REBT as a potentially valid alternative to the more traditional models of psychotherapy.

At the core of REBT is the assumption that human thinking and emotion are significantly interrelated. According to Ellis's "ABC" model, neurotic symptoms or consequences (C) are determined by a person's belief systems (B) regarding particular activating experiences or events (A). The goal of therapy is to identify and challenge the irrational beliefs that are at the root of emotional disturbance. REBT assumes that individuals possess innate and acquired tendencies to think and behave irrationally. Thus, in order to maintain a state of emotional health, individuals must constantly monitor and challenge their basic belief systems.

Ellis (1970) identified 12 basic irrational beliefs that take the general form of unrealistic or absolutistic expectations. REBT assumes that when unrealistic, overgeneralized demands are replaced with realistic desires, preferences, or wishes, major changes in emotions and behaviors can occur. However, since individuals tend to forcefully preserve their irrational thought patterns, significant and durable changes require forceful methods of intervention.

REBT employs a multidimensional approach that incorporates cognitive, emotive, and behavioral techniques. Nevertheless, the major therapeutic tool remains a "logico-empirical method of scientific questioning, challenging, and debating" (Ellis, 1979a, p. 20) designed to assist individuals in surrendering irrational beliefs. In addition to disputation, REBT therapists may selectively employ a broad variety of techniques including self-monitoring of thoughts, bibliotherapy, role playing, modeling, rational emotive imagery, shame-attacking exercises, relaxation methods, operant conditioning, and skill training (Ellis, 1979b). The theory and practice of REBT have not undergone any major reformulations since their introduction. Thus Ellis's original conceptualization of RET, as outlined in his book *Reason and Emotion in Psychotherapy* (1962), remains a primary reference for this approach. The renaming of RET as REBT did not represent a change in philosophy or emphasis so much as it reflected Ellis's desire to reflect the broad interests of REBT therapists more accurately.

One of the major differences between REBT and other cognitive-behavioral approaches lies in its philosophical emphasis. Ellis's (1980) distinctly philosophical outlook is reflected in what he identifies as the major goals of REBT: self-interest, social interest, self-direction, tolerance of self and others, flexibility, acceptance of uncertainty, commitment to vital interests, self-acceptance, scientific thinking, and a nonutopian perspective on life. REBT assumes that individuals who adopt this type of rational philosophy will experience a minimum of emotional disturbance.

REBT has generated a large body of literature (see Dryden & Ellis, 1988 and Chapter 9, this volume). Unfortunately, the majority of articles published have been authored by REBT advocates rather than researchers concerned with collecting objective data concerning the validity and utility of REBT (Mahoney, 1979). Some publications suggest, however, that REBT is beginning to receive the objective empirical scrutiny that has been notably absent in the past (Haaga & Davison, 1993; Kendall & Bemis, 1983).

Cognitive Therapy

Aaron Beck, the primary founder of cognitive therapy, was originally trained in psychoanalysis. Like Ellis, Beck began to question psychoanalytic formulations of the neuroses, and in particular with respect to depression. In a paper published in 1963, Beck observed that cognitive factors associated with depression were largely ignored, in favor of the psychoanalytic emphasis on motivational–affective conceptualizations. However, on the basis of an investigation into the thematic content of the cognitions of psychiatric patients, Beck was able to distinguish consistent differences in the ideational content associated with common neurotic disorders, including depression. He also found that patients exhibited systematic distortions in their thinking patterns. Consequently, he generated a typology of cognitive distortions to describe these systematic errors, which included the now well-known concepts of arbitrary inference, selective abstraction, over-generalization, magnification, and minimization.

The findings of a 5-year research project at the University of Pennsylvania culminated in the 1967 publication of *Depression: Causes and Treatment*. In this volume, Beck outlined his cognitive model and therapy of depression and other neuroses. A second book, *Cognitive Therapy and the*

Emotional Disorders (Beck, 1976), presented in more detail the specific cognitive distortions associated with each of the neuroses; it also described the principles of cognitive therapy, with special reference to depression. In 1979, Beck coauthored a comprehensive treatment manual for depression, which presented cognitive interventions that had been developed over the previous decade of clinical work and inquiry (Beck, Rush, Shaw, & Emery, 1979).

From the early emphasis on unipolar depression, Beck's model (Beck, 1970) was extended to other disorders and difficulties, including anxiety (Beck, Emery, & Greenberg, 1985), bipolar disorder (Basco & Rush, 1996), marital problems (Beck, 1988), personality disorders (Beck, Freeman, & Associates, 1990; Layden, Newman, Freeman, & Morse, 1993; Linehan, 1993), substance use problems (Beck, Wright, Newman, & Liese, 1993), crisis management (Dattilio & Freeman, 1994), and anger (Beck, 1999). Throughout these developments, the cognitive model has maintained an emphasis on the way in which distorted thinking and unrealistic cognitive appraisals of events can negatively affect one's feelings and behavior. Therefore, it is assumed that the way in which an individual structures reality determines his or her affective state. Furthermore, the cognitive model proposes that a reciprocal relation exists between affect and cognition such that one tends to reinforce the other, resulting in a possible escalation of emotional and cognitive impairment (Beck, 1971).

"Schemata," defined as cognitive structures that organize and process incoming information, are proposed to represent the thought patterns acquired early in an individual's development. Whereas the schemata of well-adjusted individuals allow for the realistic appraisal of life events, those of maladjusted individuals result in the distortion of reality and facilitate psychological disorders (Beck, 1976). Thus the schematic processes of depressed individuals can be characterized as a negative cognitive triad, in which the views of the self, the world, and the future are disturbed (Hollon & Beck, 1979).

Consistent with the cognitive model, the goal of cognitive therapy is to replace the client's presumed distorted appraisal of life events with more realistic and adaptive appraisals. Treatment is based upon a collaborative, psychoeducational approach, which involves designing specific learning experiences in order to teach clients to (1) monitor automatic thoughts; (2) recognize the relations among cognition, affect, and behavior; (3) test the validity of automatic thoughts; (4) substitute more realistic cognitions for distorted thoughts; and (5) identify and alter underlying beliefs, assumptions, or schemata that predispose individuals to engage in faulty thinking patterns (Kendall & Bemis, 1983).

Unlike REBT, Beck's cognitive theory of psychopathology and cognitive techniques have been subjected to a substantial degree of empirical scrutiny (Clark, Beck, & Alford, 1999; Ingram, Miranda, & Segal, 1998). Cognitive therapy of depression is now considered to be a viable alternative to behavioral and biochemical interventions (DeRubeis, Tang, & Beck, Chapter 10, this volume; Hollon & Beck, 1979; Hollon, DeRubeis, & Evans, 1996). Cognitive therapy for anxiety disorders, in fact, has been shown to have superior efficacy to pharmacotherapy. The generalizability of Beck's model and therapy, and treatment efficacy with respect to other mental disorders, require further research (Clark et al., 1999). Nonetheless, the contributions of Beck and his associates have made a significant impact on researchers and clinicians alike, and will in all probability continue to stimulate research for many years to come (Dobson & Khatri, in press).

Self-Instructional Training

Donald Meichenbaum's clinical interests developed during a period when the technology of behavior therapy was flourishing and the then-radical ideas of Ellis (1962), Beck (1963), and other advocates of cognitive treatment approaches were beginning to attract the attention of a new generation of clinicians. Amidst this climate, Meichenbaum (1969) carried out a doctoral research program that investigated the effects of an operant treatment procedure for hospitalized schizophrenic patients trained to emit "healthy talk." He observed that patients who engaged in spontaneous self-instruction to "talk healthy" were less distracted and demonstrated superior task performance on a variety of measures. This serendipitous finding became the impetus for a long-term research program focusing on the role of cognitive factors in behavior modification (Meichenbaum, 1973, 1977).

The direction of Meichenbaum's research was influenced heavily by two Soviet psychologists, Luria (1961) and Vygotsky (1962), who studied the developmental relation among language, thought, and behavior. They suggested that the development of voluntary control over one's behavior involves a gradual progression from external regulation by significant others (e.g., parental instructions) to self-regulation as a result of the internalization of verbal commands. Consequently, the relation between verbal self-instruction and behavior became the major focus of Meichenbaum's research. He proposed that covert behaviors operate according to the same principles as do overt behaviors, and that covert behaviors are thus subject to modification via the same behavioral strategies employed to modify overt behaviors (Meichenbaum, 1973).

Meichenbaum's early attempts to explore the validity of this proposal involved the development of a self-instructional training (SIT) program designed to treat the mediational deficiencies of impulsive children (Meichenbaum & Goodman, 1971). The goals of the treatment program were fourfold: (1) to train impulsive children to generate verbal self-commands and respond to them appropriately; (2) to strengthen the mediational properties of children's inner speech, in order to bring their behavior under their own verbal control; (3) to overcome any comprehension, production, or mediational deficiencies; and (4) to encourage children to self-regulate their behavior appropriately. The specific procedures employed were designed to replicate the developmental sequence outlined by Luria (1961) and Vygotsky (1962): (1) A model performed a task, talking aloud, while a child observed; (2) the child performed the same task while the model gave verbal instructions; (3) the child performed the task while instructing him- or herself aloud; (4) the child performed the task while whispering the instructions; and (5) the child performed the task covertly. The self-instructions employed in the program included (1) questions about the nature and demands of the task, (2) answers to these questions in the form of cognitive rehearsal, (3) self-instructions in the form of self-guidance while performing the task, and (4) self-reinforcement. Meichenbaum and Goodman found that their self-instructional training program significantly improved the task performance of impulsive children across a number of measures relative to attentional and control groups.

Encouraged by the results of their initial studies, Meichenbaum and his associates sought to expand and refine SIT. Additional investigations were designed to examine the ability of SIT to generalize in the treatment of a variety of psychological disorders, including schizophrenia, speech anxiety, test anxiety, and phobias (Mahoney, 1974).

The behavioral background of Meichenbaum is evident in the procedural emphasis that SIT places on graduated tasks, cognitive modeling, directed mediational training, and self-reinforcement. SIT provides a basic treatment paradigm that may be modified to suit the special requirements of a particular clinical population. In general, clients are trained in six global skills related to self-instruction: (1) problem definition, (2) problem approach, (3) attention focusing, (4) coping statements, (5) error-correcting options, and (6) self-reinforcement (Kendall & Bemis, 1983). The flexibility of SIT is perhaps one of its most attractive features, and, not surprisingly, a large literature has accumulated on the utility of SIT for a variety of psychological disorders. An interesting side note is that recently Meichenbaum's clinical interests have changed somewhat. He has developed a constructive, narrative approach to the problem of posttraumatic stress disorder (Meichenbaum, 1994), in which more traditional SIT methods do not figure largely. It will be interesting to see the extent to which interest in SIT wanes, given the conflicting forces of the apparent loss of this key figure in the field, but a solid data base to substantiate SIT's clinical utility.

Systematic Rational Restructuring

Marvin Goldfried was among the growing number of clinicians in the early 1970s who challenged the adequacy of learning theory and advocated the incorporation of cognitive processes into conceptualizations of human behavior. Like many other behaviorally oriented researchers during this period, he supported the shift in emphasis from discrete situation-specific responses and problem-specific procedures to a focus on coping skills that could be applied across response modalities, situations, and problems (Mahoney, 1974). In a 1971 paper, Goldfried proposed that systematic desensitization be conceptualized in terms of a general mediational model, in contrast to Wolpe's (1958) counterconditioning model. Goldfried interpreted systematic desensitization as a means of teaching clients a general self-relaxation skill. In his attempt to transform desensitization into a more comprehensive coping skills training program, emphasis was placed on four components: (1) the description of the therapeutic rationale in terms of skills training; (2) the use of relaxation as a generalized or multipurpose coping strategy; (3) the use of multiple-theme hierarchies; and (4) training in "relaxing away" scene-induced anxiety, as opposed to the traditional method of terminating the imaginal scene at the first indication of subjective distress (Goldfried, 1973, 1979).

Goldfried's coping skills orientation eventually led to the development of a technique called "systematic rational restructuring" (SRR; Goldfried, Decenteceo, & Weinberg, 1974). Borrowing from the work of Dollard and Miller (1950) on the development of symbolic thinking processes, Goldfried (Goldfried & Sobocinski, 1975) suggested that early social learning experiences teach individuals to label situations in different ways. He argued that emotional reactions may be understood as a response to the way an individual labels situations, as opposed to a response to the situation per se. The extent to which individuals inappropriately distinguish situational cues as personally threatening will determine their subsequent maladaptive emotional and behavioral responses. Goldfried assumed that individuals can acquire more effective coping repertoires by learning to modify the maladaptive cognitive sets that they engage automatically when faced with anxiety-provoking situations. Thus the goal of SRR is to train clients to perceive situational cues more accurately. Thus, the implementation of SRR is divided into five discrete stages: (1) exposure to anxiety-provoking situations, using imaginal presentation or role playing; (2) self-evaluation of subjective anxiety level; (3) monitoring anxiety-provoking cognitions; (4) rational reevaluation of these maladaptive cognitions; and (5) observing one's subjective anxiety level following the rational reevaluation. Techniques utilized in therapy include relaxation methods, behavioral rehearsal, *in vivo* assignments, modeling, and bibliotherapy (Goldfried & Davison, 1976). As a coping skills approach, the ultimate goal of SRR is to provide clients with the personal resources to cope independently with future life stresses.

SRR was introduced during a period when a variety of coping skills training approaches were being designed and tested by behavioral researchers. Some of these multicomponent treatment packages have received more research attention than others, and many are similar in terms of their underlying rationale and therapeutic strategies. Unfortunately, even in the period between the first edition of the present volume and the current edition, SRR has not been investigated as extensively as other coping skills training programs. Nevertheless, it represents one of the first attempts to make operational a self-control treatment model designed to enhance treatment generalization through the use of training in general coping skills believed to be applicable in a variety of stress-provoking situations.

Anxiety Management Training

Suinn and Richardson's (1971) anxiety management training (AMT) program was introduced at about the same time that Goldfried (1971) proposed a reconceptualization of systematic desensitization. In their original article, Suinn and Richardson discussed three shortcomings of desensitization procedures: (1) the time-consuming nature of constructing anxiety hierarchies for each problem presented by clients undergoing treatment, (2) the relatively long duration of treatment, and (3) the absence of generalized coping strategies to prepare clients to deal effectively with future problems. These suggested limitations of conventional systematic desensitization techniques led to the development of a nonspecific approach for anxiety control that was designed to provide clients with a short-term coping skills training program applicable to a wide range of problem areas.

The theory underlying AMT assumes that anxiety is an acquired drive that has stimulus generalization properties. Autonomic responses associated with anxiety act as cues that facilitate and maintain avoidance behavior. Clients can be conditioned to respond to these discriminative cues with responses that eliminate the anxiety through the process of reciprocal inhibition. Thus the goal of AMT is to teach clients to use relaxation and competency skills in order to control their feelings of anxiety.

AMT emphasizes the elimination of anxiety without specific attention to the particular anxiety-provoking stimulus. In the first stage of treatment, clients receive training in deep muscle relaxation. Following this, clients are instructed to visualize anxiety-arousing scenes, and then to practice their relaxation skills and/or imagine responding to stimuli in a competent fashion (Suinn, 1972). A variety of anxiety-arousing scenes that may be unrelated to clients' specific problems are incorporated into the treatment program.

Empirical data regarding AMT are emerging slowly. One early study examined the efficacy of this coping strategy (Richardson & Suinn, 1973). Unfortunately, a matched control group was not included in the design, making the data difficult to interpret. A more recent study, however, showed that AMT was superior to a defined control group in a randomized clinical trial (Suinn, 1995). Given the lack of research, AMT has remained a less well-developed cognitive-behavioral approach than it might otherwise be.

Stress Inoculation Training

Like many of his contemporaries in the 1970s, Meichenbaum developed an interest in the multicomponent coping skills approach as a potentially effective therapeutic strategy. Following a review of the stress literature, Meichenbaum, Turk, and Burstein (1975) suggested several guidelines for the development of a coping skills treatment program, which were later incorporated into Meichenbaum's 1977 volume:

1. Coping devices are complex and need to be flexible. . . . [Any] coping-skills training approach should be flexible enough to incorporate a variety of cognitive and behavioral strategies that can be differentially employed.
2. [It is necessary] for any training technique to be sensitive to individual differences, cultural differences, and situational differences.
3. Skills training should encourage the utilization of available information and the incorporation of potentially threatening events into cognitive plans. To be effective, information should stimulate mental rehearsal . . . which may "short circuit" the experience of stress or reduce its after-effects.
4. Actual exposure during training to less threatening events has a beneficial effect. (Meichenbaum, 1977, pp. 148–149)

In particular, Meichenbaum emphasized the systematic acquisition of coping skills, highlighting the importance of learning to cope with small, manageable amounts of stress as a means of facilitating treatment maintenance and generalization. Stress inoculation training is the behavioral analogue of Orne's (1965) immunization model, and incorporates the guidelines that Meichenbaum and his associates gleaned from their review of the stress literature. The rationale underlying this approach is that clients who learn ways of coping with mild levels of stress are "inoculated" against uncontrollable levels of stress.

Meichenbaum and Cameron (1973) operationalized stress inoculation training in three stages. The first stage is educational, and involves didactic training about the nature of stressful reactions. The second stage involves the presentation of a number of behavioral and cognitive coping skills, including relaxation exercises, coping self-statements, and self-reinforcement.

In the final stage of application training, the client is exposed to a variety of stressors in order to rehearse his or her newly acquired coping skills.

Since the introduction of stress inoculation training in 1973, researchers have applied this approach to a variety of problems, including anxiety, anger, and pain (Meichenbaum & Deffenbacher, 1988; Meichenbaum & Jaremko, 1983, Meichenbaum & Turk, 1976). These studies led to a detailed clinical guidebook (Meichenbaum, 1985), and a large body of studies (see Meichenbaum, 1993, for a review). However, as Jaremko (1979) has observed, investigations into stress inoculation training have introduced a considerable degree of procedural variation. In this regard, Jaremko has proposed a revised procedural model that is intended to add greater uniformity to the research, as well as to increase the "usability" of this approach as a therapeutic procedure. As in the case with other multicomponent treatment programs, there remains a need for further empirical investigations to demonstrate the utility of the individual treatment components employed in stress inoculation training. Moreover, the validity of the underlying rationale requires additional research. Nonetheless, stress inoculation training is regarded by many as a useful therapeutic approach for the development of generalized coping skills.

Problem-Solving Therapy

In 1971, D'Zurilla and Goldfried published an article that proposed the application of problem-solving theory and research in behavior modification. With the goal of facilitating "generalized" behavior change, they conceptualized problem-solving therapy as a form of self-control training, emphasizing the importance of training the client to function as his or her own therapist. D'Zurilla and Goldfried (1971) summarized the rationale underlying this approach as follows:

> Ineffectiveness in coping with problematic situations, along with its personal and social consequences, is often a necessary and sufficient condition for an emotional or behavior disorder requiring psychological treatment; . . . general effectiveness may be most efficiently facilitated by training individuals in general procedures or skills which would allow them to deal independently with the critical problematic situations that confront them in day-to-day living. (p. 109)

According to D'Zurilla and Goldfried, "problem solving" refers to an overt or cognitive process that makes available a variety of effective response alternatives for coping with a problem situation and increases the likelihood of selecting the most effective response available (1971, p. 108). Drawing upon a large body of research regarding the fundamental operations involved in effective problem solving, D'Zurilla and Goldfried identified five overlapping stages as representative of the problem-solving process: (1) general orientation or "set," (2) problem definition and formulation, (3) generation of alternatives, (4) decision making, and (5) verification. Training in problem solving involves teaching clients these basic skills and guiding their application in actual problem situations.

Spivack and Shure (1974) initiated the systematic investigation into the efficacy of a problem-solving treatment approach. The interpersonal cognitive problem-solving (ICPS) model proposed by these researchers involves essentially the same skills as those outlined by D'Zurilla and Goldfried (1971). According to Spivack, Platt, and Shure (1976), effective ICPS involves (1) the ability to recognize the range of possible problem situations in the social environment; (2) the ability to generate multiple, alternative solutions to interpersonal problems; (3) the ability to plan a series of steps necessary to achieve a given goal; (4) the ability to foresee the short-term and long-term consequences of a given alternative; and (5) the ability to identify the motivational elements related to one's actions and those of others. ICPS training has been most commonly used with preschoolers and emotionally disturbed children. In general, ICPS training programs include discussion and structured activities involving hypothetical and actual interpersonal problem situations designed to teach problem-solving skills. Despite numerous methodological problems, the work of Spivack and his colleagues has resulted in the development of a growing interest in the potential of problem-solving therapies.

D'Zurilla and Nezu (1982) reviewed applications of D'Zurilla and Goldfried's (1971) original model of problem solving in adult clinical populations. Like Spivack and Shure (1974), they concluded that the data available at that time supported the existence of a relation between problem-solving skills and psychopathology. However, the evidence regarding the importance of the individual problem-solving components was less clear. Nonetheless, the broadening of clinical intervention objectives as recommended by D'Zurilla and Goldfried (1971) stimulated the development of a number of problem-solving therapies (Mahoney & Arnkoff, 1978). Problem-solving therapies have now been developed in several areas (for a review, see D'Zurilla & Nezu, Chapter 7, this volume), including stress management and prevention (D'Zurilla, 1990), depression (Nezu, 1986), anger management (Crick & Dodge, 1994), and coping with cancer (Nezu, Nezu, Friedman, Faddis, & Houts, 1998). Furthermore, a recent excellent addition to the list of clinical publications available is the second edition of a book describing the general problem-solving approach (D'Zurilla & Nezu, 1999). It is likely that the flexibility and pragmatism of these approaches will continue to attract the attention of clinicians in search of comprehensive treatment programs.

Self-Control Therapy

The trend toward developing treatment models that promoted a philosophy of self-control influenced Rehm's (1977) development of a self-control model of depression. The work of Rehm was guided to a great extent by the general model of self-regulation proposed by Kanfer (1970, 1971), which explains the persistence of certain behaviors in the absence of reinforcement in terms of a closed-loop feedback system of adaptive self-control. Kanfer suggested that three interconnected processes are involved in self-regulation: self-monitoring, self-evaluation, and self-reinforcement. Rehm adapted this model in order to explain the multivariate nature of depressive symptomatology. Thus symptoms of depression are conceptualized as the reflections or consequences of one or some combination of six deficits in self-control behavior. In the self-monitoring phase, potential deficits include the selective monitoring of negative events and the selective monitoring of immediate versus delayed consequences of behavior. Self-evaluative deficits consist of stringent self-evaluative criteria and inaccurate attributions of responsibility. In the third phase, self-reinforcement, deficits involving insufficient self-reward and excessive self-punishment may be observed in depressed individuals. According to Rehm (1981), the varied symptom profile in clinical depression is a function of different subsets of these deficits. Furthermore, these deficits may exist in varying degrees across individuals and can be observed prior to depressive episodes. The occurrence of a depressive episode is postulated to be a joint function of the degree of stress experienced and the self-control skills available for coping with the stressful situation.

Fuchs and Rehm (1977) developed the original treatment package based on Rehm's (1977) model of depression. Self-control therapy involves the sequential application of Kanfer's (1970, 1971) three self-regulatory processes as adapted by Rehm. "The assumption is that each may be conceptualized as a therapy module and that self-evaluation builds on self-monitoring, and that self-reinforcement builds on self-evaluation" (O'Hara & Rehm, 1983, p. 69). Each of the six self-control deficits is described over the course of treatment, with an emphasis on how a particular deficit is causally related to depression and what can be done to remedy the deficit. A variety of clinical strategies are employed to teach clients self-control skills, including therapist-directed group discussion, overt and covert reinforcement, behavioral assignments, self-monitoring, and modeling.

The appeal of Rehm's (1977) self-control model lies in its integration of a range of cognitive and behavioral variables on which other models of depression focus exclusively. In addition, Rehm's framework provides a logical analysis of the manner in which each of the various symptoms of depression is associated with a particular aspect of self-control. From a broader perspective, this self-control model appears to have potential as a general model of psychopathology. Unfortunately, the ability of Rehm's theoretical approach to generalize to other clinical disorders has not been researched (see Rokke & Rehm, Chapter 6, this volume). However, efforts to develop a comprehensive self-control therapy would seem a worthwhile endeavor.

Structural and Constructivist Psychotherapy

In a book entitled *Cognitive Processes and Emotional Disorders*, Guidano and Liotti (1983) introduced a structural approach to psychotherapy. This volume represented the culmination of 10 years of clinical research and experience, which began with the observation of a significant discrepancy between the demonstrated efficacy of behavioral techniques and the limited explanatory potential of learning theory. Following an extensive study of numerous literatures, including behavior therapy, social learning theory, evolutionary epistemology, cognitive psychology, psychodynamic theory, and cognitive therapy, Guidano and Liotti concluded that in order to understand the full complexity of emotional disorders and subsequently to develop an adequate model of psychotherapy, an appreciation of the development and the active role of an individual's knowledge of self and the world is critical: "Only a consideration of the structure within which the single elements of an individual's knowledge are placed allows us to understand how these elements rule and coordinate that individual's emotions and actions" (1983, p. 34).

Guidano and Liotti's structural model of cognitive dysfunction borrowed heavily from Bowlby's (1977) attachment theory. They suggested that relationships with significant others (i.e., parents or parental figures) determine the development of a child's self-image and provide continuous confirmation and reinforcement of this self-image. The definition of self is assumed to coordinate and integrate cognitive growth and emotional differentiation. If the self-concept is distorted or rigid, the individual is unable to assimilate life experiences effectively. This in turn leads to maladjustment and subsequent emotional distress, the final product being cognitive dysfunction. Different abnormal patterns of attachment are assumed to correspond to different clinical syndromes.

Guidano and Liotti's original formulation was expanded in subsequent writings by Guidano (1987, 1991). These writings expanded the idea that problem behaviors are believed to be the consequences of an individual's cognitive organization (i.e., the causal theories, basic assumptions, and tacit rules of inference that determine thought content). The patient is perceived as struggling to maintain a particular dysfunctional cognitive organization in the face of a continuously challenging environment. Thus the ultimate goal of psychotherapy is to modify these cognitive structures. In order for therapy to be effective, the therapist begins by identifying and modifying superficial cognitive structures, and then turns to the identification and modification of deeper cognitive structures (i.e., the implicit causal theories held by the patient). This therapeutic strategy bears close resemblance to Beck's (Beck et al., 1979) cognitive therapy, which begins with the assessment of the patient's automatic thoughts and subsequently leads to the specification of the basic assumptions underlying these thoughts. A major difference between the creators of structural psychotherapy and Beck, however, is the former theorists' emphasis on a postrationalist philosophy. Whereas Beck and related authors make a philosophical assumption that there is an external world that can be perceived accurately, or distorted, Guidano's later writings in particular make it clear that he was increasingly less concerned with the "truth value" of cognitive structures, than he was with the "validity value" or coherence of these structures:

> Adaptation, therefore, is the ability to transform perturbation arising from interaction with the world into information meaningful to one's experiential order. Maintaining an adaptive adequacy essentially means reserving one's sense of self by continuously transforming the perceived world rather than merely corresponding to it. This explains why the notion of the *viability* of knowing processes has become much more important in recent evolutionary epistemology than that of their *validity*. (Guidano, 1991, p. 9; italics in original)

In discussing psychotherapy as a strategic process, structural therapists refer to the analogy between the empirical problem-solving approach of the scientist and that of the patient. "Therapists should enable patients to disengage themselves from certain engrained beliefs and judgments, and to consider them as hypotheses and theories, subject to disproof, confirmation, and logical challenge" (Guidano & Liotti, 1983, p. 144). This analogy is similar to that drawn by Mahoney (1977) in his personal science approach. Various behavioral experiments and cognitive techniques compose the therapeutic armory from which the therapist selects a range of suitable tactics for a particular patient. They include such techniques as imaginal flooding, systematic desensitization, assertiveness training, coping skills training, problem-solving procedures, and rational restructuring. The final stage of the therapeutic process is conceptualized in terms of a "personal revolution" (Mahoney, 1980; Guidano, 1991), during which the patient, having rejected his or her old view of self and the world, is in a state of transformation and is establishing a new, more adaptive belief system.

Those who are familiar with the work of Beck et al. (1979), Ellis (1962), Mahoney (1977), and other advocates of the cognitive-behavioral perspective will recognize the many parallels between their writings and the structural approach to therapy. The distinction between rational and postrational approaches, however is important, and has been further amplified in the work of individuals who refer to their work as "constructivist psychotherapy" (Mahoney, 1995; Neimeyer, 1993, 1995; Neimeyer & Raskin, Chapter 11, this volume). Constructivist therapy takes the view of the individual as an imperfect personal scientist, who uses cognitive constructs to make sense out of experiences and to order choices in the world. From this perspective, key features of treatment include identifying preferences in behavior and understanding how meaning is attached to experience. There is less focus on the content of what is being thought about (as opposed, for example, to Beck's work, in which a typology of cognitions is associated with different emotional states; Beck, 1976), and more focus on the process of making meaning and connections among experiences. Consequently, therapy is less involved with corrective exercises about what is being thought, and more about facilitative exercises that emphasis the process of thinking, as well as the generation of meaning.

It is important to note constructivist therapy's close affinity to the philosophical schools of hermeneutics, and to narrative and discourse approaches to psychology. Nonetheless, there are more or less "radical" approaches within constructivism (see Neimeyer & Raskin, Chapter 11, this volume). At the extreme perspective in constructivist therapy, which has been referred to as "discursive critique," the epistemological position is that reality *only* exists in the mind of the individual, and that the only criterion for mental health is the coherence of that mind set. Individuals are viewed as contextual, and as temporally, culturally, sexually, and otherwise positioned with respect to other persons. As such, predetermined concepts of health and illness (such as the diagnostic nomenclature traditionally associated with mental disorders) lose their meaning, and treatment is no longer a process of helping people to recover from their diagnoses. At this extreme, the relationship between constructivist therapies and other cognitive-behavioral therapies begins to break down. Some have even questioned the extent to which constructivist therapies are conceptually compatible with cognitive-behavioral therapies: " . . . we suspect that the full integration of cognitive and constructivist models advocated by some authors . . . will encounter conceptual obstacles" (Neimeyer & Raskin, Chapter 11, p. 421). Other authors (e.g., Held, 1995) have critiqued the movement toward constructivist schools of thought in psychotherapy, and have suggested that therapies need to go "back to reality."

Clearly, the final chapter on the constructivist approaches to psychotherapy has yet to be written. It is not lost upon us that many former advocates of more traditional cognitive and cognitive-behavioral therapies are now advocating, in whole or in part, the use of treatments that draw on constructivist principles (Mahoney, 1991; Meichenbaum, 1994; Young, 1994). The extent to which these therapies will continue to be considered a part of the cognitive-behavioral movement, or will move off into antithetical and alternative approaches to therapy, remains to be seen.

SIMILARITY AND DIVERSITY
IN THE COGNITIVE-BEHAVIORAL THERAPIES

As our chronology of cognitive-behavioral models of psychopathology and therapy suggests, a large number of approaches can be identified as cognitive-behavioral in nature. At their very basis, these approaches all share the three fundamental assumptions discussed earlier in this chapter related to the mediational position. Briefly stated, the mediational position is that cognitive activity mediates the individual's responses to his or her environment, and to some extent dictates the individual's degree of adjustment or maladjustment. As a direct result of the mediational assumption, the cognitive-behavioral therapies share a belief that therapeutic change can be effected through an alteration of idiosyncratic, dysfunctional modes of thinking. In addition, due to the behavioral heritage, many of the cognitive-behavioral methods draw upon behavioral principles and techniques in the conduct of therapy, and many of the cognitive-behavioral models rely to some extent upon behavioral assessment of change to document therapeutic progress.

Beyond these central assumptions regarding the mediated nature of therapeutic change, there are a number of commonalities between limited sets of cognitive-behavioral therapies. Kendall and Kriss (1983), for example, have suggested that five dimensions can be employed to characterize cognitive-behavioral therapies: the theoretical orientation of the therapeutic approach and the theoretical target of change; various aspects of the client–therapist relationship; the cognitive target for change; the type of evidence used for cognitive assessment; and the degree of emphasis on self-control on the part of the client. The scheme they have proposed is a useful one for the identification of both similarities and differences between the various cognitive-behavioral therapies. Notwithstanding the coverage of the topic by Kendall and Kriss (1983), it also appears that other commonalities between the approaches that are not theoretically central can be identified. For example, one commonality among the various cognitive-behavioral therapies is their time-limited nature. In clear distinction from longer-term psychoanalytic therapy, cognitive-behavioral therapies attempt to effect change rapidly, and often with specific preset lengths of therapeutic contact. Many of the treatment manuals that have been written for cognitive-behavioral therapies recommend treatments in the range of 12–16 sessions (Chambless et al., 1996).

Related to the time-limited nature of cognitive-behavioral therapy is the fact almost all of the applications of this general therapeutic approach are to specific problems. Although this commonality is in no way a criticism of the various cognitive-behavioral therapies, the problem-focused nature of cognitive-behavioral interventions does in part explain the time limits that are commonly set in these approaches to therapy. Indeed, the utilization of these therapies for specific disorders and problems is a direct legacy from behavior therapy's emphasis on the collection of outcome data, and the focus on the remediation of specific, predefined problems. Thus, rather than being a limitation of cognitive-behavioral therapies, the application of these therapies to specific problems serves as a further demonstration of the continuing desire for the complete documentation of therapeutic effects. Also, the focus on specific problems allows for the experimental determination of the therapeutic limits of these various approaches, and potentially to the future ability of therapists to select the most efficacious therapy for their patients' problems.

A third commonality among the various cognitive-behavioral approaches is the belief that clients are the architects of their own misfortune, and that they therefore have control over their thoughts and actions. This assumption is clearly reflected in the types of patient problems that have been identified for cognitive-behavioral interventions. The most frequently cited appropriate problems include the "neurotic" conditions (e.g., anxiety, depression, and anger problems), self-control problems (e.g., overeating, behavioral management difficulties, child dysfunction), and general problem-solving abilities. These types of problems all make the assumption of patient control tenable. Even in the more general approaches to treatment, such as the constructivist models, the emphasis on individuals as the active agents in their own lives is a predominant focus.

Related to the assumption of patient control is another element shared by a number of the cognitive-behavioral therapies. This commonality has to do with the fact that many of the cognitive-behavioral therapies are by nature either explicitly or implicitly educative. Many of the therapeutic approaches include a therapist's teaching the therapeutic model to a patient, and many also involve the explication of the rationale for any interventions that are undertaken. This type of educative interaction between the therapist and patient is one facet that the various cognitive-behavioral therapies share, and that again sets them apart from other schools of therapy. Compare this with traditional psychoanalytic therapy, in which the therapist offers interpretations to the client (Blanck, 1976; Kohut, 1971), or strategic family therapy, in which the therapist may even dictate that the client do the opposite of what the therapeutic goal is in a "paradoxical" intervention (Haley, 1976; Minuchin & Fishman, 1981).

Directly related to the educative process often seen in cognitive-behavioral therapies is the implicit goal that many cognitive-behavioral therapists set, which is that the patients will not only overcome the referral problems during the course of therapy, but that they will also learn something about the process of therapy. In the event that the patients suffer a recurrence of their problems, they will therefore have some therapeutic skills to deal with the problems themselves. In some of the cognitive-behavioral therapies, the desire to have patients learn about the process of therapy is taken to its logical conclusion, so that time is spent in therapy reviewing the therapeutic concepts and skills that the patients have learned over the course of therapy, and that they may later employ in a maintenance or preventive manner (Beck et al., 1979; DeRubeis et al., Chapter 10, this volume; D'Zurilla & Goldfried, 1971; Mahoney, 1977).

Up to this point in this review, it may appear that cognitive-behavioral therapies have so many commonalities that the distinctions among them are more illusory than real. In fact, however, Kendall and Kriss (1983) have provided an excellent framework for the identification of differences among the specific approaches. Furthermore, even the brief overview of the various cognitive-behavioral therapies provided in this chapter demonstrates the very real diversity of models and techniques that have been developed by cognitive-behavioral therapists. It is thus no more appropriate to state that there is really one cognitive-behavioral approach than it is to state that there is one monolithic psychoanalytic therapy. As the chapters in this volume demonstrate, many different facets of cognitive-behavioral processes may be attended to, identified, and altered within the overarching definition of the cognitive-behavioral approach. The diversity of the cognitive-behavioral therapies, while undeniably present, does argue for further definitional and technical discussion among the proponents of the various approaches. There are at least two areas where further theory and research are required to help further differentiate the different therapies that are labeled as "cognitive-behavioral." These areas are the targets of therapeutic change and the modality specificity of intervention techniques.

Although cognitive-behavioral therapies share the mediational approach, and therefore all target "cognitions" for change, the variety of different specific labels and descriptions of cognitions seen in the cognitive-behavioral literature is truly overwhelming. A partial list of the various terms that have been applied to cognitive constructs and processes includes "cognitions," "thoughts," "beliefs," "attitudes," "ideas," "assumptions," "attributions," "rules for living," "self-statements," "cognitive distortions," "expectancies," "notions," "stream of consciousness," "scripts," "narratives," "ideation," "private meanings," "illusions," "self-efficacy predictions," "cognitive prototypes," and "schemata." Adding further to the confusion is that a number of these constructs have been developed in a purely clinical context (e.g., "self-efficacy predictions") and therefore have relatively clear definitions, but many others are terms also employed in other areas of psychology. Where terms are shared across subdisciplines of psychology, the application may not be identical, and semantic confusion may be the result. The use of the "schema" notion, for example, is fraught with potential difficulty, since the concept was first developed within cognitive psychology (Neisser, 1967), was later applied to social cognition (Markus, 1977), and now has been applied to clinical problems (Clark et al., 1999; Dobson, 1986; Goldfried & Robins, 1983; Ingram et al., 1998; Turk & Speers, 1983). Even a quick reading of the various applications of the term reveals that while the essence of the schema concept is intact throughout its various uses, several idiosyncratic applications have been suggested by various authors. Thus, while the elaboration of various specific cognitive processes and constructs is useful, it is important for theorists to define constructs precisely, and for others in the field to subscribe to these definitions. This increase in precision would help to clarify the terrain of cognitive-behavioral theory, and also may assist the efforts of researchers whose interest is cognitive assessment (Meichenbaum & Cameron, 1981). In this latter regard, it is clear that cognitive assessment is severely hampered by the lack of clear definitions of cognitive phenomena (e.g., Genest & Turk, 1981; Glass & Merluzzi, 1981; Shaw & Dobson, 1981); it is equally clear that further efforts in the area of cognitive assessment are required, to enable clinicians to fully document the nature and process of change during cognitive-behavioral therapy (Blankstein & Segal, Chapter 2, this volume; Clark, 1997; Kendall & Bemis, 1983; Segal & Shaw, 1988; Sutton-Simon, 1981).

A second major area where the further delineation of different approaches to cognitive-behavioral therapy may be possible is with respect to modality-specific techniques. Cognitive-behavioral therapists have been extremely innovative in the development of techniques, and have thereby added to the clinical armamentarium in numerous ways. However, it has not always been made clear what manner of technique is being developed (i.e., whether it is a generic and nonspecific technique, or is a modality-specific method). Although it may be reasonably argued that such distinctions are not important at a practical level, it is important from a theoretical perspective to know what limits different theorists place upon their models of therapy. Process research, which actually records and analyzes therapeutic interventions espoused by various therapeutic models, has often been suggested (DeRubeis, Hollon, Evans, & Bemis, 1982; Mahoney & Arnkoff, 1978; Prochaska, 2000) but has not yet become well advanced. This type of research has the potential of adding greatly to our knowledge of the extent to which different descriptions of therapies translate themselves in different clinical practice.

Finally, another area of research that may be profitably expanded is that which investigates the applications of various modes of cognitive-behavioral therapy to different presenting problems (Beutler, Harwood, & Caldwell, Chapter 5, this volume). When different approaches are contrasted in the context of different problems, it may become possible to start to suggest preferred treatment methods for specific patient problems. This matching of problems to therapies would not only represent a practical advantage over current clinical practice, but would also enable a better understanding of the mechanisms of change within each type of intervention, and within different types of patient problems.

Clearly, the field of cognitive-behavioral therapy has developed dramatically since its inception in the 1960s and 1970s. There are now a number of identifiable models of a cognitive-behavioral nature, and the demonstrated efficacy of these methods is generally strong (Chambless et al., 1996; Dobson et al., 2000). The continuing emphasis on the development of an adequate data base has enabled cognitive-behavioral theorists and therapists to make steady progress in research and practice, and can be expected to lead to continued improvements in the future. Some of the most pressing areas that require further conceptualization and research include the definition of cognitive phenomena (at both construct and process levels) and the procedural overlap among the various cognitive-behavioral therapies that currently exist. The next decade is likely to see considerable advances in the field.

REFERENCES

Bandura, A. (1965). Vicarious processes: A case of no-trial learning. In L. Berkowitz (Ed.), *Advances in experimental social psychology* (Vol. 2, pp. 3–57). New York: Academic Press.

Bandura, A. (1971). Vicarious and self-reinforcement processes. In R. Glaser (Ed.), *The nature of reinforcement* (pp. 51–130). New York: Academic Press.

Bandura, A. (1977). Self-efficacy: Toward a unifying theory of behavioral change. *Psychological Review, 84,* 191–215.

Bandura, A. (1997). *Self-efficacy: The exercise of control.* New York: Freeman.

Basco, M. R., & Rush, A. J. (1996). *Cognitive-behavioral therapy for bipolar disorder.* New York: Guilford Press.

Beck, A. T. (1963). Thinking and depression: 1. Idiosyncratic content and cognitive distortions. *Archives of General Psychiatry, 9,* 36–46.

Beck, A. T. (1967). *Depression: Causes and treatment.* Philadelphia: University of Pennsylvania Press.

Beck, A. T. (1970). Cognitive therapy: Nature and relation to behavior therapy. *Behavior Therapy, 1,* 184–200.

Beck, A. T. (1971). Cognition, affect, and psychopathology. *Archives of General Psychiatry, 24,* 495–500.

Beck, A. T. (1976). *Cognitive therapy and the emotional disorders.* New York: International Universities Press.

Beck, A. T. (1988). *Love is never enough.* New York: Harper & Row.

Beck, A. T. (1999). *Prisoners of hate: The cognitive bases of anger, hostility and violence.* New York: HarperCollins.

Beck, A. T., Emery, G., & Greenberg, R. L. (1985). *Anxiety disorders and phobias: A cognitive perspective*. New York: Basic Books.

Beck, A. T., Freeman, A., & Associates. (1990). *Cognitive therapy of personality disorders*. New York: Guilford Press.

Beck, A. T., Rush, A. J., Shaw, B. F., & Emery, G. (1979). *Cognitive therapy of depression*. New York: Guilford Press.

Beck, A. T., Wright, F. D., Newman, C. F., & Liese, B. S. (1993). *Cognitive therapy of substance abuse*. New York: Guilford Press.

Berman, J. S., Miller, R. C., & Massman, P. J. (1985). Cognitive therapy versus systematic desensitization: Is one treatment superior? *Psychological Bulletin, 97,* 451–461.

Blanck, G. (1976). Psychoanalytic technique. In B. J. Wolman (Ed.), *The therapist's handbook* (pp. 61–86). New York: Van Nostrand Reinhold.

Bowlby, J. (1977). The making and breaking of affectional bonds: 1. Etiology and psychopathology in the light of attachment theory. *British Journal of Psychiatry, 130,* 201–210.

Breger, L., & McGaugh, J. L. (1965). Critique and reformulation of "learning-theory" approaches to psychotherapy and neurosis. *Psychological Bulletin, 63,* 338–358.

Cautela, J. R. (1967). Covert sensitization. *Psychological Reports, 20,* 459–468.

Cautela, J. R. (1969). Behavior therapy and self-control: Techniques and implications. In C. M. Franks (Ed.), *Behavior therapy: Appraisal and status* (pp. 323–340). New York: McGraw-Hill.

Chambless, D., & Hollon, S. D. (1998). Defining empirically supported therapies. *Journal of Consulting and Clinical Psychology, 66,* 7–18.

Chambless, D., Sanderson, W. C., Shoham, V., Bennett-Johnson, S., Pope, K. S., Crits-Cristoph, P., Baker, M., Johnson, B., Woody, S. R., Sue, S., Beutler, L., Williams, D. A., & McCurry, S., (1996). An update on empirically validated therapies. *Clinical Psychologist, 49,* 5–18.

Clark, D. A. (1997). Twenty years of cognitive assessment: Current status and future directions. *Journal of Consulting and Clinical Psychology, 65,* 996–1000.

Clark, D. A., Beck, A. T., & Alford, B. A. (1999). *Scientific foundations of cognitive theory and therapy of depression*. New York: Wiley.

Coyne, J. C. (1999). Thinking interactionally about depression: A radical restatement. In T. Joiner & J. C. Coyne (Eds.), *The interactional nature of depression* (pp. 365–392). Washington, DC: American Psychological Association.

Crick, N. R., & Dodge, K. A. (1994). A review and reformulation of social information-processing mechanisms in children's social adjustment. *Psychological Bulletin, 115,* 73–101.

Dattilio, F. M., & Freeman, A. (Eds.). (1994). *Cognitive-behavioral strategies in crisis intervention*. New York: Guilford Press.

DeRubeis, R., Hollon, S. D., Evans, M., & Bemis, K. (1982). Can psychotherapies be discriminated?: A systematic investigation of cognitive therapy and interpersonal therapy. *Journal of Consulting and Clinical Psychology, 50,* 744–756.

Dobson, K. S. (1986). The self-schema in depression. In L. M. Hartman & K. R. Blankstein (Eds.), *Perception of self in emotional disorders and psychotherapy* (pp. 187–217). New York: Plenum Press.

Dobson, K. S., Backs-Dermott, B. J., & Dozois, D. (2000). Cognitive and cognitive-behavioral therapies. In C. R. Snyder & R. E. Ingram (Eds.), *Handbook of psychological change: Psychotherapy processes and practices for the 21st century* (pp. 409–428). New York: Wiley.

Dobson, K. S., & Craig, K. S. (Eds.). (1996). *Advances in cognitive-behavioral therapy.* Thousand Oaks, CA: Sage.

Dobson, K. S., & Khatri, N. (in press). Cognitive therapy: Looking forward, looking back. *Clinical Psychology: Science and Practice.*

Dollard, J., & Miller, N. E. (1950). *Personality and psychotherapy.* New York: McGraw-Hill.

Dryden, W., & Ellis, A. (1988). Rational–emotive therapy. In K. S. Dobson (Ed.), *Handbook of cognitive-behavioral therapies* (pp. 214–272). New York: Guilford Press.

Dush, D. M., Hirt, M. L., & Schroeder, H. (1983). Self-statement modification with adults: A meta-analysis. *Psychological Bulletin, 94,* 408–422.

D'Zurilla, T. J. (1990). Problem-solving training for effective stress management and prevention. *Journal of Cognitive Psychotherapy: An International Quarterly, 4,* 327–355.

D'Zurilla, T. J., & Goldfried, M. R. (1971). Problem-solving and behavior modification. *Journal of Abnormal Psychology, 78,* 107–126.

D'Zurilla, T. J., & Nezu, A. (1982). Social problem solving in adults. In P. C. Kendall (Ed.), *Advances in cognitive-behavioral research and therapy* (Vol. 1, pp. 254–281). New York: Academic Press.

D'Zurilla, T. J., & Nezu, A. (1999). *Problem-solving therapy: A social competence approach to clinical intervention* (2nd ed.). New York: Springer.

Ellis, A. (1962). *Reason and emotion in psychotherapy.* New York: Stuart.

Ellis, A. (1970). *The essence of rational psychotherapy: A comprehensive approach to treatment.* New York: Institute for Rational Living.

Ellis, A. (1973). *Humanistic psychotherapy.* New York: McGraw-Hill.

Ellis, A. (1979a). The basic clinical theory of rational–emotive therapy. In A. Ellis & J. M. Whiteley (Eds.), *Theoretical and empirical foundations of rational–emotive therapy* (pp. 33–60). Monterey, CA: Brooks/Cole.

Ellis, A. (1979b). The practice of rational–emotive therapy. In A. Ellis & J. M. Whiteley (Eds.), *Theoretical and empirical foundations of rational–emotive therapy* (pp. 61–100). Monterey, CA: Brooks/Cole.

Ellis, A. (1980). Rational–emotive therapy and cognitive-behavior therapy: Similarities and differences. *Cognitive Research and Therapy, 4,* 325–340.

Eysenck, H. (1969). *The effects of psychotherapy.* New York: Science House.

Ferster, C. G. (1974). Behavior approaches to depression. In R. J. Friedman & M. M. Katz (Eds.), *The psychology of depression: Contemporary theory and research* (pp. 29–54). New York: Wiley.

Fuchs, C. Z., & Rehm, L. P. (1977). A self-control behavior therapy program for depression. *Journal of Consulting and Clinical Psychology, 45,* 206–215.

Genest, M., & Turk, D. C. (1981). Think-aloud approaches to cognitive assessment. In T. Merluzzi, C. R. Glass, & M. Genest (Eds.), *Cognitive assessment* (pp. 233–269). New York: Guilford Press.

Glass, C., & Merluzzi, T. (1981). Cognitive assessment of social-evaluative anxiety.

In T. Merluzzi, C. R. Glass, & M. Genest (Eds.), *Cognitive assessment* (pp. 388–438). New York: Guilford Press.

Glogcuen, V., Cottraux, J., Cucherat, M., & Blackburn, I. (1998). A meta-analysis of the effects of cognitive therapy in major depression. *Journal of Affective Disorders, 49,* 59–72.

Goldfried, M. R. (1971). Systematic desensitization as training in self-control. *Journal of Consulting and Clinical Psychology, 37,* 228–234.

Goldfried, M. R. (1973). Reduction of generalized anxiety through a variant of systematic desensitization. In M. R. Goldfried & M. Merbaum (Eds.), *Behavior change through self-control* (pp. 297–304). New York: Holt, Rinehart & Winston.

Goldfried, M. R. (1979). Anxiety reduction through cognitive-behavioral intervention. In P. C. Kendall & S. D. Hollon (Eds.), *Cognitive-behavioral interventions: Theory, research, and procedures* (pp. 117–152). New York: Academic Press.

Goldfried, M. R., & Davison, G. C. (1976). *Clinical behavior therapy.* New York: Holt, Rinehart & Winston.

Goldfried, M. R., Decenteceo, E. T., & Weinberg, L. (1974). Systematic rational restructuring as a self-control technique. *Behavior Therapy, 5,* 247–254.

Goldfried, M. R., & Merbaum, M. (Eds.). (1973). *Behavior change through self-control.* New York: Holt, Rinehart & Winston.

Goldfried, M. R., & Robins, C. (1983). Self-schema, cognitive bias, and the processing of therapeutic experiences. In P. C. Kendall (Ed.), *Advances in cognitive-behavioral research and therapy* (Vol. 2, pp. 330–380). New York: Academic Press.

Goldfried, M. R., & Sobocinski, D. (1975). Effect of irrational beliefs on emotional arousal. *Journal of Consulting and Clinical Psychology, 43,* 504–510.

Granvold, D. K. (Ed.). (1994). *Cognitive and behavioral treatment: Methods and applications.* Belmont, CA: Wadsworth.

Guidano, V. F. (1987). *Complexity of the self.* New York: Guilford Press.

Guidano, V. F. (1991). *The self in process.* New York: Guilford Press.

Guidano, V. F., & Liotti, G. (1983). *Cognitive processes and emotional disorders: A structural approach to psychotherapy.* New York: Guilford Press.

Haaga, D. A. F., & Davison, G. C. (1993). An appraisal of rational–emotive therapy. *Journal of Consulting and Clinical Psychology, 61,* 215–220.

Haley, J. (1976). *Problem solving therapy.* San Francisco: Jossey-Bass.

Hamilton, V. (1979). An information processing approach to neurotic anxiety and the schizophrenias. In V. Hamilton & D. M. Warburton (Eds.), *Human stress and cognition: An information processing approach* (pp. 383–430). Chichester, England: Wiley.

Hamilton, V. (1980). An information processing analysis of environmental stress and life crises. In I. G. Sarason & C. D. Spielberger (Eds.), *Stress and anxiety* (Vol. 7, pp. 13–30). Washington, DC: Hemisphere.

Held, B. S. (1995). *Back to reality: A critique of postmodern theory in psychotherapy.* New York: Norton.

Hollon, S. D., & Beck, A. T. (1979). Cognitive therapy of depression. In P. C. Kendall & S. D. Hollon (Eds.), *Cognitive-behavioral interventions* (pp. 153–204). New York: Academic Press.

Hollon, S. D., & Beck, A. T. (1994). Cognitive and cognitive-behavioral therapies. In A. E. Bergin & S. L. Garfield (Eds.), *Handbook of psychotherapy and behavior change* (4th ed., pp. 428–466). New York: Wiley.

Hollon, S. D., DeRubeis, R. J., & Evans, M. D. (1996). Cognitive therapy in the treatment and prevention of depression. In P. M. Salkovskis (Ed.), *Frontiers of cognitive therapy* (pp. 293–317). New York: Guilford Press.

Homme, L. E. (1965). Perspectives in psychology: XXIV. Control of coverants, the operants of the mind. *Psychological Reports, 15,* 501–511.

Ingram, R. E., & Kendall, P. C. (1986). Cognitive clinical psychology: Implications of an information processing perspective. In R. E. Ingram (Ed.), *Information processing approaches to clinical psychology* (pp. 3–21). London: Academic Press.

Ingram, R. E., Miranda, J., & Segal, Z. V. (1998). *Cognitive vulnerability to depression.* New York: Guilford Press.

Janov, A. (1970). *The primal scream.* New York: Dell Books.

Jaremko, M. E. (1979). A component analysis of stress inoculation: Review and prospectus. *Cognitive Therapy and Research, 3,* 35–48.

Jeffrey, D. B., & Berger, L. H. (1982). A self-environmental systems model and its implications for behavior change. In K. R. Blankstein & J. Polivy (Eds.), *Self-control and self-modification of emotional behavior* (pp. 29–70). New York: Plenum Press.

Kanfer, F. H. (1970). Self-regulation: Research issues and speculations. In C. Neuringer & L. L. Michael (Eds.), *Behavior modification in clinical psychology* (pp. 178–220). New York: Appleton-Century-Crofts.

Kanfer, F. H. (1971). The maintenance of behavior by self-generated stimuli and reinforcement. In A. Jacobs & L. B. Sachs (Eds.), *The psychology of private events: Perspectives on covert response systems* (pp. 39–61). New York: Academic Press.

Kazdin, A. E. (1978). *History of behavior modification: Experimental foundations of contemporary research.* Baltimore: University Park Press.

Kendall, P. C., & Bemis, K. M. (1983). Thought and action in psychotherapy: The cognitive-behavioral approaches. In M. Hersen, A. E. Kazdin, & A. S. Bellack (Eds.), *The clinical psychology handbook* (pp. 565–592). New York: Pergamon Press.

Kendall, P. C., & Hollon, S. D. (Eds.). (1979). *Cognitive-behavioral interventions.* New York: Academic Press.

Kendall, P. C., & Kriss, M. R. (1983). Cognitive-behavioral interventions. In C. E. Walker (Ed.), *The handbook of clinical psychology: Theory, research, and practice* (pp. 770–819). Homewood, IL: Dow Jones–Irwin.

Kohut, H. (1971). *The analysis of the self.* New York: International Universities Press.

Layden, M., Newman, C. F., Freeman, A., & Morse, S. (1993). *Cognitive therapy of borderline personality disorder.* Needham Heights, MA: Allyn & Bacon.

Lazarus, R. S. (1966). *Psychological stress and the coping process.* New York: McGraw-Hill.

Lazarus, R. S., & Alfert, E. (1964). Short-circuiting of threat by experimentally altering cognitive appraisal. *Journal of Abnormal and Social Psychology, 69,* 195–205.

Lazarus, R. S., & Averill, J. R. (1972). Emotion and cognition: With special reference to anxiety. In C. D. Spielberger (Ed.), *Anxiety: Current trends in theory and research* (Vol. 2, pp. 242–284). New York: Academic Press.

Lazarus, R. S., & Folkman, C. (1984). *Stress, appraisal and coping.* New York: Springer.

Lazarus, R. S., Opton, E. M., Jr., Nomikos, M. S., & Rankin, N. O. (1965). The principle of short-circuitry of threat: Further evidence. *Journal of Personality, 33,* 622–635.

Ledgewidge, B. (1978). Cognitive behavior modification: A step in the wrong direction? *Psychological Bulletin, 85,* 353–375.

Linehan, M. M. (1993). *Cognitive-behavioral treatment of borderline personality disorder.* New York: Guilford Press.

Luborsky, L., Singer, G., & Luborsky, L. (1975). Comparative studies of psychotherapies: Is it true that everyone has won and that all must have prizes? *Archives of General Psychiatry, 32,* 995–1008.

Luria, A. R. (1961). *The role of speech in the regulation of normal and abnormal behavior.* New York: Liveright.

Mahoney, M. J. (1974). *Cognition and behavior modification.* Cambridge, MA: Ballinger.

Mahoney, M. J. (1977). Personal science: A cognitive learning therapy. In A. Ellis & R. Grieger (Eds.), *Handbook of rational psychotherapy* (pp. 352–368). New York: Springer.

Mahoney, M. J. (1979). A critical analysis of rational–emotive theory and therapy. In A. Ellis & J. M. Whiteley (Eds.), *Theoretical and empirical foundations of rational–emotive therapy* (pp. 167–180). Monterey, CA: Brooks/Cole.

Mahoney, M. J. (1980). Psychotherapy and the structure of personal revolution. In M. J. Mahoney (Ed.), *Psychotherapy process* (pp. 157–180). New York: Plenum Press.

Mahoney, M. J. (1991). *Human change processes.* New York: Basic Books.

Mahoney, M. J. (1995). The continuing evolution of the cognitive sciences and psychotherapies. In R. A. Neimeyer & M. J. Mahoney (Eds.), *Constructivism in psychotherapy* (pp. 39–65). Washington, DC: American Psychological Association.

Mahoney, M. J., & Arnkoff, D. B. (1978). Cognitive and self-control therapies. In S. L. Garfield & A. E. Bergin (Eds.), *Handbook of psychotherapy and behavior change: An empirical analysis* (2nd ed., pp. 689–722). New York: Wiley.

Mahoney, M. J., & Kazdin, A. E. (1979). Cognitive-behavior modification: Misconceptions and premature evacuation. *Psychological Bulletin, 86,* 1044–1049.

Mahoney, M. J., & Thoresen, C. E. (1974). *Self-control: Power to the person.* Monterey, CA: Brooks/Cole.

Markus, H. (1977). Self-schemata and processing information about the self. *Journal of Personality and Social Psychology, 35,* 63–78.

Meichenbaum, D. H. (1969). The effects of instructions and reinforcement on thinking and language behaviours of schizophrenics. *Behaviour Research and Therapy, 7,* 101–114.

Meichenbaum, D. H. (1973). Cognitive factors in behavior modification: Modifying what clients say to themselves. In C. M. Franks & G. T. Wilson (Eds.),

Annual review of behavior therapy: Theory, and practice (pp. 416–432). New York: Brunner/Mazel.

Meichenbaum, D. H. (1977). *Cognitive-behavior modification.* New York: Plenum Press.

Meichenbaum, D. H. (1985). *Stress inoculation training: A clinical guidebook.* New York: Pergamon Press.

Meichenbaum, D. H. (1993). Stress inoculation training: A twenty-year update. In R. L. Woolfolk & P. M. Lehrer (Eds.), *Principles and practice of stress management* (2nd ed., pp. 152–174). New York: Guilford Press.

Meichenbaum, D. H. (1994). *A clinical handbook/practical therapist manual for assessing and treating adults with posttraumatic stress disorder.* Waterloo, Ontario, Canada: Institute Press.

Meichenbaum, D. H., & Cameron, R. (1973). Training schizophrenics to talk to themselves. *Behavior Therapy, 4,* 515–535.

Meichenbaum, D. H., & Cameron, R. (1981). Issues in cognitive assessment: An overview. In T. Merluzzi, C. R. Glass, & M. Genest (Eds.), *Cognitive assessment* (pp. 3–15). New York: Guilford Press.

Meichenbaum, D. H., & Deffenbacher, J. L. (1988). Stress inoculation training. *Counseling Psychologist, 16,* 69–90.

Meichenbaum, D. H., & Goodman, J. (1971). Training impulsive children to talk to themselves. *Journal of Abnormal Psychology, 77,* 127–132.

Meichenbaum, D. H., & Jaremko, M. (Eds.). (1983*). Stress management and prevention: A cognitive-behavioral perspective.* New York: Plenum Press.

Meichenbaum, D. H., & Turk, D. (1976). The cognitive-behavioral management of anxiety, anger, and pain. In P. O. Davidson (Ed.), *The behavioral management of anxiety, depression, and pain* (pp. 1–34). New York: Brunner/Mazel.

Meichenbaum, D. H., Turk, D., & Burstein, S. (1975). The nature of coping with stress. In I. G. Sarason & C. D. Spielberger (Eds.), *Stress and anxiety* (Vol. 2, pp. 337–360). New York: Wiley.

Merluzzi, T., Glass, C., & Genest, M. (Eds.). (1981). *Cognitive assessment.* New York: Guilford Press.

Miller, R. C., & Berman, J. S. (1983). The efficacy of cognitive behavior therapists: A quantitative review of the research evidence. *Psychological Bulletin, 94,* 39–53.

Minuchin, S., & Fishman, H. C. (1981). *Family therapy techniques.* Cambridge, MA: Harvard University Press.

Mischel, W. (1981). A cognitive–social learning approach to assessment. In T. Merluzzi, C. Glass, & M. Genest (Eds.), *Cognitive assessment.* New York: Guilford Press.

Mischel, W., Ebbesen, E. B., & Zeiss, A. (1972). Cognitive and attentional mechanisms in delay of gratification. *Journal of Personality and Social Psychology, 21,* 204–218.

Monat, A., Averill, J. R., & Lazarus, R. S. (1972). Anticipating stress and coping reactions under various conditions of uncertainty. *Journal of Personality and Social Psychology, 24,* 237–253.

Neimeyer, R. A. (1993). Constructivism and the problem of psychotherapy integration. *Journal of Psychotherapy Integration, 3,* 133–157.

Neimeyer, R. A. (1995). Constructivist psychotherapies: Features, foundations and future directions. In R. A. Neimeyer & M. J. Mahoney (Eds.), *Constructivism in psychotherapy* (pp. 231–246). Washington, DC: American Psychological Association.

Neisser, U. (1967). *Cognitive psychology.* New York: Appleton-Century-Crofts.

Neufeld, R. W. J., & Mothersill, K. J. (1980). Stress as an irritant of psychopathology. In I. G. Sarason & C. D. Spielberger (Eds.), *Stress and anxiety* (Vol. 7, pp. 31–56). Washington, DC: Hemisphere.

Nezu, A. M. (1986). Efficacy of a social problem solving therapy approach for unipolar depression. *Journal of Consulting and Clinical Psychology, 54,* 196–202.

Nezu, A. M., Nezu, C. M., Friedman, S. H., Faddis, S., & Houts, P. S. (1998). *Helping cancer patients cope: A problem-solving approach.* Washington, DC: American Psychological Association.

Nisbett, R. E., & Wilson, T. D. (1977). Telling more than we can know: Verbal reports on mental processes. *Psychological Review, 84,* 231–259.

Nomikos, M. S., Opton, E. M., Jr., Averill, J. R., & Lazarus, R. S. (1968). Surprise versus suspense in the production of stress reaction. *Journal of Personality and Social Psychology, 8,* 204–208.

O'Hara, M. W., & Rehm, L. P. (1983). *Self-control group therapy of depression.* New York: Plenum Press.

Orne, M. (1965). Psychological factors maximizing resistance to stress with special reference to hypnosis. In S. Klausner (Ed.), *The quest for self-control* (pp. 286–328). New York: Free Press.

Paivio, A. (1971). *Imagery and verbal processes.* New York: Holt, Rinehart & Winston.

Prochaska, J. O. (2000). Change at differing stages. In C. R. Snyder & R. E. Ingram (Eds.), *Handbook of psychological change: Psychotherapy processes and practices for the 21st century* (pp. 109–127). New York: Wiley.

Rachlin, H. (1974). Self-control. *Behaviorism, 2,* 94–107.

Rachman, S. J., & Wilson, G. T. (1971). *The effects of psychological therapy.* Oxford: Pergamon Press.

Rachman, S. J., & Wilson, G. T. (1980). *The effects of psychological therapy* (2nd ed.). Oxford: Pergamon Press.

Rehm, L. (1977). A self-control model of depression. *Behavior Therapy, 8,* 787–804.

Rehm, L. (1981). A self-control therapy program for treatment of depression. In J. F. Clarkin & H. Glazer (Eds.), *Depression: Behavioral and directive intervention strategies* (pp. 68–110). New York: Garland Press.

Richardson, F. C., & Suinn, R. M. (1973). A comparison of traditional systematic desensitization, accelerated massed desensitization, and anxiety management training in the treatment of mathematics anxiety. *Behavior Therapy, 4,* 212–218.

Segal, Z. V., & Cloitre, M. (1993). Methodologies for studying cognitive features of emotional disorder. In K. S. Dobson & P. C. Kendall (Eds.), *Psychopathology and cognition* (pp. 19–50). San Diego, CA: Academic Press.

Segal, Z. V., & Shaw, B. F. (1988). Cognitive assessment: Issues and methods. In K. S. Dobson (Ed.), *Handbook of cognitive-behavioral therapies* (pp. 39–84). New York: Guilford Press.

Shapiro, D. A., & Shapiro, D. (1982). Meta-analysis of comparative therapy outcome studies: A replication and refinement. *Psychological Bulletin, 92,* 581–604.

Shaw, B. F., & Dobson, K. S. (1981). Cognitive assessment of depression. In T. Merluzzi, C. Glass, & M. Genest (Eds.), *Cognitive assessment* (pp. 361–387). New York: Guilford Press.

Spivack, G., Platt, J. J., & Shure, M. B. (1976). *The problem-solving approach to adjustment.* San Francisco: Jossey-Bass.

Spivack, G., & Shure, M. B. (1974). *Social adjustment of young children.* San Francisco: Jossey-Bass.

Stuart, R. B. (1972). Situational versus self-control. In R. D. Rubin, H. Fensterheim, J. D. Henderson, & L. P. Ullmann (Eds.), *Advances in behavior therapy* (pp. 67–91). New York: Academic Press.

Suinn, R. M. (1972). Removing emotional obstacles to learning and performance by visuomotor behavior rehearsal. *Behavior Therapy, 3,* 308–310.

Suinn, R. M. (1995). Anxiety management training. In K. D. Craig & K. S. Dobson (Eds.), *Anxiety and depression in adults and children* (pp. 159–179). Thousand Oaks, CA: Sage.

Suinn, R. M., & Richardson, F. (1971). Anxiety management training: A nonspecific behavior therapy program for anxiety control. *Behavior Therapy, 2,* 498–510.

Sutton-Simon, K. (1981). Assessing belief systems: Concepts and strategies. In P. C. Kendall & S. D. Hollon (Eds.), *Assessment strategies for cognitive-behavioral interventions* (pp. 59–84). New York: Academic Press.

Turk, D. C., & Speers, M. A. (1983). Cognitive schemata and cognitive processes in cognitive behavioral interventions: Going beyond the information given. In P. C. Kendall (Ed.), *Advances in cognitive-behavioral research and therapy* (Vol. 2, pp. 112–140). New York: Academic Press.

Vygotsky, L. S. (1962). *Thought and language.* Cambridge, MA: MIT Press.

Wolpe, J. (1958). *Psychotherapy by reciprocal inhibition.* Stanford, CA: Stanford University Press.

Young, J. (1994). *Cognitive therapy for personality disorders: A schema-focused approach.* Sarasota, FL: Professional Resource Press.

2

Cognitive Assessment
ISSUES AND METHODS

KIRK R. BLANKSTEIN
ZINDEL V. SEGAL

There are a thousand thoughts lying within a man that he
does not know till he takes up the pen to write.
—WILLIAM MAKEPEACE THACKERAY,
Henry Esmond

ASSESSMENT VIEWED
FROM THE COGNITIVE PERSPECTIVE

This chapter addresses a number of conceptual and methodological issues
relevant to the practice of cognitive assessment. We operate on the assumptions that human cognitive functioning can be described in information-processing terms, and that this perspective can inform clinical assessment
practices (Ingram & Kendall, 1986; Williams, Watts, MacLeod, &
Mathews, 1998). Within this model, humans are portrayed as actively seeking, selecting, and utilizing information (both internal and external) in the
process of constructing the mind's view of reality (Gardner, 1985). Such activity is an essential feature of the cognitive system and is thought to produce varied contents at different levels of operation. Although the passage
of information through the system is conceived of as both a synthetic and a
reciprocal process (Neisser, 1976), most of the attention in the literature
seems directed at three distinct levels of analysis. Cognitive structures (hypothesized inaccessible schemata guiding information processing), pro-

cesses (means of transforming environmental input and inferring meaning from it), and products or content (conscious thoughts and images) have been identified by numerous writers (Hollon & Kriss, 1984; Segal & Swallow, 1994; Turk & Salovey, 1985) as representing the principles or framework through which knowledge about the world is organized, how this framework guides ongoing processing, and what the most accessible products of this processing are, respectively.

PROCESS AND METHODS OF COGNITIVE ASSESSMENT

Choosing a particular method or technique of cognitive assessment is best conceived of as a theory-guided process. The type of cognition to be studied and its relationship to performance should be tied closely to the cognitive conceptualization of the disorder utilized by the clinician. Various classification systems have been presented for the numerous methods of assessing thoughts (Glass & Arnkoff, 1982; Kendall & Hollon, 1981). In their more recent work, Glass and Arnkoff (1997) have organized the methods of cognitive assessment according to each of four dimensions: temporality or timing (retrospective, concurrent, or about future events); degree of structure (endorsement versus production); response mode (written or oral); and nature of the stimulus (thoughts in general, imagined situation, situation viewed on videotape, role play, or *in vivo* situation). To this classification, we propose adding a fifth dimension: the source of thought evaluation (respondent or independent judge; Blankstein & Flett, 1990).

The resulting scheme yields a continuum of assessment procedures ranging from concurrent evaluations to retrospective evaluations. In some instances, participants are requested to give their thoughts about the probability of events (both positive and negative) occurring at some future time. Figure 2.1 illustrates the placement of some of the more common measures on this continuum. Cognitive assessment procedures may also be organized on the basis of structure; the extent to which the assessment imposes its own limits or format on the individual determines its placement on this dimension. Although highly structured self-statement endorsement measures are most commonly used, researchers have developed numerous production strategies to complement the use of questionnaires and inventories. Production measures require participants to generate or recall their thoughts. With this classification in mind, we now introduce the reader to the various methods of assessing participants' or clients' thoughts.

Recordings of spontaneous speech have been employed in a number of studies purportedly assessing respondents' or clients' actual self-talk. These

Specific Techniques

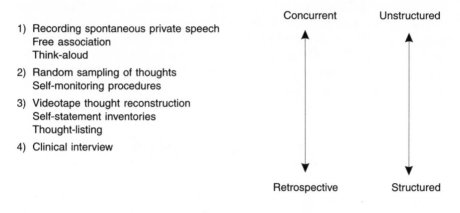

1) Recording spontaneous private speech
   Free association
   Think-aloud

2) Random sampling of thoughts
   Self-monitoring procedures

3) Videotape thought reconstruction
   Self-statement inventories
   Thought-listing

4) Clinical interview

Concurrent   Unstructured

Retrospective   Structured

FIGURE 2.1. Continuum of temporal and structural dimensions of cognitive assessment. Adapted from Glass and Arnkoff (1982). Copyright 1982 by Academic Press. Adapted by permission.

recordings can be taken unobtrusively or following specific instructions. They represent verbal behavior that can then be transcribed and coded into categories (Kendall & Hollon, 1981). This format is one of the most concurrent methods for assessing private speech, yet an investigator is limited to a subject's verbalizations and can never be fully certain that silences are synonymous with the lack of cognitive processing. The free-association method as it is used in psychoanalysis also meets the concurrence criterion, since patients are asked to verbalize their thoughts as they experience them throughout the therapy session (Bowers & Meichenbaum, 1984).

Think-aloud procedures have been used more frequently and require subjects to provide a continuous monologue of their thoughts during the performance of a specific task or in a particular situation. The exact wording of the think-aloud instructions may well influence the content of the protocol (Ericsson & Simon, 1984), but most instructions capture the spirit of this request by Duncker (1926) to his subjects:

> I am not primarily interested in your final solution, still less in your reaction time, but in your thinking behavior, in all your attempts, in whatever comes to your mind, no matter whether it is a good or less good idea or a question. Be bold. I do not count your wrong attempts, therefore speak them all out.

Davison and his colleagues (e.g., Davison, Robins, & Johnston, 1983; Davison, Vogel, & Coffman, 1997) have researched a paradigm they refer to as "articulated thoughts in simulated situations" (ATSS). Like videotape reconstruction and thought listing (see below), ATSS provides the researcher or clinician with control over stimulus situations, which are usually presented on audiotape (e.g., a social criticism tape designed to elicit thoughts associated with social anxiety). Participants are asked to imagine being in the situation and to think aloud after each 10- to 15-second segment of the 2- to 3-minute stimulus. This approach, like most cognitive production approaches, requires trained raters or judges to make inferences about the meaning of respondents' internal dialogues (usually in light of categories of interest specified by a particular cognitive theory).

At the next level on the continuum, we find methods such as random sampling of thinking in the natural environment and techniques for self-monitoring. Hurlburt (1997) recently reviewed three methods of randomly sampling thinking in participants' natural environments. Two of these methods seek to quantify thinking as it occurs as people move through their natural environment: thought sampling and the experience-sampling method. The procedures attempt to provide an unbiased estimate of cognitive activity (and sometimes affect and overt activities) by requesting people to record their current thoughts when cued either in person or, more typically, by a portable mechanical device (a beeper) at random or quasi-random intervals. On hearing the cue, participants immediately record their thoughts (and other aspects of their experience and behavior) by completing quantitative questionnaires and/or by writing narrative descriptions. This procedure enables data to be gathered over relatively long periods of time in a subject's own milieu at intervals that are not contingent on the occurrence of any particular environmental events. In an early clinical application of this method, Newton and Barbaree (1987) utilized *in vivo* random sampling to assess pain-related thoughts of individuals suffering from chronic headaches. They reported a significant shift in appraisal processes and coping strategies following a cognitive treatment program.

With self-monitoring procedures, the individual is asked to record the occurrence of specific thoughts in a particular stimulus situation or at a particular time. The utility of these procedures lies in the fact that they maximize the probability of gathering clinically relevant information concerning important but possibly infrequent situations. For example, Westling and Ost (1993) studied the nature and relation of distressing cognitions and symptoms experienced during panic attacks prospectively, via self-monitoring. Their 36 patients with panic disorder recorded a total of 285 panic attacks over the 2-week monitoring period. Over 90% of the recorded panic attacks contained catastrophic cognitions, and specific panic symptoms appeared to be associated with these catastrophic cognitions. However, a number of problems reflecting concerns about reactivity, social desirability, and evaluation apprehension are inherent in self-monitoring procedures in general.

Videotape thought reconstruction is a relatively infrequently used research strategy that allows a subject to reconstruct his or her train of thought at the time as accurately as possible by viewing a videotape of an actual or role-played problematic situation. Subjects may be asked to think aloud while watching themselves or, alternatively, to record the occurrence of specific cognitive events (Genest & Turk, 1981; Meichenbaum & Butler, 1980). With respect to temporality, these production procedures are classified as more retrospective than techniques discussed earlier since their aim is to facilitate a subject's "reliving" and reporting of a prior experience (as opposed to reporting on the original experience while it is occurring).

A methodology somewhat related to videotape thought reconstruction is thought listing, in which the subject is asked to list everything about which he or she is (or was) thinking. This production procedure can be more constrained than think-aloud methods, since the assessment typically takes place once a subject is out of a situation. The method can be likened to videotape thought reconstruction without the videotape. However, although thought listings are frequently collected retrospectively (e.g., listing what one was thinking during an examination immediately following the exam), they can also be obtained in anticipation of a task or situation (e.g., listing one's thoughts while waiting to take an exam) and even during the task or situation (e.g., listing one's thoughts at different points during the actual exam). The thought-listing technique is an open-response strategy for acquiring and categorizing the reportable products of people's cognitive processes, such as thoughts, expectations, appraisals, images, and feelings (Cacioppo, von Hippel, & Ernst, 1997). Detailed discussion of the procedures and instructions for administering the thought-listing procedure and for coding data can be found in Blankstein, Toner, and Flett (1989). A consistent finding that has emerged from various thought-listing studies conducted by Blankstein and his colleagues (e.g., Blankstein & Flett, 1990) is that test-anxious students report a preponderance of negative thoughts about the self and a relative absence of positive thoughts about the self.

Endorsement methods, such as self-report inventories or questionnaires that are designed to assess conscious self-verbalizations or thoughts, contain a predetermined set of thoughts that respondents are typically asked to rate with respect to whether or not they experienced each specific positively or negatively valenced thought in the assessment situation, as well as its frequency of occurrence (Glass & Arnkoff, 1997; Kendall & Hollon, 1981). Self-report measures have also been used to assess respondents' retrospective views of their thoughts, feelings, dysfunctional attitudes, attributions, and related cognitive activity over a long period of time. Although some skepticism has been expressed about the value of these questionnaire measures of cognition (e.g., Segal & Dobson, 1992), they undoubtedly constitute the most commonly used formal cognitive assessment method in clinical practice (Haaga, 1997). Instruments have been developed to assess cognitive contents particular to a large number of domains, such as depression (Hollon & Kendall, 1980), assertion (Schwartz & Gottman, 1976), social anxiety (Glass, Merluzzi, Biever, & Larsen, 1982), test anxiety (Blankstein, Flett, Boase, & Toner, 1990), panic attacks (Clum, Broyles, Borden, & Watkins, 1990), obsessional intrusions (Purdon & Clark, 1994), chronic headaches (Newton & Barbaree, 1987), back pain (Lefebvre, 1981), somatic problems (Moss-Morris & Petrie, 1997), nocturnal arousal (Fichten et al., 1998), and even pedophilia (Abel, Becker, Cunningham-Ratner, Rouleau, & Kaplan, 1984). A number of endorsement measures have been developed specifically for use with children (e.g., Ronan, Kendall, & Rowe, 1994). In their recent review of questionnaire methods, Glass and Arnkoff (1997) provide a description and psychometric analysis of 28 self-statement inventories that have individually been employed in at least three published studies.

The clinical interview can also be used as a retrospective cognitive assessment tool, in which case the therapist will ask the client to recall a recently upsetting situation and then recount what he or she was thinking and feeling at the time (Glass & Arnkoff, 1982). A number of other approaches to the assessment of cognitive products have been proposed and reviewed recently (see Lee & Peterson, 1997; Schwartz, 1997; Wegner & Smart, 1997). Finally, although our primary focus thus far has been on approaches that attempt to assess cognition relatively directly, via self-reports of thoughts and concurrent verbalizations, various other self-report and performance-based approaches have been used by clinical researchers to infer cognitive processes and "deep" cognitive structures such as negative self-schemata (Segal, Gemar, Truchon, Gurguis, & Hurowitz, 1995) or self-complexity (Linville, 1987; Gara et al., 1993). Segal and Cloitre (1993) have reviewed many of the methodologies available for studying the cognitive features of emotional disorders, such as attention, interpretation of ambiguous stimuli, judgments, and memory processes. Some of these experimental measures are described further in our discussion of cognitive assessment specific to anxiety and depression. It should be noted, however, that most of these measures have been used primarily in clinical-cognitive research and are not likely to be employed in clinical practice.

ADVANTAGES AND LIMITATIONS OF DIFFERENT SELF-REPORT METHODS

Structured assessments such as endorsement approaches to thought assessment, offer various benefits: economy; ease of scoring and administration; a greater potential for use in clinical practice; standardization across studies; and the accrual of normative data and psychometric information (Schwartz, 1997). The tradeoff, however, is against a potentially richer data source and the investigator's ability to uncover unexpected information about unpredicted relationships (Davison et al., 1997). Deciding on the degree of structure in an assessment often requires the specification of the extent to which an individual's ongoing cognitive activity can be "punctuated" while still providing an accurate picture of its flow. This concern has been introduced by Glass and Arnkoff (1982), who point out that as structure is added, the demand characteristics of the assessment also increase. Furthermore, structured measures typically provide only a few summary scores (Glass & Arnkoff, 1997).

Production methods such as the ATSS paradigm and related think-aloud procedures have an appeal due to their provision of the unaltered flow of subjects' thoughts (Davison et al., 1997). Constraints on ATSS data are imposed later through strategies to analyze the content, according to experimenter interest, and a virtually unlimited number of different coding schemes can be used on the same data set. Clearly, the instructions given to subjects to "think aloud" are consequential and can result in the reporting of varying contents. The rationale for videotape thought reconstruction is that providing subjects with a record of their performance will yield a richer description of what the person was thinking at the time, due to the enhancement of memory functions (Genest & Turk, 1981). Yet it is also possible that subjects are reporting what they guess they could have been thinking in the situation, rather than reporting on the basis of a visually and auditorily aided reexperience of the event (Nisbett & Wilson, 1977). In response to concerns such as these, there is a consensus within the field that a convergent-operations approach is optimal (Webb, Campbell, Schwartz, & Sechrest, 1966). Such an approach minimizes the drawbacks of relying on any one format alone, and if dissimilar measures produce similar findings, construct validity increases. As our discussion is now moving into the area of psychometrics, we turn our focus to questions of threats to the validity of the assessment process.

THREATS TO THE VALIDITY
OF COGNITIVE ASSESSMENT

In their influential book, Ericsson and Simon (1984) suggest three criteria that verbal reports should meet if they are to be validly used to infer underlying cognitive processes. The relevance criterion is that verbalization should be relevant to the given task or performance. To be considered pertinent, verbalizations should be logically consistent with those that have just preceded them, and the memory criterion is that some of the information attended to during the situation will be remembered. Ericsson and Simon then go on to illustrate how these criteria can be used as validity checks on verbal protocols:

> First, if a verbalization describes a situation that the subject can perceive directly, its correspondence with the stimulus can be checked. Second, its relevance to the task and to plausible steps toward a solution (as determined by task analysis) can be assessed. Third, its consistency with just previously verbalized information presumed to be in STM [short-term memory] can be checked. Finally, whenever there is reason to believe that verbalized information will be committed to memory, its presence in memory can be tested by subsequent demands for recall or recognition. (p. 172)

Questions regarding the construct validity of cognitive assessment focus not on the prediction of a criterion or on the match between the content of a test and a specific domain, but rather on the ability of the test itself to measure the cognitive processes of interest (Ghiselli, Campbell, & Zedeck, 1981). This issue particularly applies to questionnaire or self-report formats that supply a subject with a particular content. The subject is then asked to provide ratings on dimensions such as presence or absence, frequency, or degree of belief in the cognitions. The best example of this format is the self-statement inventory, which, as we have pointed out, remains one of the most popular formats for assessing self-talk. The question of content validity should not be confused with concerns regarding construct validity, for although we can establish that the self-statements of which the inventory is composed are a representative sample of what people in general think in the assessment situation, we are less clear on what actual meaning an endorsement of one of these statements carries for the individual. Furthermore, meaning checks or inquiries are rarely conducted in conjunction with the administration of self-statement inventories (Arnkoff & Glass, 1982; Kendall, 1982), leaving us with the assumption that self-statements have the same personal meanings for all individuals involved. One step toward remediation can be found in the "degree of belief" ratings that some inventories require in addition to the usual frequency tallies (e.g., the Automatic Thoughts Questionnaire; Hollon & Kendall, 1980).

Glass and Arnkoff (1982, 1997) provide a cogent critique of the assumption of an isomorphic relationship between cognition and its representation on self-statement inventories. They list four possibilities that reflect different processes underlying item endorsement. One possibility is that subjects who report having a thought "very frequently" may be indicating the thought's impact on or importance to them, and not necessarily its frequency. This concern is problematic for most self-statement inventories, since scores usually reflect a simple tally of items endorsed. The second possibility is that a translation process is occurring on the part of the respondents, whereby the idiosyncratic or fragmented thoughts the subjects experience in the situation are translated into grammatically correct sentences as they appear on the inventory. Alternatively, a decision to endorse a thought may reflect the view that the thought matches one's view of oneself, rather than the actual experience of that specific thought. For example, a woman who sees herself as poorly skilled at solving math problems may endorse an item such as "I'm no good at math, so why even try?" on an exam anxiety questionnaire, because it corresponds to her self-image, rather than because she necessarily had the thought. A final possibility is that endorsement may reflect the translation of affective experiences into a language-based format. Although a subject who is in a highly aroused state may or may not be aware of any ongoing cognitive activity, self-statement inventories may provide the opportunity for converting this experience into a linguistic representation of the event. In this sense, the subject may endorse a thought such as "I'm really getting worked up about this," without necessarily having experienced it at the time (Glass & Arnkoff, 1982).

Despite concerns about what endorsement measures are actually measuring and the meaning of responses, many of these questionnaires (see examples below and in the 1997 review by Glass & Arnkoff) have established criterion and predictive validity and have proved useful to researchers studying cognitive theories of adaptational outcomes. Furthermore, because they are sensitive to treatment effects, they are widely used as outcome measures by clinical researchers (Haaga, 1997). Glass and Arnkoff (1997) suggest that interpretation of frequency scores may be facilitated by rating additional aspects of each thought (e.g., intensity, salience, believability, controllability, importance, etc.), and they believe that expansion of the dimensions assessed should allow endorsement measures to approach the flexibility of production methods. They further suggest that practicing clinicians can probe their clients as to the subjective meaning of thoughts endorsed on a questionnaire.

It is clear that assessors must pay attention to the contextual cues associated with different assessment approaches. In some instances, targeted cognitions may not be available within the assessment context unless they are "primed" or activated, usually by induced mood states (Segal & Ingram, 1994). We examine this issue in greater detail below, in the context of our discussion of the cognitive vulnerability to depression. Although the use of priming appears to be particularly important in the assessment of cognitive structures or schemata, such priming may also be necessary in the assessment of conscious, "surface" cognitive products. The ATSS procedure (Davison et al., 1997) is a strategy that employs priming to elicit cognitive activity in response to hypothetical activating scenarios. This priming function probably facilitates the production of reliable and valid cognitions, and contributes to positive predictive and concurrent validity of the procedure. Although it is possible that questionnaire items used in endorsement approaches to assessing thoughts could serve as a semantic prime, Segal and Ingram (1994) argue that the use of questionnaires as primes should be used with caution. Clark (1997, p. 997) suggests that the accuracy of cognition questionnaires might be improved if "external" priming manipulations were added, such as having individuals complete a questionnaire in a situation or context that is known to elicit the relevant cognitions, or inducing a mood state that is congruent with the target cognitions.

In sum, although in the past cognitive assessment techniques have been employed with minimal attention to psychometric issues (Clark, 1988), a major development over the past decade has been increased attention to the psychometric properties of cognitive assessment measures (Clark, 1997). The psychometric status of the widely used endorsement methods is better established than that of production methods; however, in the past decade increased emphasis has been placed on psychometric evaluation of thought-listing, think-aloud, and thought-sampling approaches to cognitive assessment. In addition to issues of reliability, content validity, criterion validity, and construct validity, it is important to address the issue of clinical utility. The fact that so few of these measures are used routinely in clinical practice calls their external validity into question.

COGNITIVE ASSESSMENT OF ANXIETY

In light of the recognition that the phenomenology of anxiety is predominantly cognitive, a number of theorists posit a significant role for maladaptive cognitions in the development and maintenance of anxiety disorders (Beck, Emery, & Greenberg, 1985; Mathews & MacLeod, 1994). Cognitive assessment is therefore especially suited to this domain, yet cannot be considered as a sufficient description until it is integrated with assessment of the other response modes (behavioral, physiological) characteristic of anxiety (Nelson, Hayes, Felton, & Jarrett, 1985). In fact, the synchrony or lack thereof among the various response modes is an issue in its own (Rachman & Hodgson, 1974).

Cognitive Products

Questionnaires that purport to measure some of the general cognitive features of anxiety have been used for some time. Although the routine use of a standard test battery offers the advantage of comparability to previously published research using these measures, their relative lack of specificity and cumbersome format (e.g., true–false endorsements) often require the administration of other measures to tap more differentiated cognitive content. The Fear of Negative Evaluation (FNE) Scale (Watson & Friend, 1969) is a 30-item, true–false questionnaire designed to measure the degree of apprehension about receiving social disapproval by others in social situations, whereas the Social Avoidance and Distress (SAD) Scale (Watson & Friend, 1969) uses a similar format with 28 items, to measure the experience of distress and discomfort in social situations. Both scales show good internal consistency, with Kuder–Richardson 20 reliabilities for the FNE and SAD being .94 for both measures. Test–retest reliabilities are reported as .78 and .68, respectively, for the FNE and SAD over a 1-month interval.

Other questionnaires are available to the clinical researcher for the assessment of certain cognitive features related to anxiety. For example, according to Reiss's expectancy theory (e.g., Reiss, 1991), anxiety sensitivity is a cognitive individual-difference variable that acts as a specific risk factor in the development of anxiety disorders, especially panic disorder. Anxiety sensitivity is the fear of anxiety-related bodily sensations, based on beliefs that the sensations signal catastrophic somatic, social, or psychological consequences, It is typically assessed with the 16-item Anxiety Sensitivity Index (ASI; Peterson & Reiss, 1992). Items such as "When I am nervous, I worry that I might be mentally ill" are endorsed on a 5-point scale. The ASI has been demonstrated to have excellent psychometric properties in both clinical and nonclinical samples (Peterson & Reiss, 1992). People high in anxiety sensitivity exhibit an explicit memory bias for threatening information (McCabe, 1999). ASI scores predict who will respond anxiously to panic provocation challenges, and who is likely to develop panic attacks and panic disorder (Taylor, 1999). A growing number of studies show that anxiety sensitivity consists of multiple dimensions, structured in a hierarchical manner (e.g., Taylor & Cox, 1998). Although several studies have reported that anxiety sensitivity is also related to depression, in a recent study Schmidt, Lerew, and Joiner (1998) used a covariance analytic strategy and found that anxiety sensitivity possesses symptom specificity with respect to anxiety, but is not predictive of depression when accounting for changes in anxiety symptoms. Glass and Arnkoff (1997) have recommended that measures of internal dialogue be assessed in conjunction with cognitive "traits" such as anxiety sensitivity (and dysfunctional attitudes), in order to gain a better understanding of relations among them.

Moving toward the assessment of some of the more general features of anxiety, we find that a number of self-report measures have been developed to measure aspects of worry, obsessional thinking, and metacognitive beliefs that are predictive of, or related to, generalized anxiety disorder and obsessive–compulsive disorder. For example, the Penn State Worry Questionnaire (PSWQ; Meyer, Miller, Metzger, & Borkovec, 1990) is a widely used 16-item measure that assesses an individual's tendency to worry in general. The items reflect a tendency to worry excessively and chronically (e.g., "Once I start worrying I cannot stop"). The PSWQ provides a reliable and valid measure of worry (e.g., Brown, Antony, & Barlow, 1992). Chorpita, Tracey, Brown, Collica, and Barlow (1997) reported excellent reliability and good convergent and discriminant validity in clinical samples of an adaptation of the PSWQ for use with children and adolescents. Stober and Bittencourt (1998) recently adapted the PSWQ for monitoring changes during treatment (PSWQ—Past Week). The Anxious Thoughts Inventory (Wells, 1994) is a 22-item content and process measure of proneness to health, social, and meta- (worry about worry) dimensions of worry.

The Padua Inventory—Washington State University Revision (Burns, Keortge, Formea, & Sternberger, 1996) is a 39-item measure of obsessions and compulsions that was produced to reduce the overlap of the original Padua Inventory with worry. Cartwright-Hatton and Wells (1997) recently developed the Meta-Cognitions Questionnaire (MCQ), a 65-item questionnaire that assesses individual differences in beliefs about worry, intrusive thoughts and cognitive functioning, and the monitoring of thought processes. Beliefs about one's own thoughts, or metacognitive beliefs, have been linked to both generalized anxiety disorder and obsessive–compulsive disorder, For example, Wells (1995) proposes a cognitive model of generalized anxiety disorder in which positive and negative worry beliefs are central to the maintenance of problems. Clark and Purdon (1995) suggest that people with obsessions adhere to dysfunctional beliefs related to a need to control their thoughts. The MCQ assesses five subscales of metacognitive beliefs: Positive Worry Beliefs; Negative Beliefs about Thought Uncontrollability and Danger; Lack of Cognitive Confidence; Negative Beliefs about Thoughts in General (including themes of superstition, punishment, and responsibility); and Cognitive Self-Consciousness. Although the MCQ is a new measure, initial findings on its psychometric properties are quite positive, and the measure should prove useful in future research. In a recent study, Wells and Papageorgiou (1998) demonstrate that specific sets of metacognitive beliefs are associated with worry proneness and obsessive–compulsive symptoms.

A differentiated assessment of current (or recent) conscious thoughts is provided by self-statement inventories that sample content specific to particular problem areas, and that are constructed to reflect the typical types of thoughts subjects in the situation of interest may experience. Heterosexual social anxiety is the focus of the Social Interaction Self-Statement Test (SISST; Glass et al., 1982), in which subjects are asked to rate 15 positive and 15 negative thoughts (from 1 = "hardly ever had the thought" to 5 = "very often had the thought") after participating in a live heterosexual social interaction. Split-half reliability of the SISST, based on odd versus even items, is .73 for the positive and .86 for the negative scale. Concurrent validity, as evidenced by correlations with other measures of social anxiety, is stronger for the negative self-statements than for the positive ones (negative scale with SAD = .74, with FNE = −.58; positive scale with SAD = −.57, with FNE = −.32) when a written stimulus presentation format is used (Zweig & Brown, 1985).

The role of self-statements in assertiveness is relevant to this discussion, since high anxiety levels are among the explanatory constructs that have been proposed to account for nonassertive behavior (Goldfried & Davison, 1994). Schwartz and Gottman (1976) developed the Assertive Self-Statement Test (ASST), which asks subjects to rate on a 5-point scale the frequency of occurrence of 16 positive and 16 negative assertive responses. The self-statements represent thoughts that are believed to facilitate or inhibit the refusal of an unreasonable request, and as such represent a more detailed elaboration of cognitive content associated with a specific behavioral performance. Fiedler and Beach (1978) have adopted a different perspective, in that their interest lies in measuring the types of consequences subjects believe are associated with refusal behavior, rather than just positive or negative self-statements. Their Subjective Probability of Consequences Inventory (SPCI) lists positive and negative consequences that could result from complying with or refusing an unreasonable request. The SPCI was constructed by choosing items based on clinical experts' consensual validation of representative consequences. Bruch, Haase, and Purcell (1984) report that both the ASST and SPCI show adequate internal reliability, and that the factor structure of the ASST is more complex than was initially assumed, whereas the factor structure of the SPCI corresponds more closely to the dimensions originally outlined by Fiedler and Beach (1978).

Cognitive assessment of agoraphobia and the fear of its occurrence is the focus of a self-statement inventory developed by Chambless, Caputo, Bright, and Gallagher (1984). This measure consists of thoughts concerning negative consequences of experiencing anxiety, and its 14 items were generated through interviews with clients who had agoraphobia, as well as during imaginal and *in vivo* exposure sessions. Each item on their Agoraphobic Cognitions Questionnaire (ACQ) is rated on a 5-point scale ranging from 1 ("thought never occurs") to 5 ("thought always occurs"), and clients are asked to judge the frequency of thoughts when they are in an anxious state. Reliability data show good test–retest stability (r = .86) but low internal consistency (Cronbach alpha = .48). Validity analyses have shown this scale to be sensitive to treatment-induced changes, as well as being able to discriminate the scores of a sample with agoraphobia and a normal control sample. Together with its companion scale, the Body Sensations Questionnaire (BSQ; Chambless et al., 1984), which measures physical sensations associated with autonomic arousal, the ACQ represents the first step toward a comprehensive cognitive assessment for panic disorder with agoraphobia. When both cognitions and sensations are considered, assessment efforts will be more finely tuned to cognitive conceptualizations of panic disorder with and without agoraphobia (Clark, 1986; Goldstein & Chambless, 1978; Khawaja & Oei, 1998), which stress the fact that catastrophic thinking about anxiety in patients with panic disorder is often precipitated by catastrophic misinterpretation of arousal-mediated internal cues.

Cox (1996) has reviewed the available literature and argued that there is room for improvement in the assessment of cognitive variables related to panic attack/panic disorder. Two newer measures appear to be useful additions to the repertoire of available instruments. Khawaja and Oei (1998) note that the ACQ and BSQ do not accurately reflect cognitions with a theme of danger. Khawaja and Oei (1992) developed the Catastrophic Cognitions Questionnaire (CCQ) on student samples to reflect schemata with a content of danger. Subsequently, Khawaja, Oei, and Baglioni (1994) modified the scale and validated it on both patients and students with anxiety disorders samples. The 21-item CCQ-M consists of three factors that reflect the dimensions of catastrophic cognitions: emotional, physical, and mental catastrophes. Subsequent research may determine that the CCQ-M is a useful tool for the assessment of panic disorder; however, to date it has not been widely used.

The Panic Appraisal Inventory (PAI; Telch, Brouillard, Telch, Agras, & Taylor, 1987) also has the potential to be a valuable addition, especially if further development follows guidelines suggested recently by Feske and De Beurs (1997) in their psychometric evaluation of a 45-item version of the PAI. The PAI consists of three scales that assess the perceived likelihood of a panic attack in agoraphobic situations (Anticipated Panic), concern about possible catastrophic consequences (Panic Consequences), and confidence in coping with future panic attacks (Panic Coping). Feske and De Beurs (1997) conclude that the PAI shows excellent internal consistency and treatment sensitivity, and good convergent and divergent validity. However, tests of the measure's factorial validity, stability over time, and criterion-related validity need to be conducted. Although they conclude that the Panic Consequences scale is redundant with, and should not replace, the ACQ, they note that the Anticipated Panic and Panic Coping scales assess important features not captured by other instruments and recommend the inclusion of these scales in the assessment of panic disorder.

Several self-statement measures have been developed to assess obsessive and intrusive thoughts. The 28-item Obsessive Compulsive Thoughts Checklist (OCTC; Bouvard, Mollard, Cottraux, & Guerin, 1989) was devised to provide a measure of thoughts (past week) reported by obsessive–

compulsive clients. Bouvard et al. (1997) have recently presented new validity and factor structure findings, as well as their English translation of the OCTC. Freeston and Ladouceur (1993) developed the Cognitive Intrusions Questionnaire (CIQ) to assess intrusive thoughts, images or impulses (past month) on six proposed themes (health, embarrassing situations, unacceptable sexual behavior, etc.). Respondents choose the most frequent intrusion, and then evaluate that thought on 13 different items and answer 10 questions on strategies used when the thought occurred.

Although the CIQ is currently the most frequently used measure in this area, Glass and Arnkoff (1997) suggest that Purdon and Clark's (1994) Revised Obsessional Intrusions Inventory (ROII) may have greater potential as a measure of the frequency of intrusive obsessive thoughts. The revised measure assesses the frequency of obsessive-like thoughts, images, and impulses, and determines respondents' appraisal and thought control strategies of the most upsetting thought on 10 dimensions. The ROII has good psychometric properties; however, its sensitivity to treatment effects has not been reported.

Several other measures of anxious self-statements are worth noting. The Anxious Self-Statement Questionnaire (Kendall & Hollon, 1989) is a 32-item measure of the frequency of anxious thoughts that has excellent reliability, concurrent validity, and ability to discriminate between known groups, although Glass and Arnkoff (1997) question its discriminant validity with respect to depression. McDermut and Haaga (1994) developed a version with nonanxious thoughts in order to assess the balance of positive and negative thoughts. The Cognition Checklist (CCL) developed by Beck and his colleagues (Beck, Brown, Steer, Eidelson, & Riskind, 1987) may prove useful in the discrimination of anxiety and depression. This measure assesses the frequency of 12 cognitions related to danger and presumed to be characteristic of anxiety disorders (CCL—Anxiety) and 12 thoughts centered on loss and failure characteristic of depression (CCL—Depression). The Negative Affect Self-Statement Questionnaire (Ronan et al., 1994) also yields anxiety-specific and depression-specific subscales for children of different ages. The investigator or practitioner interested in employing thought endorsement measures with children should refer to Glass and Arnkoff's (1997) discussion of this issue.

Cognitive Processes

Moving away from self-statement inventories, we find a number of alternative structured measures of thought that have been employed in the cognitive assessment of anxiety. Some of these instruments are simply scales that have been devised to measure constructs suggested by the cognitive model of anxiety (Beck, Emery, & Greenberg, 1985), whereas others have been generated in different domains. Consistent with cognitive models of anxiety, a number of authors have assessed the constructs of perceived danger or the overestimation of personal risk as the salient cognitive processes in anxiety.

Butler and Mathews (1983) asked subjects to fill out separate questionnaires requiring interpretations of ambiguous scenarios. The subjects rated 20 threatening items in terms of their subjective cost (e.g., "How bad would it be for you?"), and rated a number of positive and negative items in terms of their subjective probability of occurrence. Anxious subjects interpreted the ambiguous material as more threatening and rated the subjective cost of the threatening events as higher than did a control group of nonanxious subjects. Anxious subjects also tended to think that negative future events, especially severe threats to their health, were more likely to happen to them than to someone else. Although it is difficult to attribute a high degree of specificity to these findings, since a control group of depressed patients scored similarly on two of these scales, the anxious group was characterized by inflated estimations of threat and personal risk. Butler and Mathews interpreted their findings as indicative of an interaction between anxiety and the availability of "danger schemata." Similarly, Williams (1985) described a measure of "perceived danger" (defined as a subject's perception of the probability of a negative event's occurring, given a specific performance). This measure is quantified as a likelihood or probability rating from 0% ("believe it is not possible") to 100% ("believe it is certain"). Williams reported that perceived danger ratings did not correlate with behavioral test performance before treatment ($r = .07$), but did correlate significantly after treatment ($r = .56$).

In the years since this important work, a series of studies has examined the relations between anxiety and/or depression, interpretation of ambiguous information, and generation of or estimates of the probability of both negative and positive future and recall of past specific situations or a range of events (Chen & Craske, 1998; MacLeod, Tata, Kentish, Carroll & Hunter, 1997). MacLeod et al. (1997) report that panic disorder was associated with generating more negative experiences but fewer positive experiences, whereas depression was associated with generating fewer positive experiences but not more negative experiences than controls. In general, it appears that both anxiety and depression are related to appraisals of both increased negative future outcomes and decreased positive future outcomes. This work supports the notion that cognitions are different in anxiety and depression; it also suggests that, when asked, anxious participants can think negatively about the past, although their negative thoughts are more commonly spontaneously centered on the future. These studies further suggest that measures of retrospective and prospective cognitions are useful in clinical cognitive research and are of potential value in clinical practice.

Less structured formats for the cognitive assessment of anxiety have ranged from attempts to sample thinking during *in vivo* (Last, Barlow, & O'Brien, 1985) or simulated (Davison et al., 1983) anxiety-arousing situations, to the random sampling of thoughts experienced by anxious individuals (Hurlburt & Spirelle, 1978). Thought listing has been used in a number of studies where the aim has been to record subjects' thoughts immediately following *in vivo* performance. Last et al. (1985), for example, had individuals with agoraphobia report what was going through their minds during an exposure session conducted at a shopping mall, while Segal and Marshall (1985) asked rapists to recall what their thoughts were in conjunction with an interaction they just had with an attractive female.

Thought sampling was employed by Williams and Rappoport (1983) in their research comparing cognitive and exposure-based treatments for agoraphobia. Each subject was provided with a beeper that would activate periodically, thus cueing the individual to record whatever he or she was thinking about on a tape recorder. The assessments had high ecological validity, as they were taken during behavioral tests of driving capability. A related approach was used by Sewitch and Kirsch (1984), who provided subjects with small booklets in which the subjects were instructed to try to recall what thoughts or feelings they were experiencing each time they felt anxious or "uptight" within a specified 24-hour interval.

When applied to anxiety-related problems, think-aloud procedures can be especially informative when the precise contents of the internal dialogue are elusive. Worry is an important case in point, especially given its link to generalized anxiety disorder (American Psychiatric Association, 1994). Borkevec and his colleagues (Molina, Borkovec, Peasley, & Person, 1998) conducted a fine-grained analysis of content of worrisome cognitive activity on stream of consciousness reports obtained from "neutral" and "worry" periods. In addition to providing a better understanding of the temporal, affective, and attentional/cognitive effects of worry (e.g., more frequent use of both words reflecting high negative affect and words reflecting potential cognitive distortions), differences were found among anxious, dysphoric, and control participants. Thus participants classified as meeting the *Diagnostic and Statistical Manual of Mental Disorders,* fourth edition (DSM-IV) criteria for generalized anxiety disorder used a higher relative frequency of statements implying catastrophic interpretations of events; statements implying a rigid, rule-bound interpretive style; and words reflecting somatic anxiety. It is of interest that dysphoric subjects made use of derivatives of the word "worry" at a very high frequency.

Cognitive Structures/Organizations

Although the majority of material covered in this section has described efforts at measuring those cognitive aspects of anxiety within an individual's awareness, attempts have also been made to assess the "deep" structure representations of anxious individuals—processes that are inferred from behavior (Landau, 1980; Rudy, Merluzzi, & Henahan, 1982). Rather than focusing on the actual cognitive content that subjects are able to report in the assessment situation, these studies aim at a level of analysis that describes the operation of certain cognitive processes or structures thought to play a key role in the experience of anxiety (Goldfried & Robins, 1983).

Multidimensional scaling has been used by a number of investigators in an attempt to map the semantic structure of social anxiety (e.g., Goldfried, Padawer, & Robins, 1984). Similarity ratings on a given dimension for a set of objects serve as the input in this approach, and yield proximity scores. The output produced is a spatial representation that reflects the data structure, so that the more dissimilar subjects' ratings are, the farther apart they will be represented on a spatial map. In this way, similarity ratings as represented by geometric distance are thought to reflect psychological space, and offer a view of the "deep" structure of a chosen data base (Merluzzi & Rudy, 1982). Goldfried et al. (1984) used multidimensional scaling with a sample of socially anxious college males and found that they weighted the dimension of "chance of being evaluated" the highest with respect to the likelihood of generating anxiety, while giving lower weights to dimensions of "intimacy" and "academic relevance." Nonanxious males, on the other hand, weighted "intimacy" twice as heavily as "chance of being evaluated," suggesting a possible difference in the saliencies that stand out for these two groups when they are confronted by an opportunity for heterosexual interaction.

Finally, several attentional paradigms have confirmed that people with anxiety disorders show selective processing of threat cues (Mathews & MacLeod, 1994; McNally, 1998). For example, Mathews and his colleagues (Butler & Mathews, 1983; MacLeod, Mathews, & Tata, 1986; Mathews & MacLeod, 1985) propose that activation of schemata biased toward the processing of information related to personal danger or other threatening input is characteristic of anxiety states. Mathews and MacLeod (1985), for example, used the Stroop Color-Naming Task and found that anxious subjects took longer than controls in color-naming words with a threatening content ("disease," "coffin") as opposed to a neutral content ("welcome," "holiday"). Studies utilizing other measures derived from cognitive science, such as the degree of visual capture associated with a particular stimulus (MacLeod et al., 1986), have reported findings in a similar direction—namely, that anxious subjects are more vigilant for or distracted by threat-related stimuli than are normal controls. The authors interpret these results as supporting the existence of cognitive "danger schemata," which when activated bias information processing at a preattentive level. Whether this bias is perceptual or attentional in nature, it is thought to play an important role in the maintenance of anxiety disorders, since it has an impact on the interpretations that individuals make at a later point in the information-processing stream.

Remaining Issues

Before we leave this section and move on to the cognitive assessment of depression, it is important to consider a number of issues that interface with both domains. Although cognitive assessment efforts in anxiety are more recent developments than those in depression, it is equally accurate to characterize both endeavors as still in their childhood. As a result, more work is needed to refine and evaluate the measures that exist in these already method-rich areas (Clark, 1997). For example, scoring criteria for thought listing or think-aloud protocols constitute a good example of an area where the injection of some degree of regularity in the dimensions or attributes scored would aid comparability among investigations. Similarly, the increasing attention being paid to cognitive structures or "deeper" levels of processing would benefit from a focus on resolving some of the definitional issues surrounding the operation of these constructs.

Readers should also bear in mind the close relationship between anxiety and depression symptoms (Clark & Watson, 1991; Watson & Kendall, 1989). Up to 90% of patients report both symptoms of anxiety and depression (Breir, Charney, & Heninger, 1984; Dobson, 1985; Swinson & Kirby, 1987). Most researchers have set out to differentiate the various syndromes of anxiety and depression using diagnostic systems or symptom inventories. Investigators have only recently made attempts to document the relative contribution of anxiety-related and depression-related cognitions within an individual diagnosed as suffering from an anxiety and/or depressive disorder (e.g., Beck et al., 1987). Considerable work is needed to clarify the value of cognition and cognitive processes for the differentiation of these disorders. Acknowledging that their resolution will no doubt be a gradual process, we now move on to consider the cognitive assessment of depression.

COGNITIVE ASSESSMENT OF DEPRESSION

The majority of cognitive assessment measures in depression are paper-and-pencil instruments designed to capture either the content of patients' thinking or their underlying attitudes or beliefs. Other significant efforts have addressed the manner in which depressed patients process information, particularly of self-referent descriptions or feedback from task performances. Only a few investigators have concerned themselves with thought-listing or think-aloud procedures, although the recall (reconstruction) of automatic thoughts or self-statements in specific situations is widely employed in the clinical interview format (Beck, Rush, Shaw, & Emery, 1979).

Cognitive Products

The Automatic Thoughts Questionnaire (ATQ; Hollon & Kendall, 1980) measures the frequency with which each of 30 negative automatic thoughts have "popped" into subjects' heads during the past week (i.e., from 1 = "not at all" to 5 = "all the time"). In addition, the extent to which subjects tend to believe each of these thoughts is rated on a 5-point scale (from "not at all" to "totally"). The 30 thoughts constituting the ATQ were derived empirically on the basis of their ability to discriminate between depressed and nondepressed subjects. Sample items include "I don't think I can go on," "No one understands me," and "It's just not worth it." The ATQ's psychometric properties have been evaluated in a number of studies. Internal-consistency estimates (i.e., split-half and coefficient alpha) have been shown to be high (in the .96–.97 range) across a range of subjects (Dobson & Breiter, 1983). In terms of construct validity, the ATQ has been found to differentiate between depressed and nondepressed subjects (Hollon & Kendall, 1980), and correlates strongly (i.e., about .63) with severity of depressive symptoms (Dobson & Breiter, 1983). Hollon and Kendall's (1980) factor analysis of the ATQ yielded four factors: (1) Personal Maladjustment and Desire for Change, (2) Negative Self-Concepts and Expectations, (3) Low Self-Esteem, and (4) Helplessness and Giving Up. Importantly, these factors are consistent with Beck's (1967, 1976) theory of depression.

More recently, investigators have emphasized the importance of assessing positive as well as negative thinking patterns in depression (e.g., Schwartz & Garamoni, 1989). Responding to this suggestion, Ingram and Wisnicki (1988) developed the Positive Automatic Thoughts Questionnaire (ATQ-P), which assesses the frequency of positive automatic thoughts. In a validation study of the ATQ-P, Ingram, Slater, Atkinson, and Scott (1990) found that depressed patients reported significantly fewer positive automatic thoughts than nondepressed controls. In addition, this study provided evidence that fewer positive thoughts may be a cognitive feature specific to individuals suffering emotional distress. Thus the ATQ-P may represent a useful counterpart to the ATQ, and serve to provide a more comprehensive picture of automatic thinking patterns in depression.

Flett, Hewitt, Blankstein, and Gray (1998) recently developed a new measure of automatic thoughts similar in format to the ATQ. However, it differs from the ATQ because of its specific focus on automatic thoughts involving perfectionism. In a series of five studies with the 25-item Perfectionism Cognitions Inventory (PCI), Flett et al. (1998) established that the

PCI has adequate levels of reliability and validity, and that high PCI scorers tend to spontaneously report perfectionistic thoughts in naturalistic settings. Additional research confirmed that the experience of frequent perfectionism thoughts is associated with dysphoria and anxiety, over and above the variance predicted by alternative measures of negative automatic thoughts and existing trait measures of perfectionism.

Developed in the framework of the reformulated learned helplessness model of depression (Abramson, Seligman, & Teasdale, 1979), the Attributional Style Questionnaire (ASQ; Peterson et al., 1982) is probably the most frequently cited measure of depressive attributions. It presents subjects with 12 hypothetical scenarios involving themes of achievement or affiliation. Six of the scenarios have positive outcomes, while the other six have negative outcomes. Subjects are asked to imagine themselves in each situation and then to identify the major cause of the event. Next, subjects rate the extent to which they believe (1) the outcome was due either to themselves or to other people or circumstances (i.e., internal vs. external factors); (2) the same cause would be operative in the future, under similar circumstances (i.e., stable vs. unstable factors); and (3) the same cause may influence a variety of life situations (i.e., global vs. specific factors).

In scoring the ASQ, Peterson et al. (1982) have recommended collapsing data across the achievement–affiliation distinction, since attributional ratings for these two types of events were significantly correlated. As such, internality, stability, and globality scores are calculated separately for good and bad outcomes (i.e., six subscales based on six items each). The internal consistency of these scales is weak, however, with alphas ranging from .44 to .58 for positive outcomes and from .46 to .69 for negative outcomes. Alternately, then, two composite "attributional style" scores can be calculated, one for good events and one for bad events (with alphas of .75 and .72, respectively). This compromise, of course, attenuates the ASQ's theoretical relevance.

The ASQ has been plagued with at least two other serious psychometric problems. One major difficulty relates to the intercorrelations among the three attributional dimensions. For good events, the ASQ is completely unable to distinguish these dimensions (Peterson et al., 1982), and does only marginally better for bad events. Indeed, a factor-analytic study (Bagby, Atkinson, Dickens, & Gavin, 1990) found that the ASQ's factor structure was best represented by a two-factor solution corresponding to the distinction between good and bad outcomes. This suggests that outcome valence has a far greater influence on causal thought than individual differences in attributional style. Another problem, more relevant to the issue of validity, is that depression-related differences on ASQ subscales reliably emerge only in attributions for negative outcomes (Seligman, Abramson, Semmel, & von Baeyer, 1979). Even there, the relationship between ASQ scores and depressed mood is relatively modest (mean r = .21; e.g., Brewin & Furnham, 1986).

In response to these problems (particularly those relating to reliability) an extended version of the ASQ has been developed (EASQ; Metalsky, Halberstadt, & Abramson, 1987). The EASQ is similar in format to the original ASQ, but its 12 scenarios describe only bad events. In addition, stability and globality subscales are averaged to create a "generality" scale. Indeed, reliability estimates for this subscale are more respectable than those reported for the ASQ (alphas for negative achievement and interpersonal outcomes are .79 and .77, respectively: Metalsky et al., 1987), and it has shown promise in predicting depressive symptoms in college students (e.g., Metalsky & Joiner, 1992). As with the ASQ, however, its relevance as a measure of cognition in more severely depressed individuals remains to be tested (Bagby et al., 1990).

One alternative approach to measuring attributions in depression involves examining individuals' attributions for negative or distressing life events that have actually occurred to them. Like studies of the ASQ, studies employing this strategy have failed to find support for the orthogonality of the three attributional dimensions (e.g., Gong-Guy & Hammen, 1980; Hammen & Cochran, 1981). However, correlations between depression and attributions about actual life events may be somewhat stronger (i.e., mean r = .29; Brewin & Furnham, 1986) than those involving hypothetical scenarios.

Negative expectancies and hopeless thoughts represent another central theme in the thinking of depressed individuals (Beck, 1976). Here we present two approaches to assessing hopeless cognitions. The Hopelessness Scale (HS; Beck, Weissman, Lester, & Trexler, 1974) is a 20-item self-report scale designed to measure the extent to which individuals harbor this kind of pessimistic outlook on the future. Sample items include "I might as well give up because I can't make things better for myself" and "The future seems dark to me." Individuals respond in a true–false format. Approximately half the items are reverse-keyed to control for acquiescence. Beck et al. (1974) have reported good internal consistency for the HS (alpha = .93). In terms of validity, the HS correlates highly with severity indices like the Beck Depression Inventory (BDI) (r's range from .68 to .84), and with clinical ratings of hopelessness (r's range from .60 to .74; Minkoff, Berhman, Beck, & Beck, 1973). HS scores have been found to differentiate depressed individuals from nondepressed or formerly depressed persons (Wilkinson & Blackburn, 1981), and, most importantly, have been shown to predict successful suicide in patients exhibiting suicidal ideation (Beck, Steer, Kovacs, & Garrison, 1985). Although some researchers have cautioned that the HS may be more sensitive to a socially undesirable response set than to suicide potential (Mendonca, Holden, Mazmanian, & Dolan

(1983), it would appear that the HS may be usefully employed as a screening instrument, with high scores (i.e., above 9) alerting clinicians to the danger of self-destructive behavior.

An emerging and less direct approach to assessing cognitions of hopelessness involves having subjects rate the probability of positive or negative outcomes in a variety of scenarios (real or hypothetical). In a study employing this procedure, Alloy and Ahrens (1987) asked depressed and nondepressed students to rate the likelihood of success or failure in a specific domain (e.g., academic) both for themselves and for others. Results suggested that depressed individuals were more pessimistic about outcomes (both for themselves and for others) than were the nondepressed (i.e., they viewed success as less likely and failure as more likely). Similar results have been reported by Pyszczynski, Holt, and Greenberg (1987). This approach may represent a somewhat less transparent strategy than the HS for assessing depressive pessimism, particularly in individuals exhibiting rather mild levels of depression. Although its use is limited to the laboratory at present, appropriate standardization may render outcome forecasting a helpful alternative to self-report measures of hopelessness.

Most cognitive accounts emphasize the role of negative or disparaging self-evaluations in depressive phenomenology. Depressed individuals typically maintain a global view of themselves as inferior, worthless, and inadequate. Traditional approaches to the assessment of global self-regard have been reviewed and evaluated elsewhere (see Demo, 1986). Here we focus on one development that is particularly salient to cognitive assessment in depression.

The Beck Self-Concept Test (BST; Beck, Steer, Epstein, & Brown, 1990) is a self-report measure designed to evaluate the negative view of self that Beck (1967, 1976) described as a central feature of depression. The BST asks subjects to evaluate themselves (relative to others with whom they are acquainted) on 25 dimensions representing personality (e.g., "good-natured," "selfish"), abilities (e.g., "knowledge," "successful"), aptitudes ("intelligent," "athletic"), virtues (e.g., "kind," "tidy") or vices (e.g., "lazy," "greed"). Ratings are made on a 5-point scale (1 = "worse than nearly anyone I know," 3 = "about the same as most people," and 5 = "better than nearly anyone I know"), and are weighted such that higher ratings always indicate a more positive self-view. The BST thus yields a single composite score reflecting global self-regard.

Beck et al. (1990) reported satisfactory internal consistency (coefficient alpha = .82) in a sample of 550 patients meeting DSM-III-R criteria for primary mood disorders and anxiety disorders. One-week test–retest reliability was .88 in a sample of 50 patients. The BST correlated highly (.51) with the well-known Rosenberg Self-Esteem Scale (Rosenberg, 1965), and significant negative correlations were reported between the BST and a variety of measures of psychopathology (i.e., measures of depression, hopelessness, suicidal ideation, depressogenic attitudes, etc.). Interestingly enough, the BST was not related to a measure of anxiety (the Beck Anxiety Inventory), thus indicating a degree of specificity to depression.

A central theme in Beck's (1967, 1976) formulation of depression is that depressive phenomenology is mediated by faulty, irrational thinking patterns. To illustrate, depressed individuals may generalize from a single event to a wide range of events (overgeneralization), exaggerate the negative impact of undesirable outcomes (magnification, catastrophizing), or jump to negative conclusions in the absence of corroborative evidence (arbitrary inference). We describe two measures of irrational thinking.

The Cognitive Bias Questionnaire (CBQ; Hammen & Krantz, 1976; Krantz & Hammen, 1979) is one instrument designed to assess the degree to which individuals exhibit these types of logical errors. It consists of six vignettes of problematic situations involving interpersonal or achievement themes. For each vignette, subjects are asked to imagine as vividly as possible what the protagonist might think and feel about the situation, and then to select from among four response alternatives the one that most closely resembles this response. The response options were constructed to reflect two dichotomous and crossed dimensions: (1) depressive (i.e., dysphoric) versus nondepressive responses; and (2) distorted (i.e., irrational) versus nondistorted. An example of a depressive–nondistorted response to a situation involving "being alone on a Friday night" would be "upsets me and makes me feel lonely." A depressive–distorted (overgeneralization) response would be "upsets me and makes me start to imagine endless days and nights by myself" (Hammen & Krantz, 1976, p. 580). Scores on the CBQ simply reflect the frequency of use of each of the four response categories. Of particular interest, in terms of both theory and practice, is the frequency of depressive–distorted responses.

Krantz and Hammen (1979) have reported relatively modest estimates of internal consistency in two student samples (alphas = .62 and .69), possibly reflecting the heterogeneity of the cognitive distortion construct (Hammen & Krantz, 1985). In addition, they report reasonable 4- and 8-week test–retest reliabilities (r's = .48 and .60, respectively). In terms of construct validity, several studies have been able to differentiate depressed and nondepressed individuals on the basis of CBQ depressive–distorted scores (Krantz & Hammen, 1979; Norman, Miller, & Klee, 1983). Mixed findings are reported concerning the CBQ's discriminant validity, with some work indicating significant correlations of depressive–distorted CBQ scores with anxiety (Krantz & Hammen, 1979) and hostility (Frost & MacInnis, 1983).

Relative to the CBQ, the Cognitive Response Test (CRT; Watkins & Rush, 1983) is a somewhat less structured measure of cognitive distortion in depression. Its 36 items are presented in an open-ended, sentence completion format. Subjects are asked to respond with the first thought that comes to mind. Sample items are "My employer says he will be making some major staff changes. I immediately think: _____," and "When I consider being married, my first thought is: _____." Although this open-ended format has the advantage of obviating the "transparency problems" of fixed-choice tests (Rush, 1984), it is also more time-consuming to score. On the basis of rules set out in a standardized test manual, responses are classified as rational, irrational, or nonscorable. Irrational responses are further classified as irrational–depressed (i.e., incorporating a negative view of the self, the past, or the future) or irrational–other.

Watkins and Rush (1983) have reported a mean interjudge correlation of .84 across subjects and response types. In terms of discriminant validity, they reported that the irrational–depressed subscale distinguished depressed individuals from a variety of nondepressed controls (e.g., psychiatric, medical, normal). Further evidence for discriminant validity derives from research indicating that CRT scores were related to the severity of depression, but not to neuroticism (Wilkinson & Blackburn, 1981).

Cognitive Processes

Various self-regulatory mechanisms have been implicated in the development and maintenance of depressive phenomenology. Unfortunately, the technology for assessing these mechanisms has often lagged behind theory. Building on work in social psychology, a number of theorists have suggested that excessive self-focused attention or rumination may be related to affective self-regulatory deficits (Carver & Scheier, 1982; Pyszczynski et al., 1987). One prominent measure of self-focused attention is the Self-Focus Sentence Completion (SFSC; Exner, 1973). The SFSC is a 30-item scale in which subjects are presented with sentence stems (e.g., "I wish . . . " or "When I look in the mirror . . . ") and asked to complete them any way they choose. In the scoring system detailed by Exner (1973), completions that reflect sole preoccupation with oneself are classified as self-focused responses. Externally focused, ambivalent, and neutral responses are also described. In addition, responses are classified as including positive, negative, and neutral content. Thus the SFSC yields 10 scores: Total Self-Focus (S); Self-Focus Positive, Negative, and Neutral; Total External Focus (E); External Focus Positive, Negative, and Neutral; Total Ambivalent (A); and Total Neutral (N). Exner (1973) has reported scoring reliabilities for the SFSC subscales ranging from .89 to .94 for experienced raters, and from .68 to .90 for novice raters (note: reliabilities for S scores were always the highest). Exner (1973) has reviewed several studies that provide evidence for the validity of the SFSC. Importantly, several more recent studies have indicated that both mildly and clinically depressed individuals generate more self-focused responses and fewer externally focused responses than non-depressives (Ingram & Smith, 1984; Ingram, Lumry, Cruet, & Sieber, 1987).

Another frequently employed measure of self-focused attention is the Self-Consciousness Scale (SCS; Fenigstein, Scheier, & Buss, 1975). The SCS consists of three factor-analytically derived subscales: Private Self-Consciousness (10 items); Public Self-Consciousness (7 items); and Social Anxiety (6 items). The Private Self-Consciousness subscale is considered the dispositional equivalent of the self-focused attention state. Items are scored on a 5-point scale (0 = "extremely uncharacteristic" to 4 = extremely characteristic). Examples of items from the Private Self-Consciousness subscale are "I'm always trying to figure myself out" and "I reflect about myself a lot." This subscale's reliability and validity has been demonstrated in several studies (e.g., Carver & Scheier, 1983; Fenigstein et al., 1975). It also has been shown to correlate significantly with depression across a number of studies (Ingram & Smith, 1984).

The Response Styles Questionnaire (RSQ; Nolen-Hoeksema & Morrow, 1991) is designed to measure dispositional responses to depressed mood by asking respondents what they generally do when they feel depressed. The RSQ consists of two subscales: the Rumination Response Scale (RRS), which is composed of 21 items, and the Distraction Response Scale (DRS), which is composed of 11 items. Items are rated on a 4-point Likert scale ranging from 1 ("almost never") to 4 ("almost always"). Respondents are asked to indicate what they do when they feel depressed. Examples of items from the RRS include "Think about how alone you feel," "Go away by yourself and think about why you feel this way," and "Think about all your shortcomings." Example of items from the DRS include "Remind myself that these feelings won't last," "Go to a favorite place to get my mind off your feelings," and "Think I'll concentrate on something other than how I feel."

The RSQ has been employed in a number of different studies, although slightly different sets of items have been employed (e.g., Nolen-Hoeksema, Morrow, & Fredrickson). The RSQ has demonstrated good internal reliability (Just & Alloy, 1997) and validity for predicting depression (e.g., Nolen-Hoeksema, Larson, & Grayson, 1999; Nolen-Hoeksema & Morrow, 1991). The RRS and DRS have also been demonstrated to be independent of one another (r = .14, n.s.; Just & Alloy, 1997) and to represent dispositional, stable styles.

In this study, the internal consistency for the RRS (alpha = .88) and the DRS (alpha = .80) was also good. A subsample of the patients (n = 34) completed the RSQ on two separate occasions with the interval ranging from 14 to 24 weeks (mean interval = 19.7 weeks, SD = 5.24). The test–

retest reliability coefficient for the RRS was .59 ($p < .01$) and for the DRS .75 ($p < .001$), supporting the contention that response styles are stable dispositions. The correlation between the RRS and DRS was nonsignificant at both Time 1 ($r = .08$) and Time 2 ($r = -.25$), replicating earlier findings (Just & Alloy, 1997).

The observation that depressed people tend to view themselves as inadequate and inferior has led some investigators to consider the possibility that certain dysfunctional patterns of social comparison may mediate depressive self-evaluations (Swallow & Kuiper, 1988). Among the more innovative measures of social comparison are those utilizing thought sampling and self-recording to study the content of naturalistic comparisons made by patients. The Rochester Social Comparison Record (RSCR; Wheeler & Miyake, 1992) includes information about the circumstances of each comparison (social interaction, visual, etc.), the comparison dimension (intellectual ability, personality, etc.), the type of relationship to the comparison target (close friend, family member, etc.), and the gender of the target. In addition, the RSCR taps pre- and postcomparison affect, and asks subjects about their motivation for engaging in each particular social comparison. Subjects complete a record for each comparison they make over a 2-week period. Wheeler and Miyake (1992) reported a test–retest reliability of .74 for the RSCR. This estimate was based on the correlation between the number of comparisons made during the first week and the second week of record keeping.

Although the RSCR was not specifically designed for use with depressed samples, Wheeler and Miyake (1992) did employ it to identify differences in social comparison that emerged as a function of self-esteem and negative affect. In addition, their study demonstrated the negative affective consequences of unfavorable social comparisons. Overall, then, the self-recording methodology holds considerable promise as a means of identifying and assessing depression-related differences in the self-evaluative process of social comparison.

Cognitive Structures/Organizations

Beck (1967; Beck et al., 1979) has proposed that schemata of negative self-referent information (i.e., negative self-schemata) become activated in depression, resulting in the tendency to view oneself unfavorably and to interpret one's experience (past, current, and future) in a predominantly negative fashion. In addition, activated negative self-schemata can facilitate the retrieval of schema-congruent information. According to Beck's formulation, negative self-schemata constitute a highly organized network of stored personal information—primarily unfavorable—along with rules for evaluating one's worth or value as a person. Measuring self-schemata, at the level of both content and organization, represents an ongoing challenge for depression investigators. Here we present several prominent paradigms.

The Dysfunctional Attitude Scale (DAS) was designed by Weissman and Beck (Weissman, 1979; Weissman & Beck, 1978) to identify the relatively stable set of attitudes associated with depressive disorders. It is now clear that these attitudes are relevant to several psychopathological conditions, although the actual DAS score may differentiate various groups (Dobson & Shaw, 1986; Hollon, Kendall, & Lumry, 1986). As dysfunctional attitudes are thought to reflect prepotent self-schemata, the DAS has been proposed as one measure of cognitive vulnerability to major depressive disorder (Ingram, Miranda, & Segal, 1998). The DAS is a self-report inventory available in three forms. The original 100-item inventory (DAS-T) is only occasionally employed in research studies. From the DAS-T, two 40-item parallel forms (DAS-A and DAS-B) have been derived, with the former being the most commonly used. Patients indicate the degree to which they agree or disagree with the stated attitudes on a 7-point scale. The scores on the DAS-T range from 100 to 700, while on the DAS-A and DAS-B the range is from 40 to 280.

The DAS items are typically stated as contingencies concerning approval from others, prerequisites for happiness, or perfectionistic standards—for example, "It is difficult to be happy unless one is good-looking, intelligent, rich, and creative," "People will probably think less of me if I make a mistake," and "If someone disagrees with me, it probably indicates he or she does not like me." Weissman (1979) developed the DAS on a sample of college students; later, Oliver and Baumgart (1985) evaluated all three forms in a sample of adult hospital workers and their spouses. A psychometric study with a nonselected normative sample remains to be completed. The DAS has been widely researched on depressed and psychiatric control patients. In the Oliver and Baumgart (1985) study, the mean score on the DAS-T was 296 ($SD = 75$), while according to Weissman (1979), the mean total score for students using either the DAS-A or the DAS-B was 117.7 ($SD = 26.8$). Depressed patients typically receive scores of 150 ($SD = 40$). Both short forms of the DAS have good internal consistency and stability over time, with coefficient alphas ranging from .89 to .92 and a test–retest correlation of .84 over an 8-week period (Weissman, 1979). Oliver and Baumgart (1985) reported alpha coefficients of .90, .85, and .81 for the DAS-T, DAS-A, and DAS-B, respectively. Their 6-week test–retest reliability for the DAS-T was .73 ($n = 43$).

One area of controversy in the research concerns the stability of DAS scores in samples of depressed patients. Some investigators report a relatively stable pattern of DAS scores, while others find a marked change in scores. The concurrent validity of the DAS has been tested in several studies, but there have been few evaluations of construct validity. It is expected that the DAS would have moderate correlations with measures of depressive severity and with measures of negative automatic thoughts, or cognitive distortions. For example, in three studies (Dobson & Shaw, 1986; Hamilton & Abramson, 1983; O'Hara, Rehm, & Campbell, 1982), the DAS correlations with the BDI were in the moderate range (i.e., .40–.65). Riskind, Beck, and Smucker (1983) found that the DAS remained significantly correlated with the HS ($r = .22$) and the BST ($r = -.15$), with the effects of depression severity partialed out. The DAS correlated .52 with the CBQ and with the ATQ, both of which are state-dependent measures of depressive cognitions (Hollon et al., 1986). Although the DAS discriminates groups of depressed and psychiatric control patients, it is not specifically associated with major depressive disorder. Patients with generalized anxiety disorder, anorexia nervosa, panic disorder, or dysthymia may manifest abnormal DAS scores (Dobson & Shaw, 1986). In addition, it is notable that approximately 15% of depressed patients do not have abnormally high scores (i.e., at least one standard deviation above the mean) scores (Hamilton & Abramson, 1983).

The DAS has been employed to evaluate attitudes hypothesized to change as a function of cognitive therapy or other treatments of depression. Several studies have found the DAS to be a sensitive measure of clinical improvement. Keller (1983) found that DAS scores were useful to predict the outcome of cognitive therapy. Simons, Garfield, and Murphy (1984) reported that DAS scores were lowered following either cognitive therapy or pharmacotherapy for depression. Silverman, Silverman, and Eardley (1984) also noted a significant reduction in DAS scores following pharmacotherapy.

The question of whether dysfunctional attitudes represent a stable self-schema component or, alternatively, another cognitive manifestation (i.e., a product) of depression has generated a good deal of controversy in the cognitive literature. The latter position is supported by earlier studies showing that dysfunctional attitudes correlate with depression (e.g., Dobson & Shaw, 1986), but do not distinguish between individuals who will go on to become depressed and those who will not (Lewinsohn, Steinmetz, Larson, & Franklin, 1981) or between persons who have recovered from depression and persons without depression (Hamilton & Abramson, 1983). Later work, however (Miranda & Persons, 1988; Miranda, Persons, & Byers, 1990), indicates that individuals prone to developing depressive symptoms do obtain higher DAS scores, but only in the presence of a negative mood. These findings suggest that transient negative mood states may serve to prime negative self-schemata, thereby increasing the accessibility of dysfunctional attitudes.

Implicit in this work is a comparison of two approaches to the cognitive assessment of patients in remission. The first suggests that markers of future risk should be detectable as residuals of the depressive episode, indicating that the patient is still at risk. The second approach suggests that such residuals may exist, but they are less likely to be detected in remission unless specific priming or activation procedures are employed prior to assessment (Teasdale, 1997). Segal and Ingram (1994) reviewed over 40 studies in which the two paradigms were employed. Positive findings of depressive cognitive processing were only obtained in 20% of studies that assessed such processing without using a prime, whereas over 80% of studies that employed a prime reported detection of depressotypic cognitions. Moreover, the lack of differences between vulnerable and nonvulnerable subjects in the various control (normal-mood) conditions of these studies closely parallels previous research that has failed to find evidence of depressive cognitive processing after the depression resolves (e.g., Lewinsohn et al., 1981); that is, under ordinary conditions, depressive cognitive processes cannot be detected after individuals are no longer depressed.

Interestingly, these differences in cognitive variables cut across several different levels of cognitive analysis (Ingram, 1990). For instance, in the presence of negative mood, dysfunctional cognition for those at risk appears evident in cognitive content (i.e., DAS scores; Miranda & Persons, 1988; Miranda et al., 1990), information encoding and retrieval (adjective recall; Teasdale & Dent, 1987; Dent & Teasdale, 1988; Williams, 1988), and attention (tracking errors in a dichotic listening task; Gata et al., 1993). This would suggest that a maladaptive cognitive structure/schema, activated as a consequence of the priming manipulation, may be the organizing construct linked to each of these more specific cognitive effects. Sad mood in these studies may serve as an analogue to potent environmental triggers: It appears to contribute to activating cognitive structures that heretofore have only minimally been involved in on-line information processing.

An important question concerns the use of questionnaires as primes. If self-report inventories offer the same capacity to activate subjects' mental representations as other types of primes do, they would confer distinct advantages in terms of convenience, standardization, and time efficiency, compared to other methods now in use. There are a number of reasons why this assumption may be unfounded. First, if questionnaire items did serve as primes, then the mathematical summation of primes over the total scale score would probably equal zero. For example, in the case of the ASQ (Peterson & Villanova, 1988), the net effects of subjects' being primed by reflecting on the positive events and negative events on the scale would cancel each other out. Second, if the ASQ were used to induce a depressogenic attributional style, then the measure that would comprise the manipulation check would probably bear too close a resemblance to the ASQ itself. This would work against being able to establish the effect independently.

Third, prime specificity would vary greatly among inventories, yielding uneven levels of construct activation. For example, if we compare the ASQ, the ATQ (Hollon & Kendall, 1980), and the CBQ (Krantz & Hammen, 1979), we find a number of differences that can mediate the degree of activation achieved. There are differences in (1) the type of response requested from subjects (a written causal attribution, circling the most descriptive item, and choosing the correct multiple-choice answer, respectively); (2) the amount of imaginal input required to respond to the item (the ASQ asks subjects to imagine their responses to a hypothetical situation, the CBQ asks subjects to choose the best response to a story about another person, and the ATQ asks for thoughts over the past week); and (3) the level of cognition being assessed (the ASQ and CBQ measure aspects of cognitive processes, while the ATQ assesses cognitive products only). For these reasons, the use of questionnaires as primes needs to be viewed with caution.

The Self-Referent Encoding Task (SRET; Kuiper & Olinger, 1986) is an adaptation of a laboratory paradigm originally developed by cognitive psychologists (Craik & Tulving, 1975) to test Craik and Lockhart's (1972) "levels-of-processing" model of memory. In the SRET, subjects are serially presented with a number of personal adjectives (positive and negative) and asked to decide, in a categorical fashion (i.e., "yes" or "no"), whether each adjective is self-descriptive. After all the adjectives have been rated, an incidental-recall test is administered.

The SRET yields several schema-related measures. First, the number of positive and negative words rated as self-descriptive may provide an index of the relative proportion of negative and positive information stored in the self-schema. Consistent with schema-based models of depression, empirical work suggests that depressed subjects endorse more negative adjectives than do nondepressed controls, who tend to rate more positive adjectives as self-descriptive (MacDonald & Kuiper, 1984).

A second and certainly less transparent index of schematic processing relates to the time required for subjects to make their "yes–no" judgments. Theoretically, schemas are thought to facilitate the processing of schema-congruent information. As such, individuals with self-schemata comprising predominantly negative information should exhibit enhanced processing of negative adjectives. This notion is supported in SRET studies demonstrating quicker rating times by nondepressed subjects for positive adjectives (Kuiper & MacDonald, 1983) and by depressed subjects for negative adjectives (MacDonald & Kuiper, 1984). The third self-schema measure yielded by the SRET relates to incidental recall. Specifically, schema-congruent information ought to be processed at a relatively deep level, and, according to the levels-of-processing model, should be better recalled. Consistent with this notion, depressed subjects have been shown to recall more negative adjectives following the SRET, whereas nondepressed subjects recall more positive ones (Kuiper & MacDonald, 1983).

Taken together, results from studies employing the SRET provide evidence for the operation of a negative self-schema in depression. They also suggest that the SRET may represent a useful strategy for mapping out the parameters of this cognitive structure. However, the SRET's validity as a measure of self-schema content and function has been questioned (see Segal, 1988, for a review). One of the more serious concerns, for example, relates to the possibility that the depression-related differences outlined above may reflect mood congruency effects rather than differences in cognitive organization. Nevertheless, despite its limitations, the SRET is a good illustration of how paradigms from cognitive psychology may be adapted to the cognitive assessment of some of the more inferred features of depression.

Another measure which has been frequently employed to assess cognitive processing in depression is the Stroop Color-Naming Task, especially a modification of this task that allows for the use of emotionally laden stimuli. On this task, depressed patients generally take longer to name the presentation color of negative words than of positive or neutral words (Gotlib & McCann, 1984; Williams & Nulty, 1986), whereas nondepressed controls show no difference in color-naming speed as a function of the valence of the word. The greater interference shown by depressed patients for negative material is thought to result from extended processing of the semantic content of stimuli, perhaps because this material is more accessible for the subject, and therefore harder to suppress in favor of rapid color naming (Williams et al., 1998).

Although the emotional Stroop paradigm can indicate the extent of semantic processing of valenced material, this particular methodology is unable to examine the more detailed question of whether material is organized in some fashion. To look at this question, some form of priming methodology can be used to advantage, by examining the effect of prior presentation of material on the processing of later-presented items. Segal et al. (1995) further modified the emotional Stroop paradigm to incorporate such a priming design, in which the color naming of a target word relevant to the individual's view of self was preceded by a prime word thought to be related or unrelated to the subject's self-concept. When one element in the depressive cognitive system is previously activated, other interconnected and related elements of the organization may also become activated, thus influencing performance on these related elements. In this way, the degree of interconnection between elements in the self-representation can be studied. Within a primed Stroop paradigm, if a prime is related to a target item presented in color, the prime's influence should be demonstrated by an increase in the time it takes to name the target's color, because the target's semantic content (activated by the prime) should interfere.

Using this approach, Segal et al. (1995) found that depressed patients showed increased interference for negative self-referent material when it was primed by similar negative information than when it was primed by negative information that was not self-descriptive. These results indicate that negative self-attributes are more highly organized in the self-concept of depressed patients than attributes that are negative but not particularly descriptive of the self.

The above-described findings are consistent with accounts of depression that emphasize the importance of cognitive organization in the maintenance of the disorder. Because cognitive-behavioral therapy (CBT) is thought to alter the negative nature of such organizations (Beck, 1967), successful treatment of this nature should reduce the strong associations between negative elements in an individual's cognitive system, and thus affect the amount of interference noted on such tasks as the primed Stroop task. Segal and Gemar (1997) found that patients who were less depressed at posttreatment following CBT showed less color-naming interference for self-descriptive negative information. This finding supports the view that negative information about the self is highly interconnected in the cognitive system of depressed patients, and suggests that possible changes to this organization may result from successful treatment for depression.

Remaining Issues

In summary, research on depression has resulted in a range of measures addressing the contents, processes, and "deep" structures of cognition. It remains to be seen whether cognitive variables are important markers of a vulnerability to depression. The clinician has many ways to assess cognitive changes during a depressive episode. Depending on his or her particular theoretical concerns, measures of cognition may be taken prior to, during, and following treatment. Most measures discussed in this chapter will be useful indicators of improvement. On the other hand, it is not easy to determine the cognitive changes that are uniquely influenced by CBT. At present, it seems that any treatment (or, for that matter, time alone) that serves to alter the state of depression will also result in substantial cognitive changes.

FUTURE DIRECTIONS

The field of cognitive assessment is now a little over 20 years old, dating from the seminal work of Kendall and Korgeski (1979) and others. It is clear that there have been many significant advances, both methodological and conceptual, over the past two decades. Nonetheless, the promise is not yet fulfilled. Clark (1997) has recently outlined a number of challenges confronting researchers and practitioners in the area of cognitive assessment, especially with respect to the assessment of cognitive products. What is evident is a strong trend toward diversification, which is a healthy development within cognitive assessment. Instead of stagnating behind rigid and narrow conceptualizations of what constitutes "acceptable" modes of assessment, cognitive clinical researchers provide a more enriched and vital armamentarium of assessment tools for the study of the relationship among cognition, emotion, and behavior.

We concur with Clark (1997), and, in addition, agree with those who recommend integration within cognitive assessment and integration with other approaches. For example, Glass and Arnkoff (1997) lament the fact that so little research has examined relations among measures of cognitive structures, processes, and products. Furthermore, the links between traditional measures (such as self-report questionnaires like the DAS) and approaches borrowed from cognitive psychology that typically employ a priming methodology (such as the Stroop Color-Naming Task; e.g., Segal et al., 1995) need to be more carefully examined, so that the convergent validity of the various cognitive assessment methods can be examined further. Clearly, a reliance on self-report methodologies is insufficient, especially when it is desirable to assess relatively automatic cognitive processes and schemata that are difficult to articulate verbally. Glass and Arnkoff (1997) and Amsel and Fichten (1998) have nonetheless outlined prescriptions for the improvement and development of self-statement inventories, and there is still much to learn about the products and processes of cognition from the judicious use of production methods, such as the thought-listing and think-aloud approaches. Thought sampling is a useful strategy, especially given its high ecological validity. Various reviewers (e.g., Glass & Arnkoff, 1997; Segal & Dobson, 1992) have pointed to the possibility of benefit from the standardization of instruments. Constructs such as automatic thoughts, schemata, and dysfunctional beliefs and assumptions have been notoriously difficult to measure; standardization would at least ensure that the accumulation of data from different studies could be brought to bear on the evaluation of any single construct.

With regard to depression, Segal and Dobson (1992) have pointed up the value of developing a typology of cognitions related to stress—particularly in the interpersonal and achievement domains, given the ongoing research on the congruency between achievement or interpersonal stress and depression onset and predictors of relapse (Segal, Shaw, Vella, & Katz, 1992). It will also be useful to examine the links between various personality constructs that have been posited as vulnerability factors for emotional disorders, especially when these are congruent with particular related life events, and the various cognitive structures, processes, and products that are hypothesized to contribute to the onset, maintenance, and relapse of psychological disorders such as anxiety and depression. For example, with respect to depression, Beck (1983) proposed two personality styles or modes as vulnerability markers for depression, which he labeled "sociotropy" and "autonomy." Sociotropic individuals have an excessive investment in interpersonal relationships, whereas autonomous individuals are excessively invested in autonomy and achievement.

Gotlib and Hammen (1992) have called for researchers in the depression area to begin to integrate cognitive and interpersonal aspects, and Segal and Dobson (1992) recommend expansion of assessment of cognitive representations of social relationships. Gotlib, Kurtzman, and Blehar (1997) have proposed that researchers should now examine the intersections of biological approaches to the study of depression, and McNally (1998) has recently surveyed points of contact between the cognitive and neurobiological perspectives with regard to anxiety disorders. These proposals will influence and enrich the field of cognitive assessment.

REFERENCES

Abel, G. G., Becker, J. V., Cunningham-Ratner, J., Rouleau, J. L., & Kaplan, M. (1984). *The treatment of child molesters*. Unpublished treatment manual, Emory University.

Abramson, K. Y., Seligman, M. E. P., & Teasdale, J. D. (1978). Learned helplessness in humans: Critique and reformulation. *Journal of Abnormal Psychology, 87*, 102–109.

Alloy, L. B., & Ahrens, A. H. (1987). Depression and pessimism for the future: Biased use of statistically relevant information in predictions for self versus others. *Journal of Personality and Social Psychology, 52*, 366–378.

American Psychiatric Association. (1994). *Diagnostic and statistical manual of mental disorders* (4th ed.). Washington, DC: Author.

Amsel, R., & Fichten, C. S. (1998). Recommendations for self-statement inventories: Use of valence, end points, frequency and relative frequency. *Cognitive Therapy and Research, 22*(3), 195–207.

Arnkoff, D. B., & Glass, C. R. (1982). Clinical cognitive constructs: Examination, evaluation, and elaboration. In P. C. Kendall (Ed.), *Advances in cognitive behavioural research and therapy* (Vol. 1, pp. 1–34). New York: Academic Press.

Bagby, R. M., Atkinson, L., Dickens, S., & Gavin, D. (1990). Dimensional analysis of the Attributional Style Questionnaire: Attributions or outcomes and events? *Canadian Journal of Behavioural Science, 22*, 140–150.

Beck, A. T. (1967). *Depression: Clinical, experimental and therapeutic aspects*. New York: Harper & Row.

Beck, A. T. (1976). *Cognitive therapy and the emotional disorders*. New York: International Universities Press.

Beck, A. T. (1983). Cognitive therapy of depression: New perspectives. In P. J. Clayton & J. E. Barnett (Eds.), *Treatment of depression: Old controversies and new approaches* (pp. 265–290). New York: Raven Press.

Beck, A. T., Brown, G., Steer, R. A., Eidelson, J. L., & Riskind, J. H. (1987). Differentiating anxiety and depression: A test of the cognitive-content specificity hypothesis. *Journal of Abnormal Psychology, 96,* 179–183.

Beck, A. T., Emery, G., & Greenberg, R. L. (1985). *Anxiety disorders and phobias.* New York: Basic Books.

Beck, A. T., Rush, A. J., Shaw, B. F., & Emery, G. (1979). *Cognitive therapy of depression.* New York: Guilford Press.

Beck, A. T., Steer, R. A., Epstein, R. A., & Brown, G. (1990). Beck Self-Concept Test. *Psychological Assessment, 2,* 191–197.

Beck, A. T., Steer, R. A., Kovacs, M., & Garrison, B. S. (1985). Hopelessness and eventual suicide: A 10-year prospective study of patients hospitalized with suicidal ideation. *American Journal of Psychiatry, 142,* 559–563.

Beck, A. T., Weissman, A., Lester, D., & Trexler, L. (1974). The measurement of pessimism: The Hopelessness Scale. *Journal of Consulting and Clinical Psychology, 42,* 861–865.

Blankstein, K. R., & Flett, G. L. (1990). Cognitive components of test anxiety: A comparison of assessment and scoring methods. *Journal of Social Behavior and Personality, 5,* 187–202.

Blankstein, K. R., Flett, G. L., Boase, P., & Toner, B. B. (1990). Thought listing and endorsement measures of self-referential thinking in test anxiety. *Anxiety Research, 2,* 103–111.

Blankstein, K. R., Toner, B. B., & Flett, G. L. (1989). Test anxiety and the contents of consciousness: Thought listing and endorsement measures. *Journal of Research in Personality, 23,* 269–286.

Bouvard, M., Cottraux, J., Mollard, E., Arthus, M., Lachance, S., Guerin, J., Sauteraud, A., & Yaoa, S. N. (1997). Validity and factor structure of the Obsessive Compulsive Thoughts Checklist. *Behavioural and Cognitive Psychotherapy, 25,* 51–66.

Bouvard, M., Mollard, E., Cottraux, J., & Guerin, J. (1989). Etude preliminaire d'une liste de pensées obsédantes: Validation et analyse factorielle. *L'Encéphale, 15,* 351–354.

Bowers, K. S., & Meichenbaum, D. (1984). *The unconscious reconsidered.* New York: Wiley.

Brewin, C. R., & Furnham, A. (1986). Attributional versus preattributional variables in self-esteem and depression: A comparison and test of learned helplessness theory. *Journal of Personality and Social Psychology, 50,* 1013–1020.

Breir, A., Charney, D. S., & Heninger, G. R. (1984). Major depression in patients with agoraphobia and panic disorder. *Archives of General Psychiatry, 41,* 1129–1135.

Brown, T. A., Antony, M. M., & Barlow, D. H. (1992). Psychometric properties of the Penn State Worry Questionnaire in a clinical anxiety disorders sample. *Behaviour Research and Therapy, 30,* 33–37.

Bruch, M. A., Haase, R. F., & Purcell, M. J. (1984). Content dimensions of self-statements in assertive situations: A factor analysis of two measures. *Cognitive Therapy and Research, 8,* 173–186.

Burns, G., Keortge, S. G., Formea, G. M., & Sternberger, L. G. (1996). Revision of the Padua Inventory of obsessive compulsive disorder symptoms: Distinctions between worry, obsessions and compulsions. *Behaviour Research and Therapy, 34,* 163–173.

Butler, G., & Mathews, A. (1983). Cognitive processes in anxiety. *Advances in Behaviour Research and Therapy, 5,* 51–62.

Cacioppo, J. T., von Hippel, W., & Ernst, J. M. (1997). Mapping cognitive structures and processes through verbal content: The thought listing technique. *Journal of Consulting and Clinical Psychology, 65,* 928–940.

Cartwright-Hatton, S., & Wells, A. (1997). Beliefs about worry and intrusions: The Meta-Cognitions Questionnaire and its correlates. *Journal of Anxiety Disorders, 11,* 279–296.

Carver, C. G., & Scheier, M. F. (1982). Control theory: A useful conceptual framework for personality–social, clinical, and health psychology. *Psychological Bulletin, 92,* 111–135.

Carver, C. S., & Scheir, M. F. (1983). A control theory approach to human behavior and implications for problems in self management. In P. C. Kendall (Ed.), *Advances in cognitive-behavioral research and therapy* (Vol. 2, pp. 127–194). New York: Academic Press.

Chambless, D. L., Caputo, G. C., Bright, P., & Gallagher, R. (1984). Assessment of fear in agoraphobics: The Body Sensations Questionnaire and the Agoraphobic Cognition Questionnaire. *Journal of Consulting and Clinical Psychology, 52,* 1090–1097.

Chen, E., & Craske, M. G. (1998). Risk perceptions and interpretations of ambiguity related to anxiety during a stressful event. *Cognitive Therapy and Research, 22,* 137–148.

Chorpita, B. F., Tracey, S. A., Brown, T. A., Collica, T. J., & Barlow, D. H. (1997). Assessment of worry in children and adolescents: An adaptation of the Penn State Worry Questionnaire. *Behaviour Research and Therapy, 35,* 569–581.

Clark, D. A. (1988). The validity of measures of cognition: A review of the literature. *Cognitive Therapy and Research, 12,* 1–20.

Clark, D. A. (1997). Twenty years of cognitive assessment: Current status and future directions. *Journal of Consulting and Clinical Psychology, 65,* 996–1000.

Clark, D. A., & Purdon, C. L. (1995). The assessment of unwanted intrusive thoughts: A review of the literature. *Behaviour Research and Therapy, 33,* 967–976.

Clark, D. M. (1986). A cognitive approach to panic. *Behaviour Research and Therapy, 24,* 461–470.

Clark, L. A., & Watson, D. (1991). Tripartite model of anxiety and depression: Psychometric evidence and taxonomic implications. *Journal of Abnormal Psychology, 100,* 316–336.

Clum, G. A., Broyles, S., Borden, J., & Watkins, P. L. (1990). Validity and reliability of the Panic Attack Symptoms and Cognitions Questionnaire. *Journal of Psychopathology and Behavioral Assessment, 12,* 233–245.

Cox, B. J. (1996). The nature and assessment of catastrophic thoughts in panic disorder. *Behaviour Research and Therapy, 34,* 363–374.

Craik, F. M., & Lockhart, R. S. (1972). Levels of processing: A framework for memory research. *Journal of Verbal Learning and Verbal Behaviour, 11,* 671–684.

Craik, F. M., & Tulving, E. (1975). Depth of processing and the retention of words in episodic memory. *Journal of Experimental Psychology: General, 104,* 268–294.

Davison, G. C., Robins, C., & Johnston, M. K. (1983). Articulated thoughts during simulated situations: A paradigm for studying cognition in emotion and behaviour. *Cognitive Therapy and Research, 7,* 17–40.

Davison, G. C., Vogel, R. S., & Coffman, S. G. (1997). Think-aloud approaches to cognitive assessment and the articulated thoughts in simulated situations paradigm. *Journal of Consulting and Clinical Psychology, 65,* 950–958.

Demo, D. H. (1985). The measurement of self-esteem: Refining our methods. *Journal of Personality and Social Psychology, 48,* 1490–1502.

Dent, J., & Teasdale, J. D. (1988). Negative cognition and the persistence of depression. *Journal of Abnormal Psychology, 97,* 29–34.

Dobson, K. S. (1985). The relationship between anxiety and depression. *Clinical Psychology Review, 5,* 307–324.

Dobson, K. S., & Breiter, H. J. (1983). Cognitive assessment of depression: Reliability and validity of three measures. *Journal of Abnormal Psychology, 92,* 107–109.

Dobson, K. S., & Shaw, B. F. (1986). Cognitive assessment with major depressive disorders. *Cognitive Therapy and Research, 10,* 13–29.

Duncker, K. (1926). A qualitative (experimental and theoretical) study of productive thinking (solving of comprehensible problems). *Pedagogical Seminary, 33,* 642–708.

Ericsson, K. A., & Simon, H. A. (1984). *Protocol analysis.* Cambridge, MA: MIT Press.

Exner, J. E. (1973). The self-focus sentence completion: A study of egocentricity. *Journal of Personality Assessment, 37,* 437–455.

Fenigstein, A., Scheier, M., & Buss, A. (1975). Public and private self-consciousness: Assessment and theory. *Journal of Consulting and Clinical Psychology, 37,* 522–577.

Feske, U., & De Beurs, E. (1997). The Panic Appraisal Inventory: Psychometric properties. *Behaviour Research and Therapy, 35,* 875–882.

Fichten, C. S., Libman, E., Creti, L., Amsel, R., Tagalakis, V., & Brender, W. (1998). Thoughts during awake times in older good and poor sleepers: The Self-Statement Test: 60+. *Cognitive Therapy and Research, 22,* 1–20.

Fiedler, R., & Beach, L. R. (1978). On the decision to be assertive. *Journal of Consulting and Clinical Psychology, 46,* 537–546.

Flett, G. L., Hewitt, P. L., Blankstein, K. R., & Gray, L. (1998). Psychological distress and the frequency of perfectionistic thinking. *Journal of Personality and Social Psychology, 75,* 1363–1381.

Freeston, M. H., & Ladouceur, R. (1993). Appraisal of cognitive intrusions and response style: Replication and extension. *Behaviour Research and Therapy, 31,* 185–191.

Frost, R. D., & MacInnis, D. J. (1983). The Cognitive Bias Questionnaire: Further evidence. *Journal of Personality Assessment, 47,* 173–177.

Gara, M. A., Woolfolk, R. L., Cohen, B. D., Goldston, R. B., Allen, L. A., & Novalany, J. (1993). Perception of self and others in major depression. *Journal of Abnormal Psychology, 102,* 93–100.

Gardner, H. (1985). *The mind's new science: A history of the cognitive revolution.* New York: Basic Books.

Genest, M., & Turk, D. C. (1981). Think-aloud approaches to cognitive assessment. In T. V. Merluzzi, C. R. Glass, & M. Genest (Eds.), *Cognitive assessment* (pp. 233–269). New York: Guilford Press.

Ghiselli, E. E., Campbell, J. P., & Zedeck, S. (1981). *Measurement theory for the behavioural sciences.* San Francisco: Freeman.

Glass, C. R., & Arnkoff, D. B. (1982). Think cognitively: Selected issues in cognitive assessment and therapy. In P. C. Kendall (Ed.), *Advances in cognitive-behavioral research and therapy* (Vol. 1, pp. 35–71). New York: Academic Press.

Glass, C. R., & Arnkoff, D. B. (1997). Questionnaire methods of cognitive self-statement assessment. *Journal of Consulting and Clinical Psychology, 65,* 911–927.

Glass, C. R., Merluzzi, T. V., Biever, J. L., & Larsen, K. H. (1982). Cognitive assessment of social anxiety: Development and validation of a self-statement questionnaire. *Cognitive Therapy and Research, 6,* 37–55.

Goldfried, M. R., & Davison, G. C. (1994). *Clinical behavior therapy* (expanded edition). New York: Wiley.

Goldfried, M. R., & Robins, C. (1983). Self-schema, cognitive bias, and the processing of therapeutic experiences. In P. C. Kendall (Ed.), *Advances in cognitive-behavioral research and therapy* (Vol. 2, pp. 330–380). New York: Academic Press.

Goldfried, M. R., Padawer, W., & Robins, C. (1984). Social anxiety and the semantic structure of heterosocial interactions. *Journal of Abnormal Psychology, 93,* 86–97.

Goldstein, A. J., & Chambless, D. L. (1978). A reanalysis of agoraphobia. *Behavior Therapy, 9,* 47–59.

Gong-Guy, E., & Hammen, C. L. (1980). Causal perceptions of stressful events in depressed and nondepressed outpatients. *Journal of Abnormal Psychology, 89,* 662–669.

Gotlib, I. H., & Hammen, C. L. (1992). *Psychological aspects of depression: Toward a cognitive-interpersonal integration.* Chichester, England: Wiley.

Gotlib, I. H., Kurtzman, H. S., & Blehar, M. C. (1997). The cognitive psychology of depression: Introduction to the special issue. *Cognition and Emotion, 5,* 497–675.

Gotlib, I. H., & McCann, C. D. (1984). Construct accessibility and depression: An examination of cognitive and affective factors. *Journal of Personality and Social Psychology, 47,* 427–439.

Haaga, D. A. (1997). Introduction to the special section on measuring cognitive products in research and practice. *Journal of Consulting and Clinical Practice, 65,* 907–919.

Hamilton, E. W., & Abramson, L. Y. (1983). Cognitive patterns and major depressive disorder: A longitudinal study in a hospital setting. *Journal of Abnormal Psychology, 92,* 173–184.

Hammen, C. L., & Cochran, S. D. (1981). Cognitive correlates of life stress in depression in college students. *Journal of Abnormal Psychology, 90,* 23–27.

Hammen, C. L., & Krantz, S. E. (1976). Effects of success and failure on depressive cognitions. *Journal of Abnormal Psychology, 85,* 577–586.

Hollon, S. D., & Kendall, P. C. (1980). Cognitive self-statements in depression: Development of an Automatic Thoughts Questionnaire. *Cognitive Therapy and Research, 4,* 383–396.

Hollon, S. D., Kendall, P. C., & Lumry, A. (1986). Specificity of depressotypic cognitions in clinical depression. *Journal of Abnormal Psychology, 95,* 52–59.

Hollon, S. D., & Kriss, M. R. (1984). Cognitive factors in clinical research and practice. *Clinical Psychology Review, 4,* 35–76.

Hurlburt, R. T. (1997). Randomly sampling thinking in the natural environment. *Journal of Consulting and Clinical Psychology, 65,* 941–948.

Hurlburt, R. T., & Spirelle, C. N. (1978). Random sampling of cognitions in alleviating anxiety attacks. *Cognitive Therapy and Research, 2,* 165–169.

Ingram, R. E. (1990). Self-focused attention in clinical disorders: Review and a conceptual model. *Psychological Bulletin, 107,* 156–176.

Ingram, R. E., & Kendall, P. C. (1986). Cognitive clinical psychology: Implications of an information processing perspective. In R. E. Ingram (Ed.), *Information processing approaches to clinical psychology* (pp. 3–21). New York: Academic Press.

Ingram, R. E., Lumry, A. B., Cruet, D., & Sieber, W. (1987). Attentional processes in depressive disorders. *Cognitive Therapy and Research, 11,* 351–360.

Ingram, R. E., Miranda, J., & Segal, Z. V. (1998). *Cognitive vulnerability to depression.* New York: Guilford Press.

Ingram, R. E., Slater, M. A., Atkinson, J. H., & Scott, W. (1990). Positive automatic cognition in major affective disorder. *Psychological Assessment, 2,* 209–211.

Ingram, R. E., & Smith, T. S. (1984). Depression and internal versus external locus of attention. *Cognitive Therapy and Research, 8,* 139–152.

Ingram, R. E., & Wisnicki, K. S. (1988). Assessment of positive automatic cognition. *Journal of Consulting and Clinical Psychology, 56,* 898–902.

Just, N., & Alloy, L. B. (1997). The response theory of depression: Test and an extension for the theory. *Journal of Abnormal Psychology, 106,* 221–229.

Keller, K. E. (1983). Dysfunctional attitudes and cognitive therapy for depression. *Cognitive Therapy and Research, 7,* 437–444.

Kendall, P. C. (1982). Behavioral assessment and methodology. In C. M. Franks, G. T. Wilson, P. C. Kendall, & K. D. Brownell (Eds.), *Annual review of behavior therapy* (Vol. 8, pp. 39–81). New York: Guilford Press.

Kendall, P. C., & Hollon, S. D. (1981). Assessing self-referent speech: Methods in the measurement of self-statements. In P. C. Kendall & S. D. Hollon (Eds.), *Assessment strategies for cognitive-behavioral interventions* (pp. 85–118). New York: Academic Press.

Kendall, P. C., & Hollon, S. D. (1989). Anxious self-talk: Development of the Anxious Self-Statements Questionnaire (ASSQ). *Cognitive Therapy and Research, 13,* 81–93.

Kendall, P. C., & Korgeski, G. P. (1979). Assessment and cognitive-behavioural interventions. *Cognitive Therapy and Research, 3,* 1–21.

Khawaja, N. G., & Oei, T. P. S. (1992). Development of a Catastrophic Cognitions Questionnaire. *Journal of Anxiety Disorders, 6,* 305–318.

Khawaja, N. G., & Oei, T. P. S. (1998). Catastrophic cognitions in panic disorder with and without agoraphobia. *Clinical Psychology Review, 18,* 341–365.

Khawaja, N. G., Oei, T. P. S., & Baglioni, A. (1994). Modification of the Catastrophic Cognitions Questionnaire (CCQ-M) for normals and patients: Exploratory and LISREL analyses. *Journal of Psychopathology and Behavioral Assessment, 16,* 325–342.

Krantz, S., & Hammen, C. L. (1979). Assessment of cognitive bias in depression. *Journal of Abnormal Psychology, 88,* 611–619.

Kuiper, N. A., & MacDonald, M. R. (1983). Schematic processing in depression: The self-consensus bias. *Cognitive Therapy and Research, 7,* 469–484.

Kuiper, N. A., & Olinger, L. J. (1986). Dysfunctional attitudes and a self-worth contingency model of depression. In P. C. Kendall (Ed.), *Advances in cognitive-behavioral research and therapy* (Vol. 5, pp. 115–142). New York: Academic Press.

Landau, R. J. (1980). The role of semantic schemata in phobic word interpretation. *Cognitive Therapy and Research, 4,* 427–434.

Last, C. G., Barlow, D. H., & O'Brien, G. T. (1985). Assessing cognitive aspects of anxiety: Stability over time and agreement between several methods. *Behaviour Modification, 9,* 72–93.

Lee, F., & Peterson, C. (1997). Content analysis of archival data. *Journal of Consulting and Clinical Psychology, 65,* 959–969.

Lefebvre, M. (1981). Cognitive distortion and cognitive errors in depressed psychiatric and low back pain patients. *Journal of Consulting and Clinical Psychology, 49,* 517–525.

Lewinsohn, P. M., Steinmetz, J. L., Larson, D. W., & Franklin, J. (1981). Depression-related cognitions: Antecedent or consequence? *Journal of Abnormal Psychology, 90,* 213–219.

Linville, P. W. (1987). Self-complexity as a cognitive buffer against stress-related illness and depression. *Journal of Personality and Social Psychology, 52,* 663–676.

MacDonald, M. R., & Kuiper, N. A. (1984). Self-schema decision consistency in clinical depressives. *Journal of Social and Clinical Psychology, 2,* 264–272.

MacLeod, A. K., Tata, P., Kentish, J., Carroll, F., & Hunter, E. (1997). Anxiety, depression and explanation-based pessimism for future positive and negative events. *Clinical Psychology and Psychotherapy, 4,* 15–24.

MacLeod, C., Mathews, A., & Tata, P. (1986). Attentional bias in emotional disorders. *Journal of Abnormal Psychology, 95,* 15–20.

Mathews, A., & MacLeod, C. (1985). Selective processing of threat cues to anxiety states. *Behaviour Research and Therapy, 23,* 563–569.

Mathews, A., & MacLeod, C. (1994). Cognitive approaches to emotion and emotional disorders. *Annual Review of Psychology, 45,* 25–50.

McCabe, R. E. (1999). Implicit and explicit memory for threat words in high and low anxiety sensitive participants. *Cognitive Therapy and Research, 23,* 21–38.

McDermut, W., & Haaga, D. A. F. (1994). Cognitive balance and specificity in anxiety and depression. *Cognitive Therapy and Research, 18,* 333–352.

McNally, R. J. (1998). Information-processing abnormalities in anxiety disorders: Implications for cognitive neuroscience. *Cognition and Emotion, 12,* 479–495.

Meichenbaum, D., & Butler, L. (1980). Cognitive ethology: Assessing the streams of cognition and emotion. In K. R. Blankstein, P. Pliner, & J. Polivy (Eds.), *Advances in the study of communication and affect: Vol. 6. Assessment and modification of emotional behavior* (pp. 139–163). New York: Plenum Press.

Mendonca, J. D., Holden, R. D., Mazmanian, D., & Dolan, J. (1983). The influence of response style on the Beck Hopelessness Scale. *Canadian Journal of Behavioural Science, 15,* 237–247.

Merluzzi, T. V., & Rudy, T. E. (1982, August). *Cognitive assessment of social anxiety: A "surface" and "deep" structure analysis in social anxiety. Social, personality, and clinical perspectives.* Paper presented at the annual convention of the American Psychological Association, Washington, DC.

Metalsky, G. I., Halberstadt, L. J., & Abramson, L. Y. (1987). Vulnerability to depressive mood reactions: Toward a more powerful test of the diathesis–stress and causal mediation components of the reformulated theory of depression. *Journal of Personality and Social Psychology, 52,* 386–393.

Metalsky, G. I., & Joiner, T. E. (1992). Vulnerability to depressive symptoms: A prospective test of the diathesis–stress and causal mediation components of the hopelessness theory of depression. *Journal of Personality and Social Psychology, 63,* 667–675.

Meyer, T. J., Miller, M. L., Metzger, R. L., & Borkovec, T. D. (1990). Development and validation of the Penn State Worry Questionnaire. *Behaviour Research and Therapy, 26,* 169–177.

Minkoff, K., Berhman, E., Beck, A. T., & Beck, R. (1973). Hopelessness, depression, and attempted suicide. *American Journal of Psychiatry, 130,* 455–459.

Miranda, J., & Persons, J. B. (1988). Dysfunctional attitudes are mood-state dependent. *Journal of Abnormal Psychology, 97,* 76–79.

Miranda, J., Persons, J. B., & Byers, C. N. (1990). Endorsement of dysfunctional beliefs depends on current mood state. *Journal of Abnormal Psychology, 99,* 237–241.

Molina, S., Borkovec, T. D., Peasley, C., & Person, D. (1998). Content analysis of worrisome streams of consciousness in anxious and dysphoric participants. *Cognitive Therapy and Research, 22,* 109–123.

Moss-Morris, R., & Petrie, K. J. (1997). Cognitive distortions of somatic experiences: Revision and validation of a measure. *Journal of Psychosomatic Research, 43,* 293–306.

Neisser, S. (1976). *Cognition and reality: Principles and implications of cognitive psychology.* San Francisco: Freeman.

Nelson, R. D., Hayes, S. C., Felton, J. L., & Jarrett, R. B. (1985). A comparison of data produced by different behavioural assessment techniques with implications for models of social-skills inadequacy. *Behaviour Research and Therapy, 23*, 1–11.

Newton, C. R., & Barbaree, H. E. (1987). Cognitive changes accompanying headache treatment: The use of a thought sampling procedure. *Cognitive Therapy and Research, 11*, 635–652.

Nisbett, R. E., & Wilson, T. D. (1977). Telling more than we can know: Verbal reports on mental processes. *Psychological Review, 84*, 231–259.

Nolen-Hoeksema, S., Larson, J., & Grayson, C. (1999). Explaining the gender differences in depressive symptoms. *Journal of Personality and Social Psychology, 77*, 1061–1072.

Nolen-Hoeksema, S., & Morrow, J. (1991). A prospective study of depression and posttraumatic stress symptoms after a natural disaster: The 1989 Loma Prieta earthquake. *Journal of Personality and Social Psychology, 61*, 115–121.

Nolen-Hoeksema, S., Morrow, J., & Fredrickson, B. L. (1993). Response styles and the duration of episodes of depressed mood. *Journal of Abnormal Psychology, 102*, 20–28.

Norman, W. H., Miller, I. W., & Klee, S. H. (1983). Assessment of cognitive distortion in a clinically depressed population. *Cognitive Therapy and Research, 7*, 133–140.

O'Hara, M. W., Rehm, L. P., & Campbell, S. B. (1982). Predicting depressive symptomatology: Cognitive behavioral models and post-partum depression. *Journal of Abnormal Psychology, 91*, 457–461.

Oliver, J. M., & Baumgart, E. P. (1985). The Dysfunctional Attitude Scale: Psychometric properties and relation to depression in an unselected adult population. *Cognitive Therapy and Research, 9*, 161–168.

Peterson, C., Semmel, A., von Baeyer, C., Abramson, L., Metalsky, G., & Seligman, M. E. P. (1982). The Attributional Style Questionnaire. *Cognitive Therapy and Research, 6*, 287–299.

Peterson, C., & Villanova, P. (1988). An expanded Attributional Style Questionnaire. *Journal of Abnormal Psychology, 97*, 87–89.

Peterson, R. A., & Reiss, S. (1992). *Anxiety Sensitivity Index manual* (2nd ed.). Worthington, OH: International Diagnostic Systems.

Purdon, C., & Clark, D. A. (1994). Perceived control and appraisal of obsessional and intrusive thoughts: Replication and extension. *Behavioural and Cognitive Psychotherapy, 22*, 269-285.

Pyszczynski, T., Holt, K., & Greenberg, J. (1987). Depression, self-focused attention, and expectancies for positive and negative future life events for self and others. *Journal of Personality and Social Psychology, 52*, 94–1001.

Rachman, S., & Hodgson, R. (1974). 1. Synchrony and desynchrony in fear and avoidance. *Behaviour Research and Therapy, 12*, 311–318.

Reiss, S. (1991). Expectancy theory of fear, anxiety, and panic. *Clinical Psychology Review, 11*, 141–153.

Riskind, J. H., Beck, A. T., & Smucker, M. R. (1983, December). *Psychometric properties of the Dysfunctional Attitude Scale in a clinical population.* Paper presented at the meeting of the World Congress of Behaviour Therapy, Washington, DC.

Ronan, K. R., Kendall, P. C., & Rowe, M. (1994). Negative affectivity in children: Development and validation of a self-statement questionnaire. *Cognitive Therapy and Research, 18,* 509–528.

Rosenberg, M. (1965). *Society and the adolescent self-image.* Princeton, NJ: Princeton University Press.

Rudy, T. E., Merluzzi, T. V., & Henahan, P. T. (1982). Construal of complex assertive situations: A multidimensional analysis. *Journal of Consulting and Clinical Psychology, 50,* 125–137.

Rush, A. J. (1984, March). *Measurement of the cognitive aspects of depression.* Paper presented at the NIMH Workshop on Measurement of Depression, Honolulu, HI.

Schmidt, N. B., Lerew, D. R., & Joiner, T. E., Jr. (1998). Anxiety sensitivity and the pathogenesis of anxiety and depression: Evidence for symptom specificity. *Behaviour Research and Therapy, 36,* 165–177.

Schwartz, R. M. (1997). Consider the simple screw: Cognitive science, quality improvement, and psychotherapy. *Journal of Consulting and Clinical Psychology, 65,* 970–983.

Schwartz, R. M., & Garamoni, G. L. (1989). Cognitive balance and psychopathology: Evaluation of an information processing model of positive and negative states of mind. *Clinical Psychology Review, 9,* 271–294.

Schwartz, R. M., & Gottman, J. (1976). Toward a task analysis of assertive behaviour. *Journal of Consulting and Clinical Psychology, 44,* 910–920.

Segal, Z. V. (1988). Appraisals of the self-schema construct in cognitive models of depression. *Psychological Bulletin, 103,* 147–162.

Segal, Z. V., & Cloitre, M. (1993). Methodologies for studying cognitive features of emotional disorder. In K. S. Dobson & P. C. Kendall (Eds.), *Psychopathology and cognition* (pp. 19–50). San Diego, CA: Academic Press.

Segal, Z. V., & Dobson, K. S. (1992). Cognitive models of depression: Report from a consensus conference. *Psychological Inquiry, 3,* 219–224.

Segal, Z. V., & Gemar, M. (1997). Changes in cognitive organization for negative self-referent material following cognitive behaviour therapy for depression: A primed Stroop study. *Cognition and Emotion, 11,* 501–516.

Segal, Z. V., Gemar, M., Truchan, C., Gurguis, M., & Hurowitz, L. M. (1995). A priming methodology for studying self-representation in major depressive disorder. *Journal of Abnormal Psychology, 104*(1), 205–213.

Segal, Z. V., & Ingram, R. E. (1994). Mood priming and construct activation in tests of cognitive vulnerability to unipolar depression. *Clinical Psychology Review, 14,* 663–695.

Segal, Z. V., & Marshall, W. L. (1985). Heterosexual social skills in a population of rapists and child molesters. *Journal of Consulting and Clinical Psychology, 53,* 55–63.

Segal, Z. V., Shaw, B. F., Vella, D. D., & Katz, R. (1992). Cognitive and life stress predictors of relapse in remitted unipolar depressed patients: Test of the congruency hypothesis. *Journal of Abnormal Psychology, 101,* 26–36.

Segal, Z. V., & Swallow, S. R. (1994). Cognitive assessment of unipolar depression: Measuring products, processes and structures. *Behaviour Research and Therapy, 32*(1), 147–158.

Seligman, M. E. P., Abramson, L., Semmel, A., & von Baeyer, C. (1979). Depressive attributional style. *Journal of Abnormal Psychology, 88,* 242–248.

Sewitch, T. S., & Kirsch, I. (1984). The cognitive content of anxiety: Naturalistic evidence for the predominance of threat-related thoughts. *Cognitive Therapy and Research, 8,* 49–58.

Silverman, J. S., Silverman, J. A., & Eardley, D. A. (1984). Do maladaptive attitudes cause depression? *Archives of General Psychiatry, 41,* 28–30.

Simons, A. D., Garfield, S. L., & Murphy, G. E. (1984). The process of change in cognitive therapy and pharmacotherapy for depression: Changes in mood and cognition. *Archives of General Psychiatry, 41,* 45–51.

Stober, J., & Bittencourt, J. (1998). Weekly assessment of worry: An adaptation of the Penn State Worry Questionnaire for monitoring changes during treatment. *Behaviour Research and Therapy, 36,* 645–656.

Swallow, S. R., & Kuiper, N. A. (1988). Social comparison and negative self-evaluations: An application to depression. *Clinical Psychology Review, 8,* 55–76.

Swinson, R., & Kirby, M. (1987). The differentiation of anxiety and depressive syndromes. In B. F. Shaw, Z. V. Segal, T. M. Vallis, & F. E. Cashman (Eds.), *Anxiety disorders: Psychological and biological perspectives* (pp. 21–34). New York: Plenum Press.

Taylor, S. (Ed.). (1999). *Anxiety sensitivity: Theory, research, and treatment of the fear of anxiety.* Mahwah, NJ: Erlbaum.

Taylor, S., & Cox, B. J. (1998). Anxiety sensitivity: Multiple dimensions and hierarchic structure. *Behaviour Research and Therapy, 36,* 37–51.

Teasdale, J. D. (1997). Assessing cognitive mediation of relapse prevention in recurrent mood disorders. *Clinical Psychology and Psychotherapy, 4,* 145–156.

Teasdale, J. D., & Dent, J. (1987). Cognitive vulnerability to depression: An investigation of two hypotheses. *British Journal of Clinical Psychology, 26,* 113–126.

Telch, M. J., Brouillard, M., Telch, C. F., Agras, W. S., & Taylor, C. B. (1987). Role of cognitive appraisal in panic-related avoidance. *Behaviour Research and Therapy, 27,* 373–383.

Turk, D. C., & Salovey, P. (1985). Cognitive structures, cognitive processes, and cognitive behaviour modification: 1. Client issues. *Cognitive Therapy and Research, 9,* 1–17.

Watkins, J., & Rush, A. J. (1983). The Cognitive Response Test. *Cognitive Therapy and Research, 7,* 425–436.

Watson, D., & Friend, R. (1969). Measurement of social-evaluative anxiety. *Journal of Consulting and Clinical Psychology, 33,* 448–457.

Watson, D., & Kendall, P. C. (1989). Common and differentiating features of anxiety and depression: Current findings and future directions. In P. C. Kendall & D. Watson (Eds.), *Anxiety and depression: Distinctive and overlapping features* (pp. 493–508). New York: Academic Press.

Webb, E. J., Campbell, D. T., Schwartz, R. D., & Sechrest, L. (1966). *Unobtrusive measures: Non-reactive research in the social sciences.* Chicago: Rand McNally.

Wegner, D. M., & Smart, L. (1997). Deep cognitive activation: A new approach to the unconscious, *Journal of Consulting and Clinical Psychology, 65,* 984–995.

Weissman, A. N. (1979). *The Dysfunctional Attitude Scale: A validation study.* Unpublished doctoral dissertation, University of Pennsylvania.

Weissman, A. N., & Beck, A. T. (1978). *Development and validation of the Dysfunctional Attitude Scale: A preliminary investigation.* Paper presented at the annual meeting of the American Educational Research Association, Toronto.

Wells, A. (1994). A multidimensional measure of worry: Development and preliminary validation of the Anxious Thoughts Inventory. *Anxiety, Stress and Coping, 6,* 289–299.

Wells, A. (1995). Meta-cognition and worry: A cognitive model of generalized anxiety disorder. *Behavioural and Cognitive Psychotherapy, 23,* 301–320.

Wells, A., & Papageorgiou, C. (1998). Relationships between worry, obsessive–compulsive symptoms and metacognitive beliefs. *Behaviour Research and Therapy, 36,* 899–913.

Westling, B. E., & Ost, L-B. (1993). Relationship between panic attack symptoms and cognitions in panic disorder patients. *Journal of Anxiety Disorders, 7,* 181–194.

Wheeler, L., & Miyake, K. (1992). Social comparison in everyday life. *Journal of Personality and Social Psychology, 62,* 760–773.

Wilkinson, I. M., & Blackburn, I. M. (1981). Cognitive style in depressed and recovered depressed patients. *British Journal of Clinical Psychology, 20,* 283–292.

Williams, J. M. G., & Nulty, D. D. (1986). Construct accessibility depression and the emotional Stroop task: Transient mood or stable structure. *Personality and Individual Differences, 7,* 485–491.

Williams, J. M. G., Watts, F., MacLeod, C., & Mathews, A. (1998). *Cognitive psychology and emotional disorders.* Chichester, England: Wiley.

Williams, R. M. (1988). *Individual differences in the effects of mood on cognition.* Unpublished doctoral dissertation, University of Oxford.

Williams, S. L. (1985). On the nature and measurement of agoraphobia. In M. Hersen, R. M. Eisler, & P. M. Miller (Eds.), *Progress in behavior modification* (Vol. 19, pp. 109–144). New York: Academic Press.

Williams, S. L., & Rappoport, A. (1983). Cognitive treatment in the natural environment for agoraphobics. *Behavior Therapy, 14,* 299–313.

Zweig, D. R., & Brown, S. D. (1985). Psychometric evaluation of a written stimulus presentation format for the Social Interaction Self-Statement Test. *Cognitive Therapy and Research, 9,* 285–296.

3

Cognitive-Behavioral Case Formulation

JACQUELINE B. PERSONS
JOAN DAVIDSON

A case formulation is a theory of a particular case. A cognitive-behavioral case formulation is an idiographic (individualized) theory that is based on a nomothetic (general) cognitive-behavioral theory (Haynes, Kaholokula, & Nelson, 2000). For example, a formulation might rely on Beck's (Beck, Rush, Shaw, & Emery, 1979) cognitive theory of psychopathology, which states that external life events activate schemata to produce symptoms and problems. A case formulation based on Beck's theory specifies *which* life events have activated *which* schemata to produce the symptoms and problems experienced by the particular patient under consideration.

The format and content of a case formulation depend on its function (Haynes & O'Brien, 2000). In this chapter we describe a format for a case formulation that has, as its chief function, helping the therapist devise an effective treatment plan (cf. Hayes, Nelson, & Jarrett, 1987).

Individualized case formulation has a long history in behavior therapy and behavior analysis and in psychodynamic psychotherapy, but it is a relatively recent development in cognitive therapy. Writings by behavior analysts are too numerous to name exhaustively, but include those by Nelson and Hayes (1986), Turkat (1985), and Wolpe (1980). Useful recent clinically oriented writings in behavioral analysis include those by Haynes, Leisen, and Blaine (1997), Haynes and O'Brien (2000), and O'Brien and

Haynes (1995). Recent writings on case conceptualization by cognitive and cognitive-behavioral therapists include those by Persons and colleagues (Persons, 1989, 1992; Persons & Tompkins, 1997), Nezu, Nezu, Friedman, and Haynes (1997), and Koerner and Linehan (1997). Eells (1997) has edited a volume that provides detailed description of conceptualization methods utilized by numerous psychotherapeutic orientations.

This chapter describes three levels of case formulation: formulation at the level of the case, at the level of the problem or syndrome, and at the level of the situation. We describe in detail the format of the cognitive-behavioral formulation at the case level, providing a clinical example (Judy). To illustrate the role of the formulation in enhancing treatment effectiveness, we offer several examples of the way the formulation was useful in Judy's therapy. We conclude with a brief discussion of the role of the individualized case formulation in an evidence-based approach to psychotherapy.

LEVELS OF CASE FORMULATION

As noted above, case formulation can occur at three levels: at the level of the case, at the level of the problem or syndrome, and at the level of the situation. In the formulation at the case level, the therapist develops a conceptualization of the case as a whole. One of the key roles of the case-level formulation is to explain the relationships among the patient's problems (see Haynes, 1992). This level of formulation can be helpful to the therapist when selecting treatment targets, as the therapist would like to focus first on problems that appear to play a causal role in other problems (e.g., depression may be causing marital problems and contributing to a child's behavior problems, and thus may merit early intervention). We strive to develop an initial case-level formulation after three to four sessions of therapy.

A formulation at the level of problem or syndrome provides a conceptualization of a particular clinical problem or syndrome, such as depressive symptoms, shoplifting, insomnia, obsessive–compulsive disorder, or bingeing and purging. Beck's cognitive theory of depression is a formulation at this level. In fact, when we use Beck's theory to conceptualize at the case level, we are extrapolating from the original theory, which was developed to explain a syndrome. The therapist's treatment plan for the syndrome or problem depends on the formulation of the problem. For example, one of us (J. B. P.) recently treated a patient who complained of severe fatigue. The assessment process yielded two possible formulations, either or both of which might explain the fatigue: abuse of sleeping medications, or negative thoughts ("There's no point in trying—I always fail") in response to a recent professional setback. The different formulations suggest different interventions.

A conceptualization at the level of situation provides a "miniformulation" of the patient's reactions in a particular situation, and this formulation guides the therapist's interventions in that situation. For developing a situation-level formulation based on Beck's theory, the Thought Record format (see Figure 3.1) is ideal, as it includes columns for the central components of Beck's theory: situation, thoughts, behaviors, and emotions. For example, a patient came to her therapy session wanting help with feelings of anxiety she had experienced in her Spanish class the previous evening. If that patient's Thought Record indicated that she had had the automatic thoughts "If I get anxious, I'll have a panic attack and pass out," and that she had responded emotionally by feeling anxious and apprehensive and behaviorally with rapid, shallow breathing and by sitting in the back of the class so as to be able to leave quickly if needed, then the therapist's interventions would focus on those problematic thoughts, behaviors, and feelings. If the patient's Thought Record indicated that she had had the automatic thoughts "I'm fat. No one will like me. I don't belong here," and that she had responded by feeling worthless and inadequate, speaking to no one, and leaving early, the therapist's interventions would address those problematic thoughts, behaviors, and feelings. The behavioral chain analyses of parasuicidal behaviors in Linehan's (1993) dialectical behavior therapy for patients with borderline personality disorder provide further examples of formulation at the level of the situation.

DATE	SITUATION (Event, memory, attempt to do something, etc.)	BEHAVIOR(S)	EMOTIONS	THOUGHTS	RESPONSES

FIGURE 3.1. Thought Record. Copyright 1998 San Francisco Bay Area Center for Cognitive Therapy. Reprinted by permission.

Case-level formulations often accrue from information collected in situation-level and problem-level formulations (J. S. Beck, 1995). All formulations are considered hypotheses, and the therapist is constantly revising and sharpening the formulations as the therapy proceeds. This chapter focuses primarily on the cognitive-behavioral formulation at the level of the case.

FORMAT OF THE COGNITIVE-BEHAVIORAL CASE FORMULATION

The cognitive-behavioral case formulation has five components: Problem List, Diagnosis, Working Hypothesis, Strengths and Assets, and Treatment Plan (see Figure 3.2). We describe each in turn, both in general and for the case of Judy, a patient treated (by J. D.) at the San Francisco Bay Area Center for Cognitive Therapy. Judy was a 35-year-old single European American woman who was living alone and working as a teacher. She sought treatment because she felt "down, dissatisfied, and discouraged about my current life and future plans."

Problem List

The Problem List is an exhaustive list of the patient's difficulties, stated in concrete, behavioral terms. We recommend that clinicians make a comprehensive Problem List that includes any difficulties the patient is having in any of the following domains: psychological/psychiatric symptoms, interpersonal, occupational, medical, financial, housing, legal, and leisure. We (and others; see Nezu & Nezu, 1993; Turkat & Maisto, 1985) recommend that the therapist make a comprehensive Problem List for several reasons. An all-inclusive list is helpful as the therapist searches for themes or speculates about causal relationships, in order to develop a Working Hypothesis (see below) that describes relationships among problems. A comprehensive list ensures that important problems are not overlooked. Simply making a comprehensive Problem List for a complex case can help the therapist feel less overwhelmed by the patient's multitudinous problems; even if all the problems cannot be tackled in the therapy or in a given session, at least they are on the list and won't be forgotten. A typical Problem List for an outpatient has five to eight items.

It is not always easy or even possible to make a comprehensive Problem List. Sometimes this is because the therapist is unassertive or does not take the time to conduct a comprehensive assessment. Sometimes it is because patients are not willing or able to acknowledge problems that they

Cognitive-Behavioral Case Formulation and Treatment Plan

Name: _____

Identifying Information: _____

Problem List

1. _____
   _____

2. _____
   _____

3. _____
   _____

4. _____
   _____

5. _____
   _____

6. _____
   _____

7. _____
   _____

8. _____
   _____

Diagnosis

Axis I: _____

Axis II: _____

Axis III: _____

Axis IV: _____

Axis V: _____

Working Hypothesis

Schemata:

(Self) _____ (Other) _____

(World) _____ (Future) _____

Precipitant/Acitivating Situations: _____

Origins: _____

Summary of the Working Hypothesis:

(continued)

FIGURE 3.2. Form for recording a cognitive-behavioral case formulation, including a Treatment Plan. Copyright 1999 by San Francisco Bay Area Center for Cognitive Therapy. Reprinted by permission.

Strengths and Assets _____

Treatment Plan

Goals (measures):

1. _____
2. _____
3. _____
4. _____

Modality: _____   Frequency: _____
Interventions: _____
_____
_____

Adjunct Therapies: _____
Obstacles: _____
_____
_____

FIGURE 3.2. *(cont.)*

consider shameful or frightening, or that they do not consider to be problems.

The use of paper-and-pencil assessment tools can be helpful in some of these situations. Because substance abuse is often a problem that patients are reluctant to discuss, we ask patients at our center to complete a standard pretreatment assessment packet that includes a substance abuse scale. We use a modification of the CAGE questionnaire (Mayfield, McLeod, & Hall, 1974), to which we have added a few items to assess what substances the patient uses and how much and how often he or she uses them.

Careful observation can also reveal problem behaviors that patients may not mention directly. Bounced checks, last-minute cancellations, or frequent requests to reschedule appointments may point to financial problems or a chaotic lifestyle. A patient who is overly accommodating and compliant may have assertion difficulties.

When the therapist observes or suspects problems that the patient does not wish to acknowledge, the therapist must use his or her judgment to determine whether it is necessary to get a particular problem out on the table right away or whether a detailed discussion might be postponed. We find the categories Linehan (1993) uses to prioritize problems of patients with borderline personality disorder to be helpful in making this judgment. Linehan proposes that problems involving suicidal and parasuicidal behaviors, therapy-interfering behaviors (e.g., noncompliance with treatment) or "quality-of-life-interfering behaviors" (e.g., significant substance abuse, shoplifting, or homelessness—problems that, unless solved, will interfere with the individual's ability to achieve any other goals) must be explicitly addressed early on. Less acute problems can be put on hold or ignored altogether.

We recommend that the format of each item on the Problem List consist of a one- to two-word description of the problem, followed by a short description of some typical behavioral, cognitive, and mood components of the problem when this is appropriate. This format is particularly important for describing psychological problems; some problems (medical, housing, legal, or financial problems, for example) are not readily described in terms of cognitions, behaviors, and moods. The behavioral component of a problem might include gross motor behaviors (e.g., avoiding driving across bridges), physiological responses (e.g., increased heart rate), or both. This format has its origins in Beck's cognitive theory, which describes clinical problems in terms of cognitive, behavioral and mood components.

Sometimes it is difficult to decide how to categorize problems on the Problem List. For example, procrastination could be categorized as a behavioral component of a psychological problem or as a work problem, because the procrastination interferes with the patient's functioning at work. Should this problem appear on the Problem List as "Procrastination," as "Work problems," or both? There is no clear-cut answer to this question; we recommend that therapists approach this situation in whatever way facilitates their work and communication with their patients. We often list a problem in both ways. For example, in the case illustration below, Judy's therapist listed a procrastination problem, as well as work and interpersonal problems. This was done because the patient herself described her problem as "procrastination," and so it was useful to state it this way on her Problem List. Then, as the therapist obtained details of the procrastination problem, it became clear that it occurred in both work and interpersonal arenas. Both these two domains were added to the Problem List, in part because procrastination was not Judy's only problem in those domains.

JUDY'S PROBLEM LIST

Here is Judy's Problem List as her therapist recorded it:

   1. *Depressed, dissatisfied, passive.* Beck Depression Inventory at intake = 16. Thoughts: "My job is boring," "I'll never find a life partner," "I'm not happy with my life and I probably never will be." Behaviors: Procrastination, poor follow-through (takes fitful steps to join a gym, see friends more, find a better job, begin dating, but does not follow through).
   2. *Disorganized, unfocused, and unproductive.* This happens daily at

work (lesson planning, grading papers) and at home (household repair projects). Judy feels overwhelmed, has difficulty concentrating, thinks "I can't handle this quite right, so I'll move on to something else," and jumps from task to task with no overall plan or direction. As a result, she accomplishes less than she wants, and frequently feels dissatisfied and discouraged at the end of the day.

3. *Job dissatisfaction.* Judy states, "I'm bored, I don't like my job," and describes the work environment as stressful and unsupportive. She has many responsibilities but little authority or administrative support. She wants to find a better, more challenging job, but does not move forward to do this.

4. *Social isolation.* Judy has many friends but spends little time with them. Behaviors: Comes home from work, grades papers, prepares the next day's lesson, watches TV, goes to bed. Mood: Tired and discouraged. Thoughts: "I'm too tired to see anyone. I just want to go home and collapse. I have work to do anyway." On weekends she meets one or two friends for dinner, but she has not seen many friends for months, and she wants to go to "more interesting" events where she can meet new people. She often sleeps late, has difficulty accomplishing errands and work tasks, and then cancels evening social plans to stay home and finish them.

5. *No relationship.* Judy states, "I want to marry and have children, but I don't think I'll ever meet anyone." Mood: Hopeless, discouraged. Behaviors: She makes plans to answer personal ads and join a dating service but does not follow through; no dating except for casual get-togethers with a man who is not interested in a long-term relationship. Thoughts: "Why bother? I won't meet anyone decent. It probably won't work out anyway."

6. *Unassertive.* Judy frequently feels angry with others for not meeting her needs, but she does not speak up to express her needs. This happens with both coworkers and friends. Thoughts: "It won't matter if I say anything. I won't get what I want anyway. It will just lead to a confrontation, and I'll feel worse than if I hadn't said anything." Recent situations include a friend who repeatedly asks her for help and two coworkers who often ask her to take on additional menial tasks. Judy agrees to such requests, but then feels resentful.

Diagnosis

Psychiatric diagnosis is not, strictly speaking, part of a cognitive-behavioral case formulation. However, we include a section for Diagnosis in our formulation for several reasons. The Diagnosis can lead to some initial formulation hypotheses. For example, Beck's cognitive theory underpins a therapy for treatment of major depression that has been shown to be effective in randomized trials. If our patient meets criteria for major depression, we might consider the hypothesis that Beck's theory can serve as the template for an idiographic formulation of her case. In addition, the diagnosis can give some information about helpful treatment interventions; the evidence-based therapist will want to rely on results of randomized trials, and randomized trials are generally organized around diagnoses.

DIAGNOSES FOR JUDY

> Axis I: Dysthymic disorder
> Axis II: None.
> Axis III: None.
> Axis IV: Socially isolated, occupational problems.
> Axis V: Global Assessment of Functioning score = 60.

Working Hypothesis

The Working Hypothesis is the heart of the formulation. Here the therapist develops a minitheory of the case, adapting a nomothetic theory to the particulars of the case at hand. After showing how to develop a Working Hypothesis based on Beck's theory, we say a bit about how to develop a Working Hypothesis based on other cognitive-behavioral theories.

The Working Hypothesis also describes the relationships among the problems on the Problem List. Some problems result not from the activation of schemata, but from other problems. For example, a depressed man's marital problems may result not from schema activation, but from the depressive symptoms themselves, which cause him to withdraw from his wife and family. And some problems result entirely or in part from biological, environmental, or other nonpsychological factors, as in the case of medical problems or financial problems resulting from an employer's bankruptcy.

WORKING HYPOTHESIS BASED ON BECK'S COGNITIVE THEORY

Beck's cognitive diathesis theory states that external life events activate schemata to produce symptoms and problems. A Working Hypothesis based on Beck's cognitive theory describes the external events and schemata that are operative in the case at hand, and offers a summary statement describing the relationships among these components and among the problems on the Problem List. Separate subheadings can be used for the Schemata, Precipitants/Activating Situations, Origins, and Summary of the Working Hypothesis, as we detail here and illustrate for the case of Judy.

Schemata. In the first section of the Working Hypothesis, the therapist offers hypotheses about the schemata, or core beliefs, that appear to be causing or maintaining the problems on the Problem List. These are generally negative beliefs. Patients may also hold positive schemata, but the negative ones are usually the ones that cause the problems on the Problem List, so they are the ones itemized in this section of the formulation.

Beck's theory emphasizes the importance of understanding patients' beliefs about self, others, world, and future. The therapist may wish to provide hypotheses about all four of these types of beliefs or to focus on only two or three (the goal is clinical utility, not exhaustive explanation). We find the patient's views of self and others to be particularly clinically useful. The patient's views of others can be helpful to the therapist because the therapist is, of course, an "other," and this component of the formulation can allow the therapist to make some predictions about distortions that may arise in the patient's views of the therapist.

A patient probably has multiple views of self, others, world, and future. For example, Judy had two prominent views of others—one apparently learned from experiences with her mother (passive/weak/helpless), and one learned from her father (angry/critical/attacking). She viewed some people as weak and fragile, others as potentially hostile and attacking, and still others as having both sets of qualities. Judy held a general belief that subsumed these two: a view of others as unsupportive of her.

The therapist may also find it useful to specify some conditional beliefs, stated in "if–then" terms, in this part of the formulation. An example is "If I speak up, others will get angry and withdraw from me" (see Beck, Freeman, & Associates, 1990).

Precipitants and Activating Situations. In the second section of the Working Hypothesis, the therapist specifies external events and situations that activate schemata to produce symptoms and problems. The term "Precipitants" refers to larger-scale, molar events that precipitated an episode of illness or the patient's decision to seek treatment. An example is a poor work evaluation that activated, for a computer salesperson, a downward spiral into a clinical depression.

The term "Activating Situations" refers to smaller-scale events that precipitate negative mood or maladaptive behaviors. Typical examples of Activating Situations for a patient whose depression had its onset following receiving a poor work evaluation included driving to work in the morning, attending meetings with his boss, and meeting with a client who was critical of him and his firm's products.

It is not always easy to draw a distinction between Precipitants and Activating Events, and this distinction is not always crucial for treatment-planning purposes. The main goal is to say something in this section of the formulation about the types of external events and situations that are problematic for the patient.

We believe it is important to assess external events and situations for several reasons. First, the cognitive theory states that psychopathological symptoms and problems are not due simply to intrapsychic events; they arise from the *activation*, by external events, of internal structures (schemata). As a result, we expect a "match" between the patient's schemata and the external events activating them. For example, Beck (1983) states that autonomous types of individuals (who believe "I must be successful in order to be a worthwhile person") are vulnerable to depression when they experience failure. If this theory is correct (and some evidence supports it; see Hammen, Ellicott, Gitlin, & Jamison, 1989), then the therapist can gain some information about what schemata the patient holds by examining the external events that appear to play a role in activating the schemata.

Information about which situations are problematic for the patient is also helpful when intervening, as it is important to design interventions that can be utilized in those situations. Finally, although it is not much discussed in the literature, we find that it is useful to work with patients not just to change their reactions to external situations, but sometimes to help them change the situations themselves. Some activity-scheduling interventions can be conceptualized in this way. For example, an engineer reported that he functioned poorly in a work environment in which he was isolated and required to function independently; he functioned much better when he worked as part of a team. An important part of treating this young man's depression involved helping him take assertive action to obtain the type of work environment in which he flourished.

Origins. In the third section of the Working Hypothesis, the clinician briefly describes one or a few incidents or circumstances in the patient's early history that account for how the patient might have learned the Schemata or functional relationships listed in the Working Hypothesis. The Origins section can also include modeling experiences, or failures to learn important skills and behaviors, as in the case of a patient who has significant social skills deficits due in part to growing up in a family in which both parents themselves had marked social skills deficits.

Summary of the Working Hypothesis. In a summary statement, the therapist tells a story that describes the relationships among the components of the Working Hypothesis (Schemata, Precipitants/Activating Situations, and Origins), tying them to the problems on the Problem List. The Working Hypothesis can be described either verbally, or in a kind of a flow chart—as illustrated in Haynes (1992) and Nezu et al. (1997), and as we demonstrate below in the case of Judy.

WORKING HYPOTHESIS FOR JUDY

Schemata. Judy's schemata about self, others, world, and future were as follows:

"*I* am undeserving, emotionally disabled, inadequate, incapable of success."
"*Others* are undependable, unsupportive, won't come through for me. They are angry/critical/attacking or passive/weak/helpless."
"The *world* is unrewarding, demanding, scary."
"The *future* is ultimately unrewarding."

Precipitants and Activating Situations. Judy's Precipitants were watching others achieve goals and make major life transitions (e.g., getting a promotion or a new job, getting married, having a child). The experience of attending the wedding of a close friend pushed Judy into therapy.

As for Judy's Activating Situations, in general these were situations in which she felt stuck and unable to take action to achieve her goals, and situations in which she felt resentful and overburdened when she did not assert herself with others. Examples included looking at the personal ads, looking at her "to-do list" for the day, and being asked for help she didn't want to give.

Origins. Judy's father was dependent on alcohol; he was prone to unpredictable angry outbursts and to verbal and occasional physical abuse directed at his wife and children. He repeatedly ridiculed Judy and told her she was stupid and crazy, especially if she tried to assert herself. Judy's mother appeared fragile and helpless; she modeled passive, avoidant behaviors.

Summary of the Working Hypothesis. Judy's Working Hypothesis proposed that when she was faced with taking actions to further her goals, her schemata that she was incapable and damaged were activated. She had learned from her mother's passive behaviors and from her father's abusive ones that she was damaged and incapable of taking action. When these schemata were activated, she became passive and inactive, with the result that she did not achieve her goals and felt dissatisfied and discouraged. This pattern occurred repeatedly in both work and social situations, and led to the difficulties she experienced in both those settings. A flow chart depicting Judy's Working Hypothesis is presented in Figure 3.3.

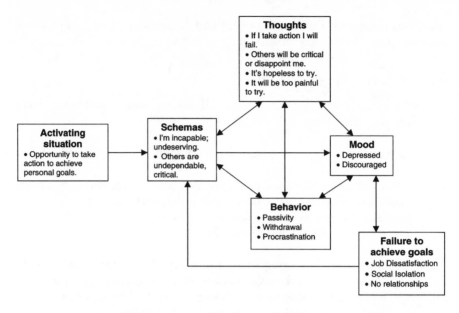

FIGURE 3.3. Judy's Working Hypothesis.

WORKING HYPOTHESES BASED ON OTHER COGNITIVE-BEHAVIORAL THEORIES

A Working Hypothesis based on Beck's cognitive theory will specify the activating events, the schemata, and some typical behaviors/automatic thoughts/moods arising when the schemata are activated. Other cognitive-behavioral theories can also serve as templates for individualized case conceptualizations (see Nezu et al., 1997; Koerner & Linehan, 1997).

Behavioral analysis offers a particularly powerful and well-developed alternative to cognitive conceptualization schemes. A functional-analytic approach to case conceptualization treats psychopathological behaviors as serving a function and as caused and controlled by contingencies in the environment (Haynes & O'Brien, 2000), in contrast to the structural view of psychopathology utilized in Beck's model, which views psychopathological symptoms as caused by underlying structures (schemata). Concretely, this means that the functional analyst attempts to understand the functions and causes of problem behaviors by collecting information about environmental antecedents and consequences, not by hypothesizing underlying causal schemata. Useful formulations often include both cognitive (structural) and functional hypotheses. In Judy's case, for example, her withdrawal and avoidance behavior could be seen, in a structural hypothesis, as a set of behaviors resulting from activation of her schemata about herself and others, and, in a functional hypothesis, as serving the function of allowing her to avoid situations she expected would be unpleasant.

Strengths and Assets

Strengths and Assets can include good social skills, the ability to work collaboratively, a sense of humor, a good job, financial resources, a good support network, regular exercise, intelligence, personal attractiveness, and/or a stable lifestyle. We recommend that therapists collect information about strengths and assets for several reasons. This type of information can assist the therapist in developing a Working Hypothesis; for example, in Judy's case, the therapist's observation that Judy had excellent social skills ruled out the possibility that a major social skills deficit might be contributing to her social isolation. Utilizing the patient's strengths can enhance the Treatment Plan; one of us (J. B. P.) recently treated a young man who made excellent use of his strong spiritual beliefs when he was learning to resist urges to perform obsessive–compulsive rituals. A clear assessment of Strengths and Assets can also assist the therapist in setting realistic treatment goals.

JUDY'S STRENGTHS AND ASSETS

The therapist listed these Strengths and Assets for Judy: Stable lifestyle; bright; excellent social skills; a good support network of girlfriends.

Treatment Plan

Strictly speaking, the Treatment Plan is not part of the formulation—it stems from and is based on the formulation, particularly the Problem List and the Working Hypothesis. We include the Treatment Plan in the case formulation to stress the point that the Treatment Plan is based directly on the formulation. For example, if the therapist hypothesizes that a patient's social anxiety is due in part to social skills deficits, the Treatment Plan for that patient will include social skills training. If, instead, the social anxiety appears to result from Schemata such as "If I speak up for myself, others will get angry and attack me" and from avoidance of social situations, the Treatment Plan will include cognitive restructuring, behavioral exposure, and behavioral experiments to test out the Schemata and automatic thoughts.

The Treatment Plan component of the formulation has six components: Goals, Modality, Frequency, Interventions, Adjunct Therapies, and Obstacles. The Goals and Obstacles sections are particularly important, and we describe each in some detail.

GOALS

The Problem List often suggests treatment goals; that is, the Goals may be seen as ways to solve the problems on the Problem List. If this is the case, is it necessary to develop both a Problem List and a list of treatment Goals? We believe it is, for two reasons. First, note that, as we have discussed earlier, patient and therapist do not always agree about the contents of the Problem List. The therapist's Problem List sometimes includes items that the patient does not view as problems. In contrast, we recommend that patient and therapist strive to develop a list of treatment Goals they can both agree on. Goals are difficult enough to reach when patient and therapist are in complete agreement about them! Second, most patients are not eager to solve all of their problems; generally they seek treatment to address one or two particularly important or distressing problems. Furthermore, most insurance companies don't want to pay for patients to solve all their problems, either. Finally, patients often have the ability to solve some problems on their own after some difficult ones are addressed in treatment.

When the therapist is specifying treatment Goals, it is important to state how progress toward the Goals will be measured. Often measurement can be done via a simple count (e.g., number of panic attacks, or number of days per week the patient exercises). Self-report inventories can also be used. At our center we routinely use the Beck Depression Inventory (Beck, Ward, Mendelsohn, Mock, & Erbaugh, 1961), the Burns Anxiety Inventory (Burns, 1998), and the Yale–Brown Obsessive–Compulsive Inventory (Goodman, Price, Rasmussen, et al., 1989) to monitor weekly progress. And, in line with our idiographic approach to treatment, we often develop idiographic measures for assessing an individual patient's problems. Self-monitoring (see Cone, 1999, devoted to self-monitoring) is ideal for this purpose. An extensive discussion of strategies for measuring patient progress is beyond the scope of this chapter (see Bloom, Fischer, & Orme, 1995).

OBSTACLES

In the last component of the Treatment Plan formulation, the therapist uses the case formulation proper—particularly the Problem List, Schemata, and Working Hypothesis—to make predictions about difficulties that might arise in the therapeutic relationship or other aspects of the treatment. Sometimes items on the Problem List, such as financial problems, major interpersonal conflicts, and difficulty working collaboratively with others, can alert the therapist to problems that are likely to occur in and interfere with therapy.

The rationale for this section of the formulation is that an early awareness of potential difficulties can help patient and therapist cope more effectively with them. For example, one of us (J. D.) recently treated Anne, a patient whose Problem List included job instability. A discussion of Anne's job difficulties in therapy led to the hypothesis that Anne had problems tolerating situations when results were not immediately gratifying. This hypothesis suggested that she might be prone to terminate therapy prematurely if results were not immediate. Anne and her therapist were able to discuss this potential obstacle to treatment very early in treatment and to address it by setting realistic therapy goals, monitoring Anne's urges to terminate therapy prematurely, and clarifying treatment expectations regularly.

JUDY'S TREATMENT PLAN

The therapist recorded Judy's Treatment Plan as follows.

Goals:

1. Reduce depressive symptoms, especially procrastination (measured via Beck Depression Inventory and a log of steps taken toward certain goals).
2. Increase ability to prioritize and organize at work and at home.
3. Find a more satisfying job (measured directly).
4. Increase time spent with friends (measured via number of social events/week with friends).
5. Begin dating in an effort to meet a husband (measured via number of dates/week with eligible men).
6. Increase assertiveness (measured via a log of assertive behaviors).

Modality: Individual cognitive-behavioral therapy.

Frequency: Weekly.

Initial Interventions:

Teach the formulation (to provide rationale for interventions).
Activity scheduling (work tasks, socializing, dating, job search).
Cognitive restructuring (Thought Records, behavioral experiments).
Assertiveness training.
Schema change interventions.

Adjunct therapies: Pharmacotherapy is an option if Judy does not respond to cognitive-behavioral therapy.

Obstacles:

Procrastination predicts problems with homework compliance.

Unassertiveness predicts Judy may have difficulty being assertive with the therapist (e.g., saying "No" to homework assignments she doesn't want to do).

"I'm incapable of succeeding" predicts Judy may have difficulty taking action to achieve her goals and may get discouraged when setbacks occur.

USING THE CASE FORMULATION IN TREATMENT

As we have indicated earlier, the role of the formulation is to assist the therapist in the treatment process. The primary role of the formulation is to guide the therapist in treatment planning and intervening. Thus treatment interventions ought to target Treatment Goals, ought to capitalize on the patient's Strengths and Assets, and should flow clearly from the Working Hypothesis.

One test of a formulation is the success of the treatment plan it drives. Judy did achieve her treatment goals. Her Beck Depression Inventory score decreased to a consistent score of 6 to 8. She learned coping strategies to follow through with initiatives she began, and to counter giving up when she had setbacks. She functioned more effectively, was more organized, and accomplished more. She resumed her previous level of interactions with her girlfriends; she found a more fulfilling job; and she began dating and married 2 years after beginning therapy. She reported feeling happier and more optimistic about her future because she was more confident in her ability to take action, even if it meant tolerating some discomfort. To accomplish these goals, Judy attended weekly therapy sessions for just over one year, followed by monthly sessions for 5 months to help her maintain her gains. After her therapy ended, she returned twice for a series of 8 to 10 sessions when she got stuck and paralyzed by demanding situations (e.g., tackling a complex legal and interpersonal problem).

We provide some detailed information about the ways in which the formulation was helpful to Judy's therapist at various points in the therapy.

1. *Constructing a Problem List clarified treatment Goals.* Judy initially described her unhappiness in vague terms, complaining of feeling "stuck, depressed, and unsatisfied with life." Judy's vague, amorphous statement of her predicament was part of what made it so hard for her to solve it. As the therapist asked questions to concretize the mood, behavioral, and cognitive com-

ponents of her complaint, the Problem List emerged. A clear Problem List led to a clear list of treatment Goals. The explicit description of Judy's difficulties was an important first step in treating them.

2. *The formulation helped the therapist maintain a clear focus while working on multiple problems.* Judy had many problems: She felt depressed and discouraged, she had interpersonal problems, and she was unhappy at work. The formulation was particularly useful in this case because it clarified the central theme of the case and helped the therapist maintain a clear focus to the therapy. Judy's Working Hypothesis proposed that when she was faced with taking actions to further her goals, her schemata that she was incapable and damaged were activated, causing her to become passive and inactive, with the result that she did not achieve her goals and felt dissatisfied and discouraged. Moreover, Judy's mood, behavioral, and cognitive responses to schemata activation led to consequences (not achieving goals) that strengthened the problematic schemata ("I'm incapable and damaged."). This pattern occurred repeatedly in both work and social situations.

Keeping this central theme in mind, the therapist sometimes used the therapy session to take up work issues and sometimes addressed interpersonal and social issues, but always focused on the maladaptive pattern described in the Working Hypothesis. Rather than seeing each of the problems on Judy's Problem List as separate and choosing unique interventions for each, the therapist used the formulation to see Judy's main task in therapy as overcoming the maladaptive pattern described in the Working Hypothesis in all of the arenas where it interfered with her functioning. The therapist used the formulation to design interventions to help Judy learn to take actions toward her Goals, and to persist and follow through even when she felt uncomfortable and believed things were hopeless. The therapist used the formulation to maintain a clear focus in the therapy, even while working on multiple problems simultaneously.

3. *The formulation helped the patient play an active and collaborative role in treatment.* With a shared formulation, patient and therapist are working collaboratively as a formidable team. Therefore, we recommend that the therapist share, as early in treatment as possible, as much of the formulation as possible. Judy's therapist laid out a key part of Judy's formulation in one of the very first sessions of therapy. In that session, when Judy learned that cognitive therapy involved learning skills to identify and change cognitions and behaviors, she became discouraged and said, "I won't be able to do this therapy. It won't help, and then I'll feel even more like a failure." The therapist used a Thought Record (a situation-level formulation) to show Judy how these thoughts caused her to feel discouraged and tempted to give up on the therapy. Using the "downward arrow" technique (see Burns, 1980), Judy identified the belief that she was "emotionally disabled" because of her childhood experiences and therefore could not succeed at anything she tried. The

therapist showed Judy how her view of herself as disabled and her tendency to feel discouraged and to give up when she encountered challenges threaded through many of her presenting problems.

Through this important therapy session and many others like it, Judy came to understand the formulation clearly. She assumed an active role in her treatment, working hard to identify and test the Working Hypothesis. Judy became adept at identifying Activating Situations, the Schemata that became activated in those situations, and the maladaptive responses she made when activated. She gained a sense of control and hope when she saw that she was capable of recognizing her maladaptive pattern when it occurred. In fact, feelings of self-efficacy engendered in this way helped Judy counter her view of herself as incapable.

4. *The case formulation helped the therapist understand and manage her own negative reactions to the patient.* The therapist found it both gratifying and frustrating to work with Judy. Judy made progress in therapy— but inconsistently. She often failed to follow through with her homework assignments and came to therapy sessions feeling discouraged and deflated, stalled and stuck. When this happened, the therapist herself sometimes felt frustrated and discouraged. Careful attention to her own reactions helped the therapist identify her own maladaptive thoughts: "Maybe Judy *is* incapable of doing better," and "Maybe she's not motivated enough to work on getting better."

To handle this maladaptive thinking, it was helpful to the therapist to review the formulation. When she did this, she noticed that she was succumbing to the patient's maladaptive Schemata ("Judy is defective and incapable," "The future is hopeless and bleak"). This recognition helped the therapist feel less frustrated when Judy did not do her homework or make smooth progress in treatment. In fact, the formulation allowed the therapist to predict (see the predicted Obstacles in Judy's Treatment Plan, above) early that Judy would have trouble doing her homework. The ability to anticipate the homework noncompliance problem made it easier for the therapist to manage the noncompliance when it occurred.

The formulation also explained why Judy had difficulty doing her homework. The formulation explained that Judy had difficulty doing her homework for the same reasons she had many of the other difficulties on her Problem List: Her Schemata about being defective and incapable became activated, and these caused her to get uncomfortable and discouraged and pull back. Remembering this formulation helped the therapist maintain her equilibrium when Judy didn't do her homework. Homework noncompliance became just another problem to work on in treatment.

To summarize, Judy's therapist used the formulation to clarify treatment goals, to help maintain a clear focus while working on multiple problems, to facilitate the patient's playing an active and collaborative role in treatment, and to help the therapist understand and manage negative reactions to working with Judy. Additional examples of the clinical utility of the formulation are provided by O'Brien and Haynes (1995), Tompkins (1999), Turkat (1980), and Turkat and Maisto (1985), among others.

ROLE OF THE INDIVIDUALIZED CASE FORMULATION IN EVIDENCE-BASED PSYCHOTHERAPY

The Tension between Formulation-Driven Treatment and Treatment Supported by Randomized Controlled Trials

We hold the value that the clinician has a professional and ethical responsibility to provide treatment that has been shown to be effective in controlled studies—ideally, in randomized controlled trials (RCTs). The thoughtful reader, however, will have noticed that most RCTs utilize standardized protocols that do not require the therapist to develop an individualized case formulation. There is a tension between RCT-validated treatment and treatment based on an individualized formulation. We propose several resolutions to this tension, and we offer guidelines for using a case formulation in an evidence-based approach to treatment.

One resolution of the tension between standardized-protocol-based and individualized-formulation-based treatment is the recognition that standardized protocols also rely on a formulation, albeit a nomothetic (general) one rather than an idiographic (individualized) one (Haynes et al., 2000). For example, Beck's cognitive therapy is based on the formulation that depression results from activation of schemata by life events, giving rise to distorted cognitions, maladaptive behaviors, and depressed mood. Cognitive therapy alleviates negative mood by changing behaviors, automatic thoughts, and schemata, as described in the protocol published by Beck et al. (1979). Moreover, as the therapist carries out the protocol, he or she individualizes it to address the particular activating events, maladaptive behaviors, automatic thoughts, and schemata that are problematic for his or her patient. Therefore, the therapist basing his or her treatment on an individualized case formulation is, in part, simply formalizing what is done informally by the therapist using a standardized protocol.

A second resolution of the tension between RCT-validated standardized treatment and individualized-formulation-driven treatment involves drawing a distinction between disorders and patients. Standardized protocols and individualized-formulation-driven treatments are complementary, not conflicting. Standardized protocols treat disorders; formulation-driven therapies treat patients. This distinction is similar to the distinction in medicine between the "disorder" and the "predicament." The "predicament" is the "social, psychological, and economic fashion in which the [medical] patient is situated in the environment" (Sackett et al., 1991, p. 4). The case formulation (particularly the Problem List component) gives the therapist a comprehensive view of the case as a whole that allows him or her to understand not just one or two of the patient's disorders, but a broad view that includes the patient's predicament.

Third, an individualized formulation facilitates the therapist's use of a standardized protocol by helping the therapist understand and manage difficulties that arise in the use of the protocol, including noncompliance, ruptures in the patient–therapist relationship, and similar problems, as we have illustrated above (see also Tompkins, 1999). The formulation allows the therapist to understand and manage these types of difficulties in a systematic, thoughtful way, rather than by applying hit-or-miss strategies.

Fourth, many patients do not meet the selection criteria utilized in the RCTs (at least those done to date). To treat these patients, the therapist extrapolates from the standardized protocol—or, in the case of patients with multiple problems, two, three, or more standardized protocols. The use of an individualized case formulation provides a systematic method for carrying out this extrapolation.

Finally, the ability to develop an individualized treatment plan based on a conceptualization is invaluable when working with patients who have not been treated successfully with the RCT-validated therapies, or who seek treatment for a disorder or problem for which no protocol is available. Without a formulation, the therapist is reduced to attempting a random series of therapy interventions. The case formulation provides a systematic method for developing a hypothesis (the formulation) about the mechanisms causing a patient's symptoms and problems, developing a treatment plan based on the formulation, and evaluating the outcome of the treatment plan. If results are poor, rather than simply attempting (blindly) some different interventions, the therapist can reformulate the case, develop a new treatment plan based on the reformulation, and again monitor outcome. Thus the case formulation method entails a hypothesis-testing approach to treatment—a systematic, scientific approach to the treatment of cases where protocols are unavailable or have proved unhelpful.

Clearly, the individualized-formulation-based approach to treatment has many advantages. However, it must be acknowledged that little empirical evidence supports the utility of developing a formal case conceptualization to guide treatment. Persons, Bostrom, and Bertagnolli (1999) have provided some initial data demonstrating the utility of the use of an individualized-formulation-driven approach to cognitive-behavioral therapy for depression. More research of this sort is needed. Haynes et al. (1997) reviewed the literature and concluded that the incremental treatment utility of the individualized formulation has been convincingly demonstrated for self-injurious behaviors, but not for other behavioral problems.

It is also important to acknowledge that the process of developing an individualized case formulation is not without risks and costs. One risk is that therapists will develop idiosyncratic formulations based on fad, lore, or unreliable clinical judgment (Wilson, 1998). These factors may explain the findings of Schulte, Kunzel, Pepping, and Schulte-Bahrenberg (1992), who reported that patients suffering from anxiety disorders who were treated with a standardized exposure-based treatment had better outcomes than those who received individualized treatment.

To reduce the risks of therapeutic work based on an case individualized formulation and to strengthen its empirical foundation, we recommend the following three procedures:

1. *Adopt an RCT-validated formulation as an initial Working Hypothesis.* We recommend that therapists adopt, as the initial Working Hypothesis for a case, one of the nomothetic formulations utilized in the RCT-validated therapies for the disorder or disorders being treated. If therapy based on these formulations fails, treatments based on untested formulations can be attempted.

2. *Have patients provide informed consent for treatment.* Before patients can provide informed consent for treatment, therapists must provide patients with information about the results of the initial assessment, treatment options and the efficacy evidence supporting each option, and treatment recommendations. In Judy's case, this meant letting her know that she met diagnostic criteria for dysthymia and describing available treatment options, including pharmacotherapy.

In many cases, especially when a patient does not meet the criteria that patients studied in RCTs met, the therapist develops a treatment plan by extrapolating from the protocols used in the RCTs. The therapist must inform the patient that this is what is being done. When the therapist extrapolates from a protocol developed for another problem or population (as in Judy's case, where interventions were drawn from Beck's protocol for treatment of major depression, as protocols for treating dysthymia have not yet been published), it is particularly important to provide informed consent for treatment. Informed consent is also particularly important if the therapist's treatment plan is based on a unique formulation that has not been studied in a controlled trial. In this case, the therapist must explain this to the patient and provide a rationale for the proposed treatment plan. The formulation can be helpful in providing a rationale for an individualized treatment plan.

3. *Monitor outcome.* RCT-validated treatments have been shown to produce a good outcome for the average case. In contrast, the clinician treats the unique, individual case. To ascertain whether the treatment is helpful to the individual patient, outcome must be carefully monitored.

In evidence-based formulation-driven psychotherapy, the clinician conducts the treatment of each case as an $n = 1$ experiment (see Barlow, Hayes, & Nelson, 1984), using a recursive process illustrated in Figure 3.4. The clinician begins by collecting data (assessment) in order to develop a hypothesis about the mechanisms causing and maintaining the patient's problems (the case formulation). The formulation is used to derive a treatment plan. As treatment proceeds, the clinician collects additional data to assess the outcome of therapy based on the formulation, and revises the formulation and treatment plan if the treatment plan based on the original formulation is unsuccessful.

The clinician who utilizes these three methods while conducting treatment guided by an individualized case formulation is, in our view, providing evidence-based formulation-driven psychotherapy. We encourage clinicians who adopt the case conceptualization methods described in this chapter to embed them in an evidence-based framework of this sort.

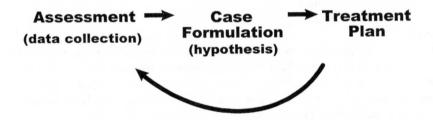

FIGURE 3.4. Recursive model linking assessment, hypothesis generation, treatment, and repeated assessment. Copyright 1999 by the San Francisco Bay Area Center for Cognitive Therapy. Reprinted with permission.

REFERENCES

Barlow, D. H., Hayes, S. C., & Nelson, R. O. (1984). *The scientist–practitioner: Research and accountability in clinical and educational settings.* New York: Pergamon Press.

Beck, A. T. (1983). Cognitive theory of depression: New perspectives. In P. J. Clayton & J. E. Barrett (Eds.), *Treatment of depression: Old controversies and new approaches* (pp. 265–288). New York: Raven Press.

Beck, A. T., Freeman, A., & Associates. (1990). *Cognitive therapy of personality disorders.* New York: Guilford Press.

Beck, A. T., Rush, A. J., Shaw, B. F., & Emery, G. (1979). *Cognitive therapy of depression.* New York: Guilford Press.

Beck, A. T., Ward, C. H., Mendelsohn, M., Mock, J., & Erbaugh, J. (1961). An inventory for measuring depression. *Archives of General Psychiatry, 4,* 561–571.

Beck, J. S. (1995). *Cognitive therapy: Basics and beyond.* New York: Guilford Press.

Bloom, M., Fischer, J., & Orme, J. G. (1995). *Evaluating practice: Guidelines for the accountable professional.* Needham Heights, MA: Allyn & Bacon.

Burns, D. D. (1980). *Feeling good: The new mood therapy.* New York: William Morrow.

Burns, D. D. (1998). *Therapist's toolkit.* (Available from David D. Burns, MD, 11987 Murietta Lane, Los Altos, CA 94022)

Cone, J. D. (Ed.). (1999). Special section: Clinical assessment applications of self-monitoring. *Psychological Assessment, 11,* 411–497.

Eells, T. D. (Ed.). (1997). *Handbook of psychotherapy case formulation.* New York: Guilford Press.

Goodman, W. K., Price, L. H., Rasmussen, S. A., Mazure, C., Fleischmann, R. L., Hill, C. L., Heninger, G. R., & Charney, D. S. (1989). The Yale–Brown Obsessive–Compulsive Scale: I. Development, use, and reliability. *Archives of General Psychiatry, 46,* 1006–1011.

Hammen, C., Ellicott, A., Gitlin, M., & Jamison, K. R. (1989). Sociotropy/autonomy and vulnerability to specific life events in patients with unipolar depression and bipolar disorders. *Journal of Abnormal Psychology, 98,* 154–160.

Hayes, S. C., Nelson, R. O., & Jarrett, R. B. (1987). The treatment utility of assessment: A functional approach to evaluating assessment quality. *American Psychologist, 42,* 963–974.

Haynes, S. N. (1992). *Models of causality in psychopathology: Toward dynamic, synthetic and nonlinear models of behavior disorders.* New York: Macmillan.

Haynes, S. N., Kaholokula, J. K., & Nelson, K. (2000). The idiographic application of nomothetic, empirically based treatments. *Clinical Psychology: Science and Practice, 6,* 456–461.

Haynes, S. N., Leisen, M. B., & Blaine, D. D. (1997). Design of individualized behavioral treatment programs using functional analytic clinical case models. *Psychological Assessment, 9,* 334–348.

Haynes, S. N., & O'Brien, W. H. (2000). *Principles and practice of behavioral assessment.* New York: Kluwer Academic/Plenum Press.

Koerner, K., & Linehan, M. M. (1997). Case formulation in dialectical behavior therapy for borderline personality disorder. In T. D. Eells (Ed.), *Handbook of psychotherapy case formulation* (pp. 340–367). New York: Guilford Press.

Linehan, M. M. (1993). *Cognitive-behavioral treatment of borderline personality disorder.* New York: Guilford Press.

Mayfield, D., McLeod, G., & Hall, P. (1974). The CAGE questionnaire: Validation of a new alcoholism screening instrument. *American Journal of Psychiatry, 131,* 1121–1123.

Nelson, R. O., & Hayes, S. C. (Eds.). (1986). *Conceptual foundations of behavioral assessment.* New York: Guilford Press.

Nezu, A. M., & Nezu, C. M. (1993). Identifying and selecting target problems for clinical interventions: A problem-solving model. *Psychological Assessment, 5,* 254–263.

Nezu, A. M., Nezu, C. M., Friedman, S. H., & Haynes, S. N. (1997). Case formulation in behavior therapy: Problem-solving and functional analytic strategies. In T. D. Eells (Ed.), *Handbook of psychotherapy case formulation* (pp. 368–401). New York: Guilford Press.

O'Brien, W. H., & Haynes, S. N. (1995). A functional analytic approach to the conceptualization, assessment, and treatment of a child with frequent migraine headaches. *In Session: Psychotherapy in Practice, 1,* 65–80.

Persons, J. B. (1989). *Cognitive therapy in practice: A case formulation approach.* New York: Norton.

Persons, J. B. (1992). The patient with multiple problems. In A. Freeman & F. Dattilio (Eds.), *Casebook of cognitive-behavior therapy* (pp. 241–247). New York: Plenum Press.

Persons, J. B., Bostrom, A., & Bertagnolli, A. (1999). Results of randomized controlled trials of cognitive therapy for depression generalize to private practice. *Cognitive Therapy and Research, 23,* 535–548.

Persons, J. B., & Tompkins, M. A. (1997). Cognitive-behavioral case formulation. In T. D. Eells (Ed.), *Handbook of psychotherapy case formulation* (pp. 314–339). New York: Guilford Press.

Sackett, D. L., Haynes, R. B., Guyatt, G. H., & Tugwell, P. (1991). *Clinical epidemiology: A basic science for clinical medicine.* Boston: Little, Brown and Company.

Schulte, D., Kunzel, R., Pepping, G., & Schulte-Bahrenberg, T. (1992). Tailor-made versus standardized therapy of phobic patients. *Advances in Behaviour Research and Therapy, 14,* 67–92.

Tompkins, M. A. (1999). Using a case formulation to manage treatment nonresponse. *Journal of Cognitive Psychotherapy: An International Quarterly, 13,* 317–330.

Turkat, I. D. (Ed.). (1985). *Behavioral case formulation.* New York: Plenum.

Turkat, I. D., & Maisto, S. A. (1985). Personality disorders: Application of the experimental method to the formulation and modification of personality disorders. In D. H. Barlow (Ed.), *Clinical handbook of psychological disorders: A step-by-step treatment manual* (pp. 502–570). New York: Guilford Press.

Wilson, G. T. (1998). Manual-based treatment and clinical practice. *Clinical Psychology: Science and Practice, 5,* 363–375.

Wolpe, J. (1980). Behavioral analysis and therapeutic strategy. In A. Goldstein & E. B. Foa (Eds.), *Handbook of behavioral interventions* (pp. 7–37). New York: Wiley.

4

Cognition and Clinical Science

FROM REVOLUTION TO EVOLUTION

RICK E. INGRAM
GREG J. SIEGLE

In 1986, Ingram and Kendall wrote that "the 'cognitive revolution' is over. No longer is it rebellious to argue for the existence of cognition, defend its importance in human functioning, or justify it as a legitimate and productive focus of study" (p. 3). They further noted that "cognitive concepts have become firmly entrenched in the vernacular of clinical researchers and clinicians alike. Indeed, cognitive psychology has become mainstream psychology" (p. 3). In the intervening years, little evidence has emerged to contradict this conclusion. With but a few exceptions (e.g., Hawkins, 1994), the field is not engaging in behaviorally motivated debates about the scientific legitimacy of cognition; nor has it again become fashionable to argue that cognition makes little meaningful contribution to either functional or dysfunctional behavior. Although other approaches to understanding behavior have gained, or regained, enthusiasm among theorists and researchers (e.g., Baldwin, 1992; Bowlby, 1988; Westin, 1991), they have served to complement the cognitive approach (Ingram, Miranda, & Segal, 1998; Safran & Segal, 1990) rather than to replace it as an important factor in psychological science. Efforts to understand the link between cognition and behavior thus remain strongly embedded in the mainstream of psychology.

Although cognitive approaches are no longer revolutionary in the scientific pursuit of clinical psychology, no discussion of the nexus of cognition and psychotherapy can be complete without at least some historical reference to the cognitive revolution. Mahoney (1988) traced these issues in the inaugural edition of the *Handbook of Cognitive-Behavioral Therapies*, and in the seminal 1974 *Cognition and Behavior Modification* volume that arguably launched the cognitive revolution in clinical psychology. He noted that cognitive perspectives in clinical psychology arose from a growing disenchantment with a behavioral paradigm that frequently did not recognize any meaningful role for cognition in human functioning. As Mahoney (1974) argued, "only a very small percentage of a person's behaviors are publicly observable. Our lives are predominately composed of private responses to private environments" (p. 1). It had become clear that any clinical approach that failed to take such "private events" seriously missed an important opportunity both to understand and to change maladaptive behavior. Exploration of the nature, structure, and functional relevance of cognition in psychological disorders was the natural outcome of restoring scientific relevance to private events.

As would be expected, however, the growing interest in cognition as a way to understand important aspects of both function and dysfunction did not escape harsh criticism. Indeed, as Mahoney (1988) suggested, behaviorist responses ranged from denial to diminishment, with the sometimes implicit (and other times explicit) suggestion that any attempt to conceptualize or study cognitive variables represented a retreat from both scientific psychology and scientific values. Although Mahoney noted that some behaviorists acknowledged a subsidiary role for cognition in behavior therapy (e.g., in the form of images), these cognitive concepts were treated for the most part as merely covert behaviors governed by the same laws as overt behaviors (e.g., Cautela, 1970). As Scott (1995) has observed, in other cases cognitive approaches were labeled merely as vague and mentalistic concepts lacking either legitimate scientific status or a theoretical basis, or both. Nevertheless, and despite the advances of behavioral approaches to the treatment of some problems (e.g., phobias), the disenchantment over the limits of behavioral approaches led to the "revolutionary" acceptance of the idea that cognition is one of the important forces driving behavior.

In some respects, the present chapter takes up where Mahoney left off. Although Mahoney described the cognitive revolution, we believe that the revolution has become an evolution both within clinical psychology and in more basic psychological science. Clinical psychology has evolved to a remarkable degree in developing and refining the cognitive components of effective treatment (of which evidence can be seen in the majority of chapters in this volume). If anything, the evolution in basic cognitive psychology has been even more remarkable; cognitive psychology has evolved into a distinct yet diverse cognitive science that, in addition to basic psychological concepts and empirical methods, has incorporated concepts and empirical methods from basic physiology and neuroanatomy, computer science, artificial intelligence, linguistics and language research, anthropology, and philosophy (Gardner, 1987).

Despite the fact that cognitive-behavioral therapists explicitly recognize an important role for cognition in the creation and amelioration of behavior problems, as Stein (1992) has noted, most of the concepts that characterize cognitive science have yet to make their way into cognitive-clinical science (e.g., computer modeling of hypothesized neural networks). Indeed, in many respects cognitive science and cognitive-behavioral therapy have taken separate evolutionary paths. Although this disconnection is unfortunate, it is also understandable. For the most part, cognitive scientists have been concerned with understanding the functioning of cognition, without much consideration of how cognition might be changed to improve quality of life. On the other hand, cognitive-behavioral therapists have naturally focused on empirically verifying the most effective ways to change cognitions to improve lives (Ingram, Hayes, & Scott, 2000), without devoting as much attention to developments in the expanding field of cognitive science. Yet the conceptual bridge that links basic cognitive science and clinical cognitive science is obvious. Indeed, as Ingram and Kendall (1986) argued in a volume explicitly devoted to bridging the gap between clinical psychology and basic cognitive psychology, the bridge carries a two-way street. Certainly cognitive scientists and clinical cognitive scientists have much to learn from each other.

Because this chapter appears in a volume devoted to cognitive-behavioral therapy, we focus on basic cognitive science and examine several key elements in this rapidly growing discipline. In general, we believe that cognitive science theory and data have a powerful potential to inform clinical treatment by enhancing the understanding of basic functions in both adaptive and maladaptive behavior. Our hope is that this understanding may suggest new insights for cognitive-behavioral therapists in how to approach changing behavior. Both to provide a brief historical context, and to clarify the separate paths of cognitive science and cognitive clinical science, we start by chronicling the development of cognitive-behavioral therapy and then of cognitive science. We next examine some current trends and developments in cognitive science. Where appropriate, we note theory or data that may instruct treatment efforts, either by helping to understand basic cognitive functioning in a given disorder, or by offering suggestions for refining some elements of treatment. We conclude by speculating on some future directions in cognitive science.

WHO PUT THE COGNITIVE
IN COGNITIVE-BEHAVIORAL THERAPY?:
A SHORT HISTORY

For a full appreciation of the link between cognitive psychology and psychotherapy, it is helpful to consider the origins of cognitive-behavioral therapy from the explicit perspective of clinical psychology. As we have previously noted, and as Ingram, Kendall, and Chen (1991) have also argued, the evolution of cognitive-behavioral therapy did not parallel the evolution of cognitive psychology. For example, as behaviorism was taking hold in experimental psychology, clinical psychology was more in the process of shifting from a fascination with Freudian constructs to an emphasis on humanistic concepts, most notably those developed by Carl Rogers. The behavioral domination of clinical psychology, however, was not far behind, and at some point after this approach had become established in experimental psychology, it took root in clinical psychology. Ironically, this was the case even as behaviorism itself had began to decline in experimental psychology. Nevertheless, in the clinical arena empirical research was beginning to suggest that behavioral interventions might be effective in alleviating behavioral problems. Clinical application of behavioral concepts thus promised, and found, substantial success (see Bergin & Garfield, 1971; Garfield & Bergin, 1978; Hammerlynck, Handy, & Mash, 1973; each includes reviews of the efficacy of behavior modification).

Buoyed by early applied successes and by the mantle of scientific status that behaviorism had claimed, behavioral researchers sought to uncover the stimulus–response links that would fully explicate behavior, particularly disordered behavior, and thus point the way toward its increasingly effective modification (e.g., Ullmann & Krasner, 1965). It was in such a milieu that journals devoted to behavioral concepts, interventions, and applied behavioral analysis arose, as did professional organizations intended to promote the advancement of behavior therapy (Mahoney, 1974).

Although the behavioral paradigm had been instrumental in basic experimental psychology, and had in fact predated the behaviorist shift in clinical psychology (Kanfer & Hagerman, 1985), a chorus of disenchantment eventually began to be heard about the limits of behavioral concepts in explaining, and modifying, complex behavior. Although there were several outcomes of this disenchantment, one of the more important was that basic psychological scientists began to revisit the role of cognition as a meaningful factor in human behavior. Unlike some of their predecessors, who had relied on inherently unreliable methods such as introspection, this time the visit was couched firmly in the context of a scientific perspective. Consequently, the "revelation" that cognition is important could be seen in the expanding development of cognitive constructs and methods in experimental, developmental, and social psychology (Ingram & Kendall, 1986). Perhaps because of the clinical treatment success that behaviorists had enjoyed, however, the acknowledgment as well as the incorporation of cognition into mainstream clinical psychology proceeded at a significantly slower pace.

It is impossible to pinpoint all of the factors that were involved in the movement of cognition into the clinical arena. There do, however, seem to be at least three discernible stages of development in the gradual blending of cognitive and clinical perspectives. First was the development of social learning theory and the emphasis on vicarious learning processes developed by such theorists as Bandura (1969) and Mischel (1973). They argued that cognitive variables are important, but placed them squarely in the theoretical context of "covert behaviors." Given our current state of knowledge about the functioning and structure of cognition, it may be difficult to appreciate the need for such a subtle introduction of cognitive variables into the clinical domain. It is important to note, however, that at that time behavioral approaches not only dominated clinical psychology and applied journals, but also correspondingly eschewed as unscientific any concepts incorporating cognition or other phenomena that were not directly observable. Shifts to a cognitive perspective were thus of necessity quite subtle, and had to be couched in the dominant vernacular of the times (e.g., "cognitive behaviors," "covert events"). Placing cognition within a behavioral vernacular allowed access to scientific legitimacy. Social learning approaches relying on vicarious learning and covert behavior thus constituted perhaps the earliest clinical predecessors of current cognitive approaches to clinical problems.

The incremental inclusion of cognitive perspectives into scientific respectability stimulated what can be considered a second phase in the linkage between cognition and practice: an explicit move toward the incorporation of cognition into clinical treatment and assessment paradigms. This move was evident in the work of a number of pioneering researchers whose primary interest was in developing effective treatment procedures. Because most of these researchers had emerged from a behavioral background, they used the term "cognitive-behavioral," perhaps for the first time, to describe the explicit focus on cognition as an appropriate and important focus of treatment efforts. This group included Kendall and Hollon (1979, 1981), Mahoney (1974), and Meichenbaum (1977). Similar pioneering perspectives on cognitive treatment processes also appeared in the work of Beck (1976; Beck, Rush, Shaw, & Emery, 1979) and Ellis (1962), although these approaches emerged from traditions that were not behaviorist in nature; their traditions were more humanistic and psychodynamic. Together, however, these researchers helped bring legitimacy to a focus on cognition in the context of treatment efforts.

The emphasis at this stage of development in cognitive-behavioral treatment was clearly on the development of effective treatment strategies, rather than on the conceptual understanding of the cognitive system as a whole. Nevertheless, this work moved away from the notion that cognitions are best represented as just another class of behaviors (cognitive behaviors), and suggested that cognition can be assigned causal status in its own right. Thus cognitive systems came to be thought of not only as causing dysfunction and mediating behavior, but also as operating according to principles that are different in important respects from those espoused by the types of learning theories at the core of behaviorist conceptions. The underlying theoretical premise of much of this work was a relatively straightforward assumption that dysfunctional thoughts cause dysfunctional behavior. The years since the explosion of cognitive-behavioral theories have done much to clarify the complexity of these early theoretical premises, but the initial reasons for the development of these therapies (to effectively treat psychological problems by targeting cognitive processes) has been borne out in the extensive volume of therapy outcome work (see Bergin & Garfield, 1994; Snyder & Ingram, 2000). Indeed, much of the work in the current book attests to the efficacy of targeting cognitions in efforts to induce positive change.

The third phase of the inclusion of cognition into clinical psychology is represented by much of the work that is currently occurring in the field. A recurring theme in contemporary activities is an increased emphasis on the development of conceptual models of cognition in psychological dysfunction. Given that much of the conceptualization of cognition in cognitive-behavioral therapy developed independently of theory and research in cognitive psychology (Winfrey & Goldfried, 1986), much of the this work has focused on developing conceptualizations that are more in line with basic psychological science (Ingram, 1986).

COGNITIVE SCIENCE

The preceding section has noted some of the major historical features of the development of cognitive-behavioral therapy. To complete our historical perspective on the interface between cognitive science and cognitive clinical science, we also need to consider the historical antecedents of cognitive science.

A Brief History of Cognitive Science

As we have noted, cognitive science is an inherently integrative discipline encompassing aspects of not only cognitive psychology, but artificial intelligence, neuroanatomy, philosophy of knowledge, linguistics, and anthropology (Gardner, 1987). The common goal of each of these fields is to understand the mind. Their integration has provided a rich theoretical foundation on which the effects of cognitive therapies can be understood and perhaps enhanced. A number of factors led to the integration of these separate fields with the rapidly emerging discipline of cognitive science.

The beginning of the decline of behaviorism in the basic science of the 1950s left psychologists open to input from other disciplines. Among the goals of these psychologists was to understand aspects of complex cognitive events—such as how long chains of actions, or planning and organization, could occur (Gardner, 1985). Without denying that stimuli and responses are important, this pursuit often centered on the question of what cognitive events occur between a stimulus and a response. There were many possible answers from a variety of sources.

As summarized by Stein (1992), several disciplines had much to offer to the nascent field of cognitive science. For instance, for hundreds of years philosophers had addressed the question of cognition from the perspective of what is "knowable," and it was therefore natural that "philosophy of mind" was incorporated into developing models of cognitive psychology. At about the same time, the advent of computers led to computer metaphors of mind that embodied information processing as a way to conceptualize cognition (Newell & Simon, 1972). Alternatively, theorists such as Minsky and McCarthy suggested that understating psychological processes is useful for making computers act like humans, and therefore established the field of artificial intelligence. Computer science and neuroscience were becoming integrated as well, as luminaries such as Von Neumann and McCullogh equated the same logic circuits used in building computers to the functioning of biological neurons (Jeffress, 1951). As Stein (1992) notes, because linguists had long held clinical interests in disorders such as dyslexia, it made sense to include the insights from this field into a developing cognitive science. Thus the disciplines of computer science, artificial intelligence, neuroscience, linguistics, and philosophy of knowledge were closely enough tied to the questions posed by cognitive psychology that an integrated field of cognitive science was born.

Current Trends and Developments in Cognitive Science

As we have noted, a number of disciplines have contributed to the integrated field that is now commonly known as cognitive science. In this section we review recent developments in philosophy, neuroscience, and artificial intelligence that are particularly applicable to understanding and improving cognitive-behavioral therapy. We note also that while linguistics and anthropology also contribute to cognitive science, their implications are not as well articulated for cognitive-behavioral therapy. We thus only note these areas briefly.

PHILOSOPHY

Epistemology, the philosophy of what can be known, has been linked to understanding mental disorder since Aristotle, who believed in interactions between the bodily humors and mental faculties. As early as the 12th century, Maimonides used Aristotelean theory to suggest that changing thoughts can be associated with changes in mood (Pies, 1997)—a concept that is fundamental to cognitive-behavioral therapy. As noted by Mahoney (1988), more recent philosophical foundations of cognitive-behavioral therapy can be seen in the tension between rationalist versus developmental schools of thought. The former expresses more reliance on a certain, absolute, and objective reality that is obtained through sensory data; the latter is more convinced that within broad physical parameters, reality is embodied in knowledge that is dynamic, subjective, and constructed by the individual's experience. Beyond developmental ideas, constructivism holds that reality is a socially constructed phenomenon and exists as a function of the observer who is creating it. Although not all of the current versions of cognitive-behavioral therapy were developed explicitly from these philosophical perspectives, these perspectives do form the basis of the "founding" cognitive-behavioral therapies of Beck and Ellis. Hence the conceptual links to philosophy are clear in the premises of all of Beck's and Ellis's therapeutic descendants (Lyddon, 1992).

Rationalism has explained the etiology of psychopathology as the expression of irrational beliefs (Mahoney, 1990). As a consequence, systems of cognitive therapy such as rational–emotive therapy (Ellis, 1962, 1980) were founded on the idea that irrational beliefs can be rationally refuted, and that such refutation leads to the development of more healthy affect and behavior. Ellis's approach, now known as rational emotive behavior therapy, has undergone several incarnations (e.g., Ellis, 1994, 1996), but it remains a fundamental and inherently a rationalist approach to behavior change.

Alternatively, the approach to treatment pioneered by Beck (see Beck, 1967, 1996) relies more on a developmental/constructivist perspective and explicitly recognizes the philosophical roots of this perspective. For instance, Bedrosian and Beck (1980) noted that the philosophical roots of Beck's approach reside in the philosophical arguments of individuals such as Kant and Marcus Aurelius, to the latter of whom the statement "If thou are pained by any external thing, it is not this thing that disturbs thee, but thine own judgment about it" is widely attributed. The modification of thought as a way to modify behavior is the natural theoretical consequence of this view.

NEUROSCIENCE

Neuroscience, the study of the brain and of brain–behavior relationships, has fueled the emerging interest in the biological basis of psychopathology. Traditionally, neuroscience has been concerned with the building blocks of cognition—how individual neurons operate and interact in concert to perform cognitive functions. The development of ways to measure brain correlates of cognitive processes may eventually pave the way for understanding the biological basis of change in cognitive therapy. Indeed, although the study of changes in brain structure and chemistry during cognitive therapy is still in its infancy, Tartaryn, Nadel, and Jacobs (1989) have suggested that advances in understanding the neuroscience of learning may lead to a better understanding of change processes in therapy. In principle, enhanced understanding of these changes may provide insight for the practice of cognitive-behavioral therapy. We thus describe the focus of much of the contemporary work in neuroscience, and provide some speculation on possible roles that neuroscience may play in inducing cognitive change.

Brain Structure. Cognitive-behavioral treatment of any given disorder assumes some knowledge of the factors that underlie the disorder. Brain-imaging techniques such as magnetic resonance imaging (MRI) allow identification of brain structures associated with a disorder to be identified. In the case of depression, for example, research has shown this disorder to be associated with volume changes in a number of different structures, including frontal and basil ganglia lesions as well as ventricle-to-brain ratio anomalies (Videbech, 1997) and temporal lobe asymmetries (Amsterdam & Moseley, 1992). As information is gained about structures that are active in maintaining mood disorders, and upon which structures cognitive-behavioral therapies seem to act, more precise treatments may be geared to target functions that are assumed to be disrupted by physiological anomalies. For example, the amygdala is thought to be responsible for assigning emotional valences to information. Emerging evidence suggests that the right amygdala responds to positive and negative information, while the left amygdala only responds to negative information (Davidson, 1998). Functional asymmetries in these structures could lead to an understanding of mood disorders as involving the relative perception of either positive and negative information, or primarily negative information. In addition, preliminary studies have suggested that some of these structural abnormalities correlate with treatment response to antidepressants (e.g., Pillay et al., 1997), which might then be potentially used to predict response to cognitive-behavioral treatment.

Brain Activation. Brain-imaging techniques such as positron emission tomography (PET) and functional MRI (fMRI), as well as traditional physiological measurement techniques (e.g., electroencephalography) and neuropsychological assessment techniques, allow localization of brain activity. PET scanners measure the amount of a radioactive isotope present in brain tissue. When an isotope that binds to the same places as substances found in the brain (e.g., dopamine) is used, the rate at which these quantities are being used can be determined. PET scanning has been used to understand the rate at which glucose and oxygen are metabolized, cerebral blood flow, and the quantities of such substances as dopamine, opiates, serotonin, and glutamate that are used (Powledge, 1997). fMRI examines proton radio signal generation, a factor that has been observed to correlate with brain activity. Thus fMRI can be used to examine where in the brain activity occurs during cognitive tasks.

Such localization may be important for understanding the mechanisms behind symptom remission during cognitive-behavioral treatment, and in fact may be useful in targeting cognitive procedures toward functionally relevant brain areas. For example, recent fMRI data reported by Schwartz (1998) suggest that obsessive–compulsive disorder is characterized by abnormal activation in the orbito-frontal complex. After cognitive-behavioral therapy, changes were found in left orbito-frontal activation in only treatment responders, suggesting that cognitive therapy may operate directly on the parts of the brain most affected by the disorder. Schwartz (1998) has used this information to inform cognitive-behavioral therapy in two ways. First, compliance with particularly difficult aspects of therapy is improved by showing patients changes in brain activation as they practice the therapeutic techniques. Second, Schwartz has modified some of the techniques of cognitive-behavioral therapy to specifically address the caudate and orbito-frontal brain areas. In particular, he helps patients change behaviors while uncomfortable urges are still present; this technique appears to allow adaptation in the caudate and orbito-frontal circuits.

Results are similarly promising for other disorders. For example, depression has been associated with left frontal hypoactivation (e.g., Henriques & Davidson, 1991). As the dorsolateral prefrontal cortex seems responsible for inhibiting emotional reactions, the research suggests that emotional responses may become especially uninhibited in depression. Bruder et al. (1997) have shown, using neuropsychological tasks, that cognitive-behavioral therapy is associated with a disappearance of these hemispheric asymmetries; this finding suggests that treatment might increase emotional inhibition processes that reverse the effects of depression. Through this type of analysis, neuroanatomical models can thus be used to help understand the mechanisms by which cognitive-behavioral therapy helps depressed individuals.

The correlates of brain activity can also be obtained via traditional physiological assessment techniques. For example, measurement of event-related potentials (ERPs) can be used to measure brain activity milliseconds after a stimulus is presented, allowing investigation of the time course of variables relevant to cognitive therapy (e.g., shifts in attentional allocation). Dipole localization techniques (e.g., Wood, 1982) are mathematical interpolation techniques for finding where brain activity associated with ERPs originates, allowing approximate identification of the sources of brain activity. Similarly, general cognitive activity can be measured physiologically by other indices derived from activity in structures innervated by multiple brain areas of interest. For example, pupil dilation has frequently been used as an index of overall cognitive load (Beatty, 1982).

The ways in which variables targeted in therapy, such as attentional style or stress, contribute to the onset and maintenance of disorder can be gauged by measuring these physiological variables in response to the presentation of affective or feared stimuli. Consequently, theoretically derived physiological response profiles may be used to predict who will be more or less amenable to therapy. Moreover, because these techniques are often relatively noninvasive and inexpensive, physiological measurement may be incorporated during therapy sessions to gauge aspects of cognition during techniques such as role plays and thought challenging.

Neurochemistry. In addition to structural and localization information, understanding how diffuse hormones and neurotransmitters function in the brain is playing an increasing role in understanding psychopathology. For example, McEwen, DeKloet, and Rostene (1986) have shown that the hippocampal system, responsible for memory formation, is populated with stress hormone receptors. Jacobs and Nadel (1985) speculate that the hippocampal system may allow stress to be associated with particular stimuli, leading to phobias. They thus suggest psychological treatments for phobias based on presumed hippocampal activity.

Similarly, diffuse neurotransmitters such as dopamine, norepinephrine, and serotonin have been implicated in the maintenance of a number of disorders, including depression (e.g., Klimek et al., 1997; Stockmeier, 1997), schizophrenia (e.g., Cohen & Servan-Schreiber, 1993), and anxiety disorders (e.g., McCann et al., 1995). To understand the role of these neurochemicals in therapeutic change, it will be useful to examine relationships among affective state, cognitive function, and neurochemical metabolism. To this end, a great deal of recent interest has been directed toward techniques that allow real-time measurement of the rate at which neurochemicals are metabolized, via magnetic resonance spectroscopy (MRS; e.g., Frangou & Williams, 1996). MRS is a noninvasive method for measuring neurochemical concentrations, using the same tools as those used for fMRI. MRS has been used to implicate changes in chemical quantities in depression, including membrane phospholipid metabolism, high-energy phosphate metabolism, and intracellular pH (Kato, Inubushi, & Kato, 1998). Such methodologies have been applied to understanding the role of pharmacotherapies, by examining the role that drugs can play in changing these quantities (e.g., Kato et al., 1998; Renshaw et al., 1997). MRS has also been applied to understanding diffuse neurochemical metabolism and pharmacotherapy response in disorders amenable to cognitive therapy, such as social phobia (Tupler, Davidson, Smith, & Lazeyras, 1997). Although studies using MRS to understand the effects of cognitive-behavioral therapy on neurochemical concentrations have yet to be published, this work in pharmacotherapy suggests a number of promising possibilities.

Comparing Cognitive and Pharmacological Therapies. Research has suggested that similar efficacy rates for disorders such as depression can be achieved through either cognitive or pharmacological therapies (e.g., Hollon, DeRubeis, Evans, & Wiemer, 1992). Yet, it is unclear whether the mechanisms behind these treatments are the same, and, consequently, what the relative tradeoffs are in long-term effects of each type of treatment. Neuroimaging data, physiological measurements, or spectrographic analysis of neurochemical metabolism, taken before and after different types of treatment, may help elucidate some of the mechanisms behind any differential treatment effects of cognitive and pharmacological therapies. Similarities and differences in the mechanisms responsible for change in cognitive and pharmacological treatments can be derived from similarities and differences in measured physiological quantities.

Creation of Pharmacological Mood Primes. One method for evaluating aspects of change and subsequent vulnerability to recurrence after therapy involves the use of priming (e.g., Segal & Ingram, 1994). When individuals are placed in a state reminiscent of their disorder, their responses to aspects of the state can be determined. As Segal and Ingram (1994) note, several psychological procedures have been used effectively to create such states. Moreover, more purely pharmacological challenges have been created as a way of simulating brain conditions involved in states associated with various disorders. For example, tryptophan depletion modifies serotonin availability; it is associated with decreases in mood, as well as with symptoms of other psychological phenomena associated with serotonin, such as anxiety and aggression (Reilly, McTavish, & Young, 1998). Cholecystokinin tetrapeptide may be used to induce threat-related cognitions associated with panic attacks (Koszycki, Bradwejn, & Cox, 1995; Koszycki, Cox, & Bradwejn, 1993). Other pharmacological challenges (e.g., clomipramine) may be useful in evaluating differential change in relevant physiological variables in anxious and nonanxious groups (e.g., Sallee, Koran, Pallanti, Carson, & Sethuraman, 1998). The continued exploration of neurological correlates of psychopathology may reveal new and useful ways of priming aspects of disorder to evaluate vulnerability after cognitive or pharmacological challenges. When it becomes clearer how pharmacological challenges affect symptom presentation after therapy, the mechanisms underlying the efficacy of cognitive-behavioral therapy may be further understood.

ARTIFICIAL INTELLIGENCE

Artificial intelligence (AI) involves programming a computer to perform tasks that model human behavior, often with the goal of making the computer's performance indistinguishable from that of a human (e.g., Jacquette, 1993; Turing, 1936, 1950). Two aspects of this pursuit have been applied to the evolution of cognitive-behavioral therapy. The first comes from a camp of AI researchers who consider humans to be conceptually analogous to extraordinarily efficient computers, and therefore try to program computers to perform tasks in the ways people perform them. Learning about performance in computer models of aspects of disorder may make it possible to learn about ways to cognitively remediate a disorder. The second involves using computers to actively perform therapy with people.

Learning about Therapeutic Change by Examining Computers That Act Like People with Psychopathology. As greater understanding is gained of mechanisms behind psychopathology, analogues of these mechanisms can be formalized as computer programs. Such computer programs behave in accordance with their programmers' directions about mechanisms of disorders, but can produce responses to inputs that were not considered by the programmers. The procedure is similar to understanding a statistical formula, but not knowing the result of applying the formula on a particular data set until the analysis is performed. Formalizing theories about cognition in disorder on computers may thus reveal some of the implications of theories, as well as contradictions that had not been considered before the theories were formalized (e.g., Cohen & Servan-Schreiber, 1992; Siegle, 1997).

AI modeling of cognitive variables relevant to cognitive-behavioral therapy can serve as a heuristic mechanism for testing aspects of cognitive theories (Siegle, 1997). Starting with a program that generates behaviors (i.e., outputs) similar to people with a disorder, researchers can incorporate analogues of change processes associated with therapy to see whether specific interventions can be predicted to produce changes in behaviors. This technique has an advantage over pure theory because, as many of the systems underlying cognition are quite complex and nonlinear, they are hard to predict without simulating them in a computer program. In addition, models of disorder implemented as AI systems can be used to refine cognitive-behavioral treatment by experimenting with how modifications to simulated cognitive change processes affect a program's simulated behaviors.

By modeling aspects of cognition and emotion on computers, AI researchers may add unique perspectives to concepts central to cognitive-behavioral therapy. For example, cognitive-behavioral therapy is often concerned with helping individuals plan and solve problems. AI modeling has long dealt with problems of planning sequences of events and solving problems (e.g., Charniak & McDermott, 1985). By creating computer programs to solve problems, often as simple as solving mathematical equations or arranging blocks in specified sequences, AI researchers have learned a great deal about how people solve problems (Newell & Simon, 1972). Webster (1995) has shown through simulations using traditional computational problem solvers that techniques such as storing and repeatedly examining past problem-solving failures can lead to the creation of an especially effective problem solver. He suggests that such a process can be likened to adaptive aspects of negative thinking and rumination in disorders such as mood disorders, but that taking such adaptive strategies to extremes may lead to nonadaptive problem-solving deficits. There are many potential implications of this research for cognitive-behavioral therapists, such as understanding that rumination may sometimes be adaptive, and that finding a client's optimal level of rumination may be a useful pursuit.

AI models of reasoning can also be applied to understanding change in cognitive-behavioral therapy. A central goal of many AI programs involves reasoning about situations that an artificially intelligent agent (e.g., a robot) could experience in the world. The notion of a schema, on which cognitive-behavioral therapies are often based, has been formalized in this literature (e.g., Schank & Abelson, 1977). Schemata have traditionally been useful to AI researchers as efficient concepts for representing collections of information typically associated with a behavioral context. Beck's original cognitive therapy was based partly on the notion that depressed individuals have negative schemata relating to themselves. Since that time, AI researchers have begun to be concerned about representing emotions in schema-based systems. Using Ortony, Collins, and Clore's (1988) theory of emotions, Elliott (1992) has built an "affective reasoner" that allows artificially intelligent agents to react emotionally to each other in a simulated world. Elliott has used the system to model individuals' emotional reactions to each other in business settings. Such a system may be used to refine cognitive-behavioral therapies by examining how emotions are generated in response to other people's actions. Current cognitive-behavioral psychotherapy aims to change an individual's schemata; practitioners hope that individuals with changed schemata will interact more adaptively with other people who may have very different schemata. Simulations may thus be used to determine whether attempted changes to schemata will have predictable effects on individuals' interactions with other people, at least within the parameters (i.e., the current knowledge and sophistication) of the simulation program.

A final area in which traditional AI can be useful for modeling the substrates of therapy is that of theoretical logic. A frequent goal of cognitive-behavioral therapy is to help individuals to reconcile inconsistent beliefs (e.g., the belief that they are guilty of something over which persons also believe that they have no control). The discipline of logic programming addresses questions of how a system should behave when it holds inconsistent beliefs. Grant and Subrahmanian (1995a) have shown that when inconsistent beliefs are central to a network of beliefs forming a data base, few conclusions can be drawn from the data base. The implication is that the more central or "core" an individual's inconsistent beliefs are, the less able the individual will be to make decisions (Dombeck, Siegle, & Ingram, 1996). Because so many beliefs depend on these central beliefs, they are very difficult to change without disrupting the entire network of beliefs. Subrahmanian (Grant & Subrahmanian, 1995a, 1995b; Pradhan, Minker, & Subrahmanian, 1995) shows that when a data base is constrained so that inconsistent beliefs cannot be considered together, the data base can again be used to draw conclusions. Based on Subrahmanian's logic, helping individuals to consider pockets of mutually consistent beliefs, and to prioritize which beliefs are held in which situations, may be useful to cognitive therapists in cases in which individuals' inconsistent beliefs are so central to their cognitive network that they cannot easily change them.

Computer-Based Therapy. Another way in which AI techniques may be used to improve cognitive-behavioral therapy is through the development of interactive systems that can perform some aspects of therapy. Techniques such as books and videotapes are often considered to be of marginal utility in cognitive therapy because they cannot interact with patients. In contrast, AI techniques can be used to create computer programs in which patients interact with a computer program as if it were a therapist (e.g., Colby, 1995).

Although interaction with a machine will never replace human interaction in the therapy enterprise, such patient–computer interactions may provide a helpful adjunct to therapy. When a person interacts with such a program, it responds based on the information the person has typed, providing exactly the types of collaborative investigation (i.e., dialogue between patient and therapist regarding the nature and resolutions of a patient's problems) central to the cognitive-behavioral therapies. Preliminary experiments designed to assess computer-based therapies incorporating artificially intelligent therapists have suggested that these techniques are promising, if somewhat limited by current difficulties in modeling the intricacies of natural language interactions (Stuart & LaRue, 1996). Such techniques that allow collaboration between computer programs and patients may prove especially valuable additions to the often noncollaborative computer-based cognitive and behavioral therapies emerging in the field.

CONNECTIONISM AND NEURAL NETWORKS: SYNTHESIS OF COGNITIVE PSYCHOLOGY, AI, AND NEUROSCIENCE

"Connectionism" is a term given to theoretical models arising from cognitive psychology and AI in which cognition is assumed to involve activation spreading between nodes. For example, the nodes can represent propositions, and activation can represent memory processes associating one belief with another. Bower (1981) used such semantic networks to understand relationships between emotion and cognition by suggesting that beliefs and emotions can be similarly represented as connected nodes in such a system. Theorists such as Ingram (1984) have explained psychopathologies as involving particularly strong connections, being created between certain thoughts and emotions in semantic networks. In this way, many thoughts can lead to the experience of a sad emotion. Such explanations have been used to understand cognitive therapies as changing connections within semantic networks (e.g., Ingram & Hollon, 1986).

Recent connectionist models have been created within the parallel-distributed-processing framework, in which patterns of information processing are theorized to result from networks of simple connected neuron-like units. These so-called "neural network" models have advantages over other connectionist models, in that they can be designed as analogues of biological systems. Such physiologically informed models bridge a gap between cognitive and neuroscientific research. Possible mechanisms of disorders derived from neuroscientific research can be embodied in neural networks designed to mimic known brain circuits. Knowledge in a neural network is acquired through learning mechanisms developed in cognitive psychology. As the networks are constructed of individually meaningless units that perform simple computations, they can be readily implemented on a computer. This process allows inputs to simulated systems to be processed by a computational neural network, generating outputs representing behavior, as in all AI simulation. Possible mechanisms underlying both psychological disorders and cognitive change can be simulated in such systems (Siegle, 1997, 1999). Conclusions about therapy derived from neural network models are thus inherently integrative, uniting behavioral, cognitive, and physiologically based views of change (Tryon, 1993a).

Because neural network models address physiological, cognitive, and behavioral aspects of change, conclusions from these models can be useful to psychologists, psychiatrists, cognitive scientists, and neuroscientists. Neural network models preserve a number of other advantages over other modeling techniques that do not have such interdisciplinary appeal. For example, many processes in nature are chaotic (i.e., future states of a system cannot be theoretically predicted from its current state). Neural network models allow observation of the effects of theoretical chaotic processes, which are difficult or impossible to predict theoretically (Movellan & McClelland, 1994). Caspar, Rosenfluh, and Segal (1992) point out specific advantages of using neural networks instead of other, more symbolic AI models to understand psychopathology, including the ability of neural networks to represent gradations of phenomena, and their ability to capture aspects of slow and fast change.

Based on these ideas, Tryon (1993b) proposes that the principles of neural networks can be incorporated into cognitive-behavioral therapies as a way to bridge gaps between cognitive and behavioral perspectives. Tryon (1993b) suggests that therapy can be thought of as affecting connection weights, so that stimuli (represented as activations of inputs to a network) are associated with different consequent responses (represented as functions of activations of a network's outputs). The role of cognition in such behavioral change can be understood by examining changes inside the network that are associated with changes in stimulus–response pairings.

Accounting for principles of learning as implemented in neural networks, Tryon suggests, could create an integrative, biologically motivated cognitive-behavioral therapy. For instance, one idea borrowed from neuroscience is that repeated associations of input and output stimuli can strengthen associations between them (Hebb, 1949). Tryon (1993b) argues that many psychopathologies can be thought of as involving especially high levels of association between a stimulus and an emotional or cognitive response. As one example, to the extent that many inputs (environmental stimuli) trigger activation of the output (mental representation) associated with a fear stimulus, posttraumatic stress disorder can be conceptualized as especially strong learning of associations with a feared stimulus. Tryon proposes that therapies based on this principle should involve helping individuals to learn new cognitive or emotional reactions to stimuli for which connections lead to activation of pathological states.

Neural network models of aspects of psychopathologies amenable to cognitive therapy have been created. For example, Siegle (1999; Siegle & Ingram, 1997) has developed a model of the cognitive processes involved in recognizing emotional features (e.g., sadness) and nonemotional features (e.g., knowledge that a birthday is the day on which a person is born) of environmental stimuli (e.g., hearing the word "birthday"). This model also incorporates rumination, which is operationalized as excessive feedback between brain areas responsible for representing emotional and nonemotional aspects of information. Computer simulations with this model suggest that once individuals are depressed, it is difficult to for them to learn new positive information if they ruminate excessively. A clinical implication of this finding is that such depressive rumination may be important to address in cognitive therapy before helping an individual to experience positive thoughts.

Caspar et al. (1992) show that theorizing about neural network models can lead to advances in therapy for other clinically relevant phenomena. They consider a neural network model of repetition compulsion, a debilitating condition characterized by repetition of actions. They reason that neural network models can learn nonoptimal associations. Under certain conditions, relevant connections may become very strong, leading to a state in which such associations are hard to unlearn. Stimuli can be repeatedly associated with responses without achieving a desirable goal. Caspar et al. generalize from techniques used to break neural networks out of such nonoptimal learning to propose mechanisms for change in cognitive therapy for repetition compulsion.

The preceding discussion suggests that connectionism can play an important role in the emerging role of cognitive science in cognitive therapy. Although basic cognitive science integrates research from cognitive psychology, AI, and neuroscience, the contributions from these disciplines to advancing cognitive therapy have largely been separate. When intuitions from these disciplines are combined via connectionist modeling techniques, the integrated field of cognitive science can be appealed to en masse for advancement of cognitive therapy.

LINGUISTICS AND CULTURAL ANTHROPOLOGY

As noted by Gardner (1987), linguistics and cultural anthropology also contribute to cognitive science. The contribution of these disciplines to advancing cognitive therapy is not as immediately apparent as are the contributions of cognitive psychology, AI, and neuroscience. Yet their foci are closely tied to current concerns in the development of cognitive therapy. The roles of cultural variables in cognitive therapy have engendered a great deal of recent research. Cultural anthropology is devoted to understanding how cultures differ. It seems natural to appeal to this discipline for an understanding of the role of culture in behavioral and cognitive change. Similarly, cognitive-behavioral therapy is founded on the idea that language (i.e., discussion) can be used to change cognition. Linguistics, which is devoted to understanding how the mind processes language, is thus an important field to appeal to in understanding the precise role of language in changing thoughts. Future research may make links between cognitive therapy and the fields of anthropology and linguistics apparent.

SOME FUTURE DIRECTIONS

Having examined the current status of cognitive science as it may apply to cognitive-behavioral therapy, we briefly address some future directions that may be helpful in facilitating the integration of basic and applied clinical science. In particular, we comment on the integration of cognition and affect in cognitive science, as well as the importance of emphasizing change processes in the continuing expansion and refinement of the models of cognitive science.

Integration of Cognition and Affect

This chapter has focused on the contributions of cognitive science to cognitive-behavioral therapy. Cognitive-behavioral therapy can also inform and advance cognitive science (Ingram & Kendall, 1986). One of the areas in which cognitive-behavioral therapy provides continuing information to cognitive scientists is the need to understand the interplay between cognition and affect. As noted previously, the incorporation of affect into traditional cognitive notions such as semantic networks has occurred only in the last two decades (e.g., Bower, 1981). Problems with early efforts such as Bower's model have been made apparent by attempts at clinically applying these models. For example, Teasdale and Barnard (1993) have shown that nodes in Bower's model have no direct neural correlates, and that there is no provision in Bower's model for representing thinking about an emotion without feeling that emotion. Partly in response, they have developed an integrative model that brings together current research on emotion with research on memory, attention, and cognition. They have applied this model toward understanding mechanisms of cognitive therapy in the context of change in global patterns of the interaction between cognitive and affective processing systems. Similar investigations have led to more complex understandings of the possible roles of constructs such as emotional appraisal and construal processes in the relationship between emotions and cognitions (e.g., Ortony et al., 1988), as well as the use of physiologically motivated neural network models to explain cognitive–affective interactions (e.g., Armony, Servan-Schreiber, Cohen, & LeDoux, 1995; Siegle, 1999).

Change Processes

Cognitive science has often focused on cognition as if it were a static phenomenon, such as investigating a person's (presumably unchanging) attentional style. Cognitive-behavioral therapy, in contrast, is devoted to modifying affect and behavior by changing people's cognitions. For example, Beutler and Guest (1984) specifically contrasted how changes in static cognitive products (e.g., beliefs) could lead to differential effects in cognitive therapy from changes in cognitive processes (e.g., appraisals leading to those beliefs). In addition, a review by Ingram and Hollon (1986) has shown how collaborative empirical investigations of cognitive processes can be used to change cognitive phenomena in belief systems and cognitive operations. Other authors have tried to clarify the role of cognitive therapy in changing key cognitive variables such as schemata (e.g., Goldfried & Robins, 1983; Hollon & Kriss, 1984), encoding (Greenberg & Safran, 1980, 1981), and the integration of multiple data streams in the production of a cognition (Teasdale & Barnard, 1993). Research on cognitive therapy may thus contribute to basic cognitive science research by elucidating the role of dynamic cognitive variables in modifying ongoing cognitive processes.

Clinical research on cognitive change processes has often resulted in notions of change that might not have been derived if cognitive-behavioral therapy had not been specifically examined. For example, Teasdale and Barnard (1993) have evaluated Beck's idea that changing an individual's specific "automatic" negative thoughts spurs recovery from depression. Their model suggests that such automatic thoughts are products of a more global impairment in which diverse stimuli are too often associated with some prototypical negative thought. As such, they suggest that changing this more global associational strategy, rather than specific automatic thoughts, should obviate many of an individual's automatic negative thoughts and may thus be a better treatment for depression.

Another example of how research on cognitive-behavioral therapy can lead to insights about change processes involves Safran and Segal's (1990) analysis of interpersonal processes in cognitive-behavioral therapy. Although many current proponents of cognitive science analyze only the role of individuals, Safran and Segal use evidence from experiments in traditional cognitive psychology to suggest that alliances with other people (e.g., therapists) may be involved in cognitive change processes. In discussing how to cognitively treat disorders characterized by interpersonal deficits, Saffron and Segal suggest that individuals who develop in interpersonal contexts are likely to develop schemata related not only to the self but to others as well (see also Ingram et al., 1998). An interpersonal schema, Saffron and Segal suggest, can serve as "a program for maintaining relatedness" (1990, p. 68). As clinical disorders often involve disrupted interpersonal relationships, they suggest that the interpersonal schema can be targeted for cognitive interventions. The notion that cognitive change can be analyzed by understanding interpersonal relationships is still in its infancy in cognitive science.

A final noteworthy example involves recent efforts to understand roles that therapies derived from other cultures (e.g., mindfulness meditation derived from Tibetan Buddhism) can play in changing cognitions (e.g., Teasdale, Segal, & Williams, 1996) and their biological substrates (e.g., Davidson, 1998). Both Teasdale's and Davidson's cross-cultural research programs start from the idea that processing is parallel and distributed, and use concepts from cognitive science to understand ideas such as awareness of self. For example, Teasdale et al. (1996) suggest, based on Teasdale and Barnard's (1993) integrative model, that meditative techniques may be useful in interrupting cyclic activations linking negative thoughts to negative emotions. Although this research is conducted to help solve clinical problems, it opens cognitive science to integration with an entirely different discipline from those that have been traditionally included under its umbrella.

SUMMARY AND CONCLUSIONS

Although Beck's original (1967) cognitive therapy was based on the best cognitive science of its day, it left much room for advancement derived from the integration of contemporary cognitive science. We hope that this chapter has illustrated the power of cognitive science to elucidate mechanisms that drive cognitive phenomena associated with psychopathology. As noted by MacLeod (1987),

> our ultimate ability to refine cognitive treatment approaches such that they comprise the most useful therapeutic techniques, will therefore depend upon our ability to identify the precise nature of the actual processing biases which underlie any particular disorder, or indeed any specific patient, and our ability to sensitively measure the effectiveness of those techniques in overcoming such biases. (p. 180)

We believe that cognitive science models represent especially useful tools for clarifying the flow of information through cognitive systems. Incorporating a cognitive science perspective into cognitive-behavioral therapies can provide a theoretically driven platform for understanding the nature of clinical change in a multitude of disorders. Appeals to philosophy of mind root this quest in a tradition with a thousand-year history of investigating similar issues. Integrating recent data from AI research can make the foundations of cognitive-behavioral therapy internally consistent with contemporary cognitive science, and hypotheses regarding possible advances in cognitive therapy can be generated. Likewise, using neuroscience data regarding brain mechanisms underlying psychological disorders can direct cognitive therapies to target specific brain areas and patterns of activation. In short, this chapter argues that each of the subdisciplines of cognitive science can be used to make cognitive-behavioral therapy stronger, more rigorous, broader, and thus more useful in treating the disorders that affect the human condition.

REFERENCES

Amsterdam, J. D., & Mozley, P. D. (1992). Temporal lobe asymmetry with iofetamine (IMP) SPECT imaging in patients with major depression. *Journal of Affective Disorders, 24,* 43–53.

Armony, J. L., Servan-Schreiber, D., Cohen, J. D., & LeDoux, J. E. (1995). An anatomically constrained neural network model of fear conditioning. *Behavioral Neuroscience, 109,* 246–257.

Baldwin, M. W. (1992). Relational schemas and the processing of social information. *Psychological Bulletin, 112,* 461–484.

Bandura, A. (1969). *Principles of behavior modification.* New York: Holt, Rinehart & Winston.

Beatty, J. (1982). Task-evoked pupillary responses, processing load, and the structure of processing resources. *Psychological Bulletin, 91,* 276–292.

Beck, A. T. (1967). *Depression: Clinical, experimental, and theoretical aspects.* New York: Hoeber.

Beck, A. T. (1976). *Cognitive therapy and the emotional disorders.* New York: International Universities Press.

Beck, A. T. (1996). Beyond belief: A theory of modes, personality, and psychopathology. In P. M. Salovskis (Ed.), *Frontiers of cognitive therapy* (pp. 1–25). New York: Guilford Press.

Beck, A. T., Rush, A. J., Shaw, B. F., & Emery, G. (1979). *Cognitive therapy of depression.* New York: New York: Guilford Press.

Bedrosian, R. C., & Beck, A. T. (1980). Principles of cognitive therapy. In M. J. Mahoney (Ed.), *Psychotherapy process* (pp. 127–152). New York: Plenum Press.

Bergin, A. E., & Garfield, S. L. (Eds.). (1971). *Handbook of psychotherapy and behavior change.* New York: Wiley.

Bergin, A. E., & Garfield, S. L. (Eds.). (1994). *Handbook of psychotherapy and behavior change* (4th ed.). New York: Wiley.

Beutler, L. E., & Guest, P. D. (1984). The role of cognitive change in psychotherapy. In A. Freeman, K. Simon, L. E. Beutler, & H. Arkowitz (Eds.), *Comprehensive handbook of cognitive therapy* (pp. 123–142). New York: Plenum Press.

Bower, G. (1981). Mood and memory. *American Psychologist, 36,* 129–148.

Bowlby, J. (1988). *A secure base: Parent–child attachment and healthy human development.* New York: Basic Books.

Bruder, G. E., Stewart, J. W., Mercier, M. A., Agosti, V., Leslie, P., Donovan, S., & Quikin, F. M. (1997). Outcome of cognitive-behavioral therapy for depression: Relation to hemispheric dominance for verbal processing. *Journal of Abnormal Psychology, 106,* 138–144.

Caspar, F., Rosenfluh, T., & Segal, Z. (1992). The appeal of connectionism for clinical psychology. *Clinical Psychology Review, 12,* 719–762.

Cautela, J. R. (1970). Covert reinforcement. *Behavior Therapy, 1,* 273–278.

Charniak, E., & McDermott, D. (1985). *Introduction to artificial intelligence.* Reading, MA: Addison-Wesley.

Cohen, J. D., & Servan-Schreiber, D. (1992). Introduction to neural network models in psychiatry. *Psychiatric Annals, 22,* 113–118.

Cohen, J. D., & Servan-Schreiber, D. (1993). A theory of dopamine function and its role in cognitive deficits in schizophrenia. *Schizophrenia Bulletin, 19,* 85–104.

Colby, K. M. (1995). A computer program using cognitive therapy to treat depressed patients. *Psychiatric Services, 46,* 1223–1225.

Davidson, R. J. (1998). Affective style and affective disorders: Perspectives from affective neuroscience. *Cognition and Emotion, 12,* 307–330.

Dombeck, M., Siegle, G., & Ingram, R. E. (1996). Cognitive interference and coping strategies in vulnerability to negative affect: The threats to identity model. In I. G. Sarason, B. Sarason, & G. Pierce (Eds.), *Cognitive interference: Theories, methods, and findings* (pp. 299–323). Hillsdale, NJ: Erlbaum.

Elliott, C. (1992). *The affective reasoner: A process model of emotions in a multiagent system* (Technical Report No. 32). Evanston, IL: Northwestern University, The Institute for the Learning Sciences.

Ellis, A. (1962). *Reason and emotion in psychotherapy.* New York: Stuart

Ellis, A. (1980). Rational–emotive therapy and cognitive behavior therapy: Similarities and differences. *Cognitive Therapy and Research, 4,* 325–340.

Ellis, A. (1994). *Reason and emotion in psychotherapy* (2nd ed.). Secaucus, NJ: Carol.

Ellis, A. (1996). *Better, deeper and more enduring brief therapy: The rational emotive behavior therapy approach.* New York: Brunner/Mazel.

Frangou, S., & Williams, S. C. (1996). Magnetic resonance spectroscopy in psychiatry: Basic principles and applications. *British Medical Bulletin, 52,* 474–485.

Gardner, H. (1985). *The mind's new science: A history of the cognitive revolution.* New York: Basic Books.

Gardner, H. (1987). Cognitive science characterized. In P. K. Moser & A. vannder Nat (Eds.), *Human knowledge: Classical and contemporary approaches* (pp. 375–393). New York: Oxford University Press.

Garfield, S. L., & Bergin, A. E. (Eds.). (1978). *Handbook of psychotherapy and behavior change: An empirical analysis* (2nd ed.). New York: Wiley.

Goldfried, M. R., & Robins, C. (1983). Self-schema, cognitive bias, and the processing of therapeutic experiences. In P. C. Kendall (Ed.), *Advances in cognitive-behavioral research and therapy* (Vol. 2, pp. 330–380). New York: Academic Press.

Grant, J., & Subrahmanian, V. S. (1995a). Reasoning in inconsistent knowledge bases. *Transactions on Knowledge and Data Engineering, 7,* 177–189.

Grant, J., & Subrahmanian, V. S. (1995b). The optimistic and cautious semantics for inconsistent knowledge bases. *Acta Cybernetica, 12,* 37–55.

Greenberg, L. S., & Safran, J. D. (1980). Encoding, information processing and the cognitive behavioural therapies. *Canadian Psychology, 21,* 59–66.

Greenberg, L. S., & Safran, J. D. (1981). Encoding and cognitive therapy: Changing what clients attend to. *Psychotherapy: Theory, Research and Practice, 18,* 163–169.

Hammerlynck, L. A., Handy, L. C., & Mash, E. J. (Eds.). (1973). *Behavior change: Methodology, concepts and practice.* Champaign, IL: Research Press.

Hawkins, R. P. (1994). The cognitive-behavioral debate: Perspectives of doctoral students. *The Behavior Therapist, 17,* 85.

Hebb, D. O. (1949). *The organization of behavior: A neuropsychological theory.* New York: Wiley.

Henriques, J. B., & Davidson, R. (1991). Left frontal hypoactivation in depression. *Journal of Abnormal Psychology, 100,* 535–545.

Hollon, S. D., DeRubeis, R. J., Evans, M. D., & Wiemer, M. J. (1992). Cognitive therapy and pharmacotherapy for depression: Singly and in combination. *Archives of General Psychiatry, 49,* 774–781.

Hollon, S. D., & Kriss, M. R. (1984). Cognitive factors in clinical research and practice. *Clinical Psychology Review, 4,* 35–76.

Ingram, R. E. (1984). Toward an information processing analysis of depression. *Cognitive Therapy and Research, 8,* 443–478.

Ingram, R. E. (Ed.). (1986). *Information processing approaches to clinical psychology.* Orlando, FL: Academic Press.

Ingram, R. E., Hayes, A., & Scott, W. (2000). Empirically-supported treatments: A critical analysis. In C. R. Snyder & R. E. Ingram (Eds.), *Handbook of psychological change: Psychology processes and practices for the 21st century* (pp. 40–60). New York: Wiley.

Ingram, R. E., & Hollon, S. D. (1986). Cognitive therapy of depression from an information processing perspective. In R. E. Ingram (Ed.), *Information processing approaches to clinical psychology* (pp. 261–284). Orlando, FL: Academic Press.

Ingram, R. E., & Kendall, P. C. (1986). Cognitive clinical psychology: Implications of an information processing perspective. In R. E. Ingram (Ed.), *Information processing approaches to clinical psychology* (pp. 3–21). Orlando, FL: Academic Press.

Ingram, R. E., Kendall, P. C., & Chen, A. H. (1991). Cognitive-behavioral interventions. In C. R. Snyder & D. R. Forsyth (Eds.), *Handbook of social and clinical psychology: The health perspective* (pp. 509–522). New York: Pergamon Press.

Ingram, R. E., Miranda, J., & Segal, Z. V. (1998). *Cognitive vulnerability to depression.* New York: Guilford Press.

Jacobs, W. J., & Nadel, L. (1985). Stress-induced recovery of fears and phobias. *Psychological Review, 92,* 512–531.

Jacquette, D. (1993). Who's afraid of the Turing Test? *Behavior and Philosophy, 20,* 63–74.

Jeffress, L. A. (1951). Cerebral mechanisms in behavior. *The Hixon symposium.* New York: Wiley.

Kanfer, F. H., & Hagerman, S. M. (1985). Behavior therapy and the information processing paradigm. In S. Reiss & R. R. Bootzin (Eds.), *Theoretical issues in behavior therapy* (pp. 3–35). New York: Academic Press.

Kato, T., Inubushi, T., & Kato, N. (1998). Magnetic resonance spectroscopy in affective disorders. *Journal of Neuropsychiatry and Clinical Neurosciences, 10,* 133–147.

Kendall, P. C., & Hollon, S. D. (1979). *Cognitive-behavioral interventions: Theory, research, and procedures.* New York: Academic Press.

Kendall, P. C., & Hollon, S. D. (1981). *Assessment strategies for cognitive-behavioral interventions.* New York: Academic Press.

Klimek, V., Stockmeier, C., Overholser, J., Meltzer, H. Y., Kalka, S., Dilley, G., & Ordway, G. A. (1997). Reduced levels of norepinephrine transporters in the locus coeruleus in major depression. *Journal of Neuroscience, 17,* 8451–8459.

Koszycki, D., Bradwejn, J., & Cox, B. J. (1995). Anxiety sensitivity and cholecystokinin tetrapeptide challenge: Reply. *American Journal of Psychiatry, 152,* 300–301.

Koszycki, D., Cox, B. J., & Bradwejn, J. (1993). Anxiety sensitivity and response to cholecystokinin tetrapeptide in healthy volunteers. *American Journal of Psychiatry, 150,* 1881–1883.

Lyddon, W. J. (1992). Cognitive science and psychotherapy: An epistemic framework. In D. J. Stein & J. E. Young (Eds.), *Cognitive science and clinical disorders* (pp. 173–187). San Diego, CA: Academic Press.

MacLeod, C. (1987). Cognitive psychology and cognitive therapy. In H. Dent (Ed.), *Clinical psychology: Research and developments* (pp. 175–181). London: Croom Helm.

Mahoney, M. J. (1974). *Cognition and behavior modification.* Cambridge, MA: Ballinger.

Mahoney, M. J. (1988). The cognitive sciences and psychotherapy: Patterns in a developing relationship. In K. S. Dobson (Ed.), *Handbook of cognitive–behavioral therapies* (pp. 357–386). New York: Guilford Press.

Mahoney, M. J. (1990). *Human change processes.* New York: Basic Books.

McCann, U. D., Thorne, D., Hall, M., Popp, K., Avery, W., Sing H., Thomas, M., & Belenky, G. (1995). The effects of L-dihydroxyphenylalanine on alertness and mood in alpha-methyl-para-tyrosine-treated healthy humans: Further evidence for the role of catecholamines in arousal and anxiety. *Neuropsychopharmacology, 13,* 41–52.

McEwen, B. S., DeKloet, E. R., & Rostene, W. (1986). Adrenal steroid receptors and actions in the nervous system. *Physiological Review, 66,* 1121–1188.

Meichenbaum, D. (1977). *Cognitive behavior modification.* New York: Plenum Press.

Mischel, W. (1973). Toward a cognitive social learning conceptualization of personality. *Psychological Review, 80,* 252–283.

Movellan, J. R., & McClelland, J. L. (1994). *Stochastic interactive processing, channel separability, and optimal perceptual interference: An examination of Morton's law.* Technical report, Department of Psychology–Carnegie Mellon University.

Newell, A., & Simon, H. A. (1972). *Human problem solving.* Englewood Cliffs, NJ: Prentice-Hall.

Ortony, A., Collins, A., & Clore, G. (1988). *The cognitive structure of emotions.* Cambridge, England: Cambridge University Press.

Pies, R. (1997). Maimonides and the origins of cognitive-behavioral therapy. *Journal of Cognitive Psychotherapy, 11,* 21–36.

Pillay, S. S., Yurgelun-Todd, D. A., Bonello, C. M., Lafer, B., Fava, M., & Renshaw, P. F. (1997). A quantitative magnetic resonance imaging study of cerebral and cerebellar gray matter volume in primary unipolar major depression: Relationship to treatment response and clinical severity. *Biological Psychiatry, 42,* 79–84.

Powledge, T. M. (1997). Unlocking the secrets of the brain. *Bioscience, 47,* 403–409.

Pradhan, S., Minker, J., & Subrahmanian, V. S. (1995). Combining databases with prioritized information. *Journal of Intelligent Information Systems, 4,* 231–260.

Reilly, J. G., McTavish, S. F. B., & Young, A. H. (1998). Rapid depletion of plasma tryptophan: A review of studies and experimental methodology. *Journal of Psychopharmacology, 11,* 381–392.

Renshaw, P. F., Lafer, B., Babb, S. M., Fava, M., Stoll, A. L., Christensen, J. D., Moore, C. M., Yurgelun-Todd, D. A., Bonello, C. M., Pillay, S. S., Rothschild, A. J., Nierenberg, A. A., Rosenbaum, J. F., & Cohen, B. M. (1997). Basal ganglia choline levels in depression and response to fluoxetine treatment: An *in vivo* proton magnetic resonance spectroscopy study. *Biological Psychiatry, 41,* 837–843.

Safran, J. D., & Segal, Z. V. (1990). *Interpersonal processes in cognitive therapy.* New York: Basic Books.

Sallee, F. R., Koran, L. M., Pallanti, S., Carson, S. W., & Sethuraman, G. (1998). Intravenous clomipramine challenge in obsessive–compulsive disorder: Predicting response to oral therapy at eight weeks. *Biological Psychiatry, 44,* 221–227.

Schank, R. C., & Abelson, R. P. (1977). *Scripts, plans, goals, and understanding.* Hillsdale, NJ: Erlbaum.

Schwartz, J. M. (1998). Neuroanatomical aspects of cognitive-behavior therapy response in obsessive–compulsive disorder. *British Journal of Psychiatry, 173,* 38–44.

Scott, W. (1995). Cognitive behavior therapy: Two basic cognitive research programs and a theoretically based definition. *The Behavior Therapist, 18,* 122–124.

Segal, Z. V., & Ingram, R. E. (1994). Mood priming and construct activation in tests of cognitive vulnerability to unipolar depression. *Clinical Psychology Review, 14,* 663–695.

Siegle, G. J. (1997). Why I make models (or what I learned in graduate school about validating clinical causal theories with computational models). *The Behavior Therapist, 20,* 179–184.

Siegle, G. J. (1999). A neural network mode of attention biases in depression. In J. Reggia & E. Ruppin (Eds.), *Neural network models of brain and cognitive disorders* (Vol. 2, pp. 415–441). Amsterdam: Elsevier.

Siegle, G. J., & Ingram, R. E. (1997). Modeling individual differences in negative information processing biases. In G. Matthews (Ed.), *Cognitive science perspectives on personality and emotion* (pp. 302–353). Amsterdam: Elsevier.

Snyder C. R., & Ingram, R. E. (Ed.). (2000). *Handbook of psychological change: Psychotherapy processes and practices for the 21st century.* New York: Wiley.

Stockmeier, C. A. (1997). Neurobiology of serotonin in depression and suicide. *Annals of the New York Academy of Sciences, 836,* 220–232.

Stein, D. J. (1992). Clinical cognitive science: Possibilities and limitations. In D. J. Stein & J. E. Young (Eds.), *Cognitive science and clinical disorders* (pp. 3–17). San Diego, CA: Academic Press.

Stuart, S., & LaRue, S. (1996). Computerized cognitive therapy: The interface between man and machine. *Journal of Cognitive Psychotherapy, 10,* 181–191.

Tataryn, D., Nadel, L., & Jacobs, W. (1989). Cognitive therapy and cognitive science. In A. Freeman, K. Simon, L. Beutler, & H. Arkowitz (Eds.), *Comprehensive handbook of cognitive therapy* (pp. 83–98). London: Plenum Press.

Teasdale, J. D., & Barnard, P. (1993). *Affect, cognition, and change: Remodeling depressive thought.* Hillsdale, NJ: Erlbaum.

Teasdale, J. D., Segal, Z. V., & Williams, M. G. (1996). How does cognitive therapy prevent depressive relapse and why should attentional control (mindfulness) training help? *Behaviour Research and Therapy, 33,* 25–39.

Tryon, W. W. (1993a). Neural networks: I. Theoretical unification through connectionism. *Clinical Psychology Review, 13,* 341–352.

Tryon, W. W. (1993b). Neural networks: II. Unified learning theory and behavioral psychotherapy. *Clinical Psychology Review, 13,* 353–371.

Tupler, L. A., Davidson, J. R. T., Smith, R. D., & Lazeyras, F. (1997). A repeat proton magnetic resonance spectroscopy study in social phobia. *Biological Psychiatry, 42,* 419–424.

Turing, A. M. (1936). On computable numbers, with an application to the Entscheidungs-Problem. *Proceedings of the London Mathematical Society, 42,* 230–265.

Turing, A. M. (1950). Computing machinery and intelligence. *Mind, 59,* 236.

Ullmann, L., & Krasner, L. (1965). *Case studies in behavior modification.* New York: Holt, Rinehart Winston.

Videbech, P. (1997). MRI findings in patients with affective disorder: A meta-analysis. *Acta Psychiatrica Scandinavica, 96,* 157–168.

Webster, C. (1995). Computer modeling of adaptive depression. *Behavioral Science, 40,* 314–330.

Westin, D. (1991). Social cognition and object relations. *Psychological Bulletin, 109,* 429–455.

Winfrey, L. L., & Goldfried, M. R. (1986). Information processing and the human change process. In R. E. Ingram (Ed.), *Information processing approaches to clinical psychology* (pp. 241–258). Orlando, FL: Academic Press.

Wood, C. C. (1982). Application of dipole localization methods to source identification of human evoked potentials. *Annals of the New York Academy of Sciences, 388,* 139–155.

5

Cognitive-Behavioral Therapy and Psychotherapy Integration

LARRY E. BEUTLER
T. MARK HARWOOD
ROSLYN CALDWELL

The history of psychotherapy is one of conflict and change. The evolution of theory and practice has both produced and precipitated rivalry and discord between those who would instigate change and those who espouse the accepted theory of the day or of the group (Freedheim, Freudenberger, Kessler, & Messer, 1992). Early theories evolved and diverged largely via disagreements among the practitioners of the "talking cure." Freud's disciples broke with him because of theoretical disagreements regarding both the nature of psychopathology and the techniques of treatment. This form of progress was understandable in the beginning of this new field, given the limited access to objective methods and findings. At a point in time when scientific findings were sparse and when the major means of discovery in psychotherapy was individual case analysis, changes in the field and in theory were inevitably stimulated by personal disagreements and differences in interpretation.

In the 1950s, when the research methods that were applied to psychotherapy became more objective, standard, and rigorous, hope arose that empirical "facts" and objective observations would replace speculation and interpretation as the bases of advancements in the field. Unexpectedly, there has been a decided lag in the acceptance of scientific findings among practicing therapists as the basis for setting new directions or as the basis for deciding what is factual. Indeed, among many who practice, the true test of a psychotherapy continues to rest in the logic of its theory and in the power of a clinician's personal observations rather than in findings from sound scientific methods, even when the latter are available (Beutler, Williams, & Wakefield, 1993; Beutler, Williams, Wakefield, & Entwistle, 1995).

Particularly in its early development, the disagreements that occurred between theorists and practitioners were founded inextricably in the fundamental question of what constitutes evidence of truth. In many instances throughout the history of psychotherapy, theoretical positions became sacrosanct, and scientific findings were readily rejected because they did not fit the canons of one or another theoretical position. This situation created a virtual Tower of Babel among psychotherapists when the number of theories began to expand with unchecked abandon during the 1970s. When the proliferation of different theoretical viewpoints and positions reached its peak in the 1980s, one would have been hard put to find any position about the nature or effectiveness of psychotherapy that would have earned majority, let alone consensual, agreement among either practitioners or scientists.

Although the remnants of this discordant state have not disappeared, there seems to be more acceptance of scientific findings in contemporary practice than has been present previously, and "evidence-based" practice has become the norm in medicine and other treatment professions (Roth & Fonagy, 1996). Scientific inquiry and evidence derived through the scientific method are gaining ground as change agents for the field. In today's world, the arguments that arise among practitioners and between academic and practitioner communities are less frequently addressed to the value of scientific evidence itself, as the basis of knowledge, than they are on what constitutes "good" science. Most psychotherapists accept (at least overtly) the value of scientific inquiry for establishing what works in their field, but they differ widely in what they consider to be acceptable scientific methods. And it is likely that the distinction between which findings practitioners will accept as valid and which they will not hinges both on how they view the methods used to derive these findings, and on the strength of their contrasting, preexisting opinions. Practitioners tend to value naturalistic research designs over randomized clinical trials, $n = 1$ studies over group designs, and individualized over group measures of outcome (Heppner & Anderson, 1985; Fava, 1986; Morrow-Bradley & Elliott, 1986). It is safe to assume that they also tend to believe findings that favor the particular brand of psychotherapy they practice over those that support alternative approaches, or those that demonstrate that all approaches yield equivalent effects. Given that most research on psychotherapy fails to comply with these values, modern psychotherapists, like practitioners of the past, are often quick to reject scientific findings that disagree with their own theoretical value systems. Thus, although the reasons given for rejecting scientific evidence may be more sophisticated today than in yesteryear, such rejection may be no less likely to occur.

THE EMERGENCE OF ECLECTIC AND INTEGRATIONIST VIEWS

In the early days of psychotherapy theory development, once a theorist departed from the mainstream views of a mentor, the theorist was frequently treated as a pariah. A wall of intellectual isolation developed between those who held different points of view. Thus it was not unusual to find that a practitioner of a given theoretical orientation was quite ignorant of the principles and practices of those in another theoretical school. Indeed, psychotherapists of a given theoretical position were often unfamiliar with the people and viewpoints that characterized contrasting theories; they remained blind to alternative conceptualizations and theoretical approaches. Although this early theoretical isolation may have motivated therapists and clinicians to refine and enhance the skills and techniques espoused by their respective theoretical orientations, it also severely limited their horizons and perspectives (Safran & Messer, 1997).

Since the 1980s, the field of psychotherapy has been changing in response to the emergence of integrationist and eclectic views. This change was stimulated only partially by the status of scientific evidence. Most of the sound empirical evidence to support the shift toward eclecticism has accumulated since the development of eclectic psychotherapy as a set of coherent treatment models. It was in the 1980s that practitioners began to become suspicious of theory and developed a profound disaffection for narrow theoretical orientations. With over 400 different theories represented on the psychotherapy landscape, the conclusion was inescapable that there was no single truth about psychopathology or psychotherapy. Dissatisfaction was compounded by the failure of scientific studies to indicate firmly that any of the psychotherapies were superior to the others. Indeed, evidence indicated that none of the psychotherapies were especially successful at generating the comprehensive interventions that would result in the effective treatment of patients presented with complex and serious problems (Goldfried, 1995).

The mental health professions have made dramatic shifts in both the directions and the bases of their growth during the past 20 years. Their growth is no longer determined by the presence of competitive theories and arguments among theorists. More often, changes are made in order to integrate new findings or perspectives more comprehensively, and in turn, this integration is designed as an ostensible effort to better fit the treatment to the needs of the individuals who are seeking services (Safran & Messer, 1997). In the last several years, practitioners from a variety of orientations have been borrowing theories, techniques, and interventions from other schools of thought in an effort to enhance their own overall clinical efficacy.

Although the eclectic and integrationist movement caught on during the 1980s, its nucleus was in the early work of Thorne (1962) and Goldstein and Stein (1976). Thorne's "eclectic" psychotherapy arose from a relationship perspective in counseling theory. He argued that therapists' training doomed them to a single-method perspective that was ill suited to the varying conditions, personalities, and needs of different patients. He observed that such single-mindedness left psychotherapists poorly armed to address the complexity of people's problems, in much the same way that a carpenter who had only a screwdriver would be poorly equipped to build a house.

Thorne offered a conceptual argument for eclecticism, but few direct guidelines for when to apply different procedures. In contrast, Goldstein and Stein (1976) suggested that the procedures selected should be based on scientific evidence of efficacy, and presented examples of treatments that worked for a variety of problems. Given their scientific bent, it is not a surprise that these latter recommendations were largely drawn from the behavior therapy literature, since behaviorism was the dominant approach in research at that time. Modern conceptualizations of eclecticism have become more broad-ranging, but have retained some of the values inherent both in Thorne's admonition to accept procedures from a variety of perspectives, and in Goldstein and Stein's admonition to let scientific evidence rather than theory dictate the methods of application.

At least four systematic views within the integrationist movement can be identified in contemporary psychotherapy practice (Goldfried, 1995; Goldfried & Padawar, 1992; Norcross, 1987): (1) "common-factors eclecticism," (2) "theoretical integrationism," (3) "technical eclecticism," and (4) "strategic eclecticism." These approaches exist in addition to the unsystematic form of "haphazard eclecticism" to which many adhere (e.g., Norcross, 1987). Haphazard eclecticism is founded in some of the general beliefs and scientific "facts" that characterize the more systematic movements within the eclectic tradition, most notably the empirical observation that different approaches seem to be best suited for different people. However, within this unsystematic perspective, there is little effort to define the principles that govern the merging of viewpoints or to define a replicable procedure for selecting and applying treatments. This approach to eclecticism is probably widespread, but its effectiveness is hard to identify because it varies from therapist to therapist and from moment to moment. Its effectiveness is inextricably bound to the judgment and skill of the particular therapist who applies it.

Among the more systematic approaches, "common factors eclecticism" relies on the identification of factors that are common or similar across approaches. The common-factors approach to understanding psychotherapy is quite distinct from the way one usually thinks of eclecticism. Common-factors eclecticism accepts the position that all effective psychotherapies rely on a common core of basic ingredients, beyond which their distinctive effects are inconsequential or unpredictable. Practitioners of this approach attempt to apply techniques or interventions that appear common in all successful treatments, and propose that these techniques be applied to everyone. They suggest that scientific study be directed to explorations of ways that particular interventions and psychotherapeutic interactions promote and contain these common factors or qualities (Arkowitz, 1995). This posture stands in contrast to the general tenet of eclecticism that embodies tailoring the interventions to the unique needs of each patient.

The therapist who works within the framework of common-factors theory is seldom concerned with specific techniques or strategies beyond those that result in a congenial and caring relationship. Common-factors therapists, like most relationship-oriented therapists, work to convey an accepting and nonthreatening atmosphere in which the patient may explore problems. But whereas relationship-oriented therapies are driven by particular theories of psychopathology and change, a certain type of relationship in common-factors therapy is considered to be necessary and sufficient, and no more specific techniques or procedures are thought to be useful (e.g., Garfield, 1981).

The preponderance of systematic eclectic theories have endeavored to address patient complexity and variability by providing structure and systematizing the therapeutic procedures recommended, in the hope of maximizing clients' exposure to the unique combination of therapeutic factors that will best improve the clients' problems (Stricker & Gold, 1996). Several of these efforts are anchored on one end by what is referred to as "theoretical integrationism" and at the other by "technical eclecticism." Between these extremes is "strategic eclecticism," espoused by those who purport to integrate both theoretical concepts and techniques at the level of intervention strategies and principles of therapeutic influence. All three of these approaches are more systematic and specified than either haphazard eclecticism or common-factors eclecticism. They are bound together by the common hope of directing the therapist through decisions about what procedures to apply, to whom, and when. They identify both the range of procedures to be used and the patient or temporal and situational cues that index the point of their maximal impact.

At the broadest level, theoretical integrationism attempts to amalgamate two or more extant theoretical viewpoints, leaving the definition of specific techniques and procedures to the imagination of the clinician. These approaches view good theory as the avenue to the development of good techniques; they contrast with those approaches that are often referred to as either "technical eclecticism" or "strategic eclecticism" (Goldfried, 1995; Stricker & Gold, 1996).

The term "integration" has a variety of meanings beyond that applied to the interdigitation of psychotherapy theories. It can refer to the status of one's personality—for example, when one refers to an "integrated" personality, in which the component traits, needs, wants, perceptions, values, emotions, and impulses are in a stable state of harmony and communication. Likewise, an "integrated" person is one who is whole with regard to overall functioning and well-being. As applied to psychotherapy, "integration" refers to harmoniously bringing together affective, cognitive, behavioral, and systems approaches to psychotherapy under the roof of one theory, and applying this theory and associated techniques to the treatment of an individual, couple, or family. This systematic notion goes beyond any single theory or set of techniques by taking into account many views of human functioning: primarily psychodynamic, client-centered, experiential, and cognitive-behavioral, with each approach being enhanced when integrated with the others (Goldfried, 1995).

At least at a superficial level, theoretical integrationism requires the translation of concepts and methods from one psychotherapeutic system into the language and procedures of another (Stricker & Gold, 1996). What often emerges is a new theory that embodies parts of each of the former ones. This theory not only encompasses the processes of identifying and standardizing the most effective concepts, terms, and methods, but includes the application of the resulting theoretical concepts to the grist mill of research and application. Within a framework of integration, theoretical linkages have been made among psychodynamic, behavioral, and cognitive approaches (Arkowitz & Messer, 1984; Safran & Messer, 1997; Stricker & Gold, 1996; Wachtel, 1978).

Theoretical integrationism is the most theoretically abstract of the various systematic approaches. It attempts to bring various theories together through the medium of a new theoretical framework that can better explain, in interactional or causal terms, the environmental, motivational, cognitive, and affective domains of an individual that influence or are influenced by change efforts. That is, approaches based on theoretical integration blend two or more traditional theoretical orientations to yield a new model of personality functioning, psychopathology, and psychological change. Such approaches have led to new forms of therapies that capitalize on the strengths of each of the therapeutic elements (Safran & Messer, 1997).

In comparison to theoretical integrationism, technical and strategic eclecticism are considered by many to be more clinically oriented and practical as methods of applying psychotherapy. These two types of approaches to therapy are less abstract than models of theoretical integration, and are more reliant on the use of specific techniques, procedures, or principles. They attempt to define strategies (strategic eclecticism) or to develop menus of techniques (technical eclecticism), quite independently of the theory that gave birth to these procedures in the first place. These types of integration are accomplished either by remaining unbound to a specific theory of change when constructing treatment objectives and plans, or by adopting a superordinate theory to replace or supplant the original.

Neither technical eclecticism nor strategic eclecticism is strongly concerned about the validity of theories of psychopathology and personality that often give rise to particular procedures. They are concerned primarily with the clinical efficacy of these procedures. These approaches draw techniques and interventions from two or more psychotherapeutic systems and apply them systematically and successively to patients who have indicating qualities, using guidelines that are based on either demonstrated or presumed clinical efficacy (Beutler, 1983; Lazarus, 1996; Safran & Messer, 1997; Stricker & Gold, 1996). They use techniques from cognitive, behavioral, psychodynamic, experiential, humanistic, and any other workable theoretical framework, as long as these procedures have been demonstrated to be effective by means of scientific study. The techniques are then applied, independently of their founding theories. This is not to say that the several approaches within the tradition of technical eclecticism are devoid of theory, but to the degree that theories are used, they are seldom theories of psychopathology or even theories of change. They are theories that link numerous empirical observations, and thus seldom require the level of abstractness inherent in most traditional theories.

The distinction between technical eclecticism and strategic eclecticism lies mainly in the degree to which specific procedures and techniques are recommended. In technical eclecticism, a menu of specific procedures is often defined to fit a given person (Beutler, 1983; Lazarus, 1996). In contrast, strategic eclecticism identifies principles and goals, but leaves the selection of the techniques used to accomplish these goals to the proclivities of each individual therapist. The fact that these interventions do not focus in techniques distinguishes them from approaches based on technical eclecticism. The implicit or working assumption of technical eclecticism is that all techniques have a finite range of applicability and use, whereas strategic eclecticism assumes that all techniques can be used in many different ways and can serve several different ends, depending on the person who applies them.

The first and best-known of the approaches within technical eclecticism is multimodal therapy (Lazarus, 1996). Multimodal therapy represents an effort to apply a variety of different theoretical approaches and models at the same time or in a coordinated sequence, depending on the "firing order" of the patient's symptoms. In other types of technical eclecticism, prescriptive matching is devoted to integrating a host of specific procedures selected from a wide variety of menus into a coherent and seamless treatment (e.g., Beutler, 1983).

In contrast, strategic eclecticism offers a middle ground between the technique focus of technical eclecticism and the abstractness of theoretical integrationism. That is, it bridges the levels of theory and technique. These approaches seek to articulate principles of therapeutic change that lead to general strategies of intervention. The strategies are designed to implement the guiding principles, but the objective is to remain true to the principles rather than focusing on the selection of specific techniques (Beutler & Clarkin, 1990; Beutler & Harwood, 2000; Norcross, Martin, Omer, & Pinsof, 1996). In this process, these approaches seek to preserve the individual therapist's flexibility in selecting among a variety of specific techniques. They also seek to maximize the use of techniques with which the therapist is both familiar and skilled, while not forsaking the use of patient factors as reliable cues for the selective application of different interventions. These approaches usually include an explicit definition of guiding principles that are designed to facilitate relationship qualities as well as to evoke symptomatic and structural changes. Thus, of the various approaches to integration, strategic eclecticism is probably the most flexible and practical, though not as complex and elaborate as theoretical integrationism and not as simplistic as technical eclecticism.

Prescriptive matching, a form of eclecticism also known as prescriptive therapy (PT) (Beutler & Harwood, 2000), can at times resemble technical eclecticism; however, it goes beyond the latter by constructing principles of change. The objective is a more coherent treatment, based upon a comprehensive view of the patient's presentation, than one might get by moving from technique to technique and from symptom to symptom (Stricker & Gold, 1996). Treatments based on explicit principles of change, like those based on elaborate theories of psychopathology, are most usefully integrated if they are researchable, are not reliant on abstract concepts for which no measurement exists, and place few theory-driven proscriptions on the use of various therapeutic techniques.

Although most systematic eclectic psychotherapies span multiple theories, another option is to use the principles to guide the use of specific theories. Cognitive therapy, for example, may be quite amenable to the use of eclectic principles because it is reliant on research findings; is not dependent on abstract theories of causation; and values sound measurement of patient characteristics, change, and treatment processes. Specifically, while offering insights into the nature of psychopathology, cognitive therapy is not dependent on the validity of these insights for effectiveness in the therapeutic arena. Cognitive theory postulates the presence of levels of cognition, but without extending beyond empirical observations to postulate how these levels are related to therapeutic change. Cognitive theory, first and foremost, has a tradition of emphasizing the importance of reliable observation and measurement in the assessment of the effects of treatment.

Thus cognitive theory offers a reasonable platform from which one might begin a process of integration based on principles of change and the definition of strategies—a process that includes, but is not limited by, an already known array of technical interventions.

COGNITIVE THERAPY
AS AN INTEGRATIVE FRAMEWORK

From its inception, cognitive theory has been empirically based. It has used findings from formal research to establish its theoretical principles. Likewise, it allows for a flexibility of viewpoints and applications. Both cognitive therapy and behavior therapy have always shared a commitment to the scientific method, and both have placed an emphasis on the patient's ability to learn new and adaptive ways of functioning. Originally, cognitive-behavioral therapy was simply an integration of cognitive and behavioral theories and techniques.

Behavior therapy became a formal approach to the treatment of psychological disorders in the late 1950s (Wilson, 1989). From its early beginnings, behavior therapy has continued to grow in complexity and scope. The behavior therapies of today encompass four main areas: (1) behavioral analysis (focusing on observable behavior); (2) a neobehavioristic, mediational stimulus–response model (applying the principles of classical and avoidance conditioning); (3) social learning theory (according to which the influence of environmental events is mediated by cognitive processes); and (4) cognitive-behavior modification (cognitive-behavioral therapy, based on the principle that an individual's interpretation of events determines his or her behaviors).

Cognitive therapy (CT), a specific form of more general cognitive-behavioral or cognitive therapies, was formulated by Aaron T. Beck and colleagues at the University of Pennsylvania. (Note that from here on in this chapter, we use the abbreviation "CT" to refer to this specific form of treatment, and "cognitive therapy" and/or "cognitive-behavioral therapy" to refer to the more general classes of procedures. Although rooted in a tradition of behaviorism, CT has now extended beyond this perspective and is recognized as an approach in its own right. CT was developed in the early 1960s as a result of Beck's research on the psychodynamic theory of depression (i.e., the hypothesis that depression is retroflected anger; Beck & Weishaar, 1989). Instead of validating Freud's theory, Beck observed that depressed individuals had predictable cognitive patterns involving negative views of self, the world, and the future (i.e., the depressive triad). This led Beck to the realization that faulty cognitive patterns—typically incorrect and untested assumptions, misperceptions, or dysfunctional belief systems—were responsible for many patients' difficulties.

CT may best be defined as the application of a cognitive model of how a certain disorder is manifested and changed via a variety of techniques that focus on the dysfunctional beliefs and maladaptive information-processing systems characteristic of that disorder (Beck, 1993). The CT of today is the result of a continuing evolutionary process, partially due to the recognition by practitioners that, in the clinical application of this therapy, the integration of techniques characteristic of therapies other than behavioral ones often enhances the overall effectiveness of this treatment (Robins & Hayes, 1993). Beck (1991) emphasizes that CT is the epitome of an integrative psychosocial treatment, because it addresses the operative common factor that cuts across all effective therapies—cognitive change. This integration allows a CT therapist to select interventions from a variety of theoretical viewpoints.

The broader collections of procedures and microtheories constituting the cognitive-behavioral and cognitive therapy traditions have also always included techniques and theoretical perspectives from other psychosocial orientations (Andrews, Norcross, & Halgin, 1992). Indeed, neither cognitive-behavioral therapy in general nor its more specific and widely known representative, CT, has remained a closed system. Cognitive-behavioral therapy as a general class of procedures has always evolved by integrating techniques and theoretical concepts from other approaches (Robins & Hayes, 1993). Thus, through the incorporation of schemata, it allows for the influence of conflicts developed early in development and to the development of personality styles. Moreover, its birth was a process of expanding on extant behavioral theory and recognizing the need to consider patients' inner lives.

The refinements that have occurred through integration of diverse research and theoretical principles have allowed for the inclusion of concepts and techniques consistent with the application of relationship therapy, behavior therapy, interpersonal therapy, and other traditions. The concept of dysfunctional cognitions/schemata/behaviors remains at the core of cognitive theory and is an integrative principle compatible with concepts from numerous other theories that reflect on the roles of early experience and unconscious processes. Recently integrated components of cognitive and cognitive-behavioral therapies include the role of defensive processes, an emphasis on the exploration of the therapeutic relationship and the patient's interpersonal dynamics, facilitative aspect of affective arousal, and the developmental experiences in the formation of maladaptive schemata (Robins & Hayes, 1993).

Defensive processes constitute a theoretical component most often associated with psychodynamic theories. These defensive processes are thought by some (e.g., Young, 1990) to help the patient avoid schema-related material through cognitive processes such as denial, repression of memories, or depersonalization. Emotional avoidance of painful schema-related material may take the form of defensive numbing, dissociation, or minimization of negative experiences. Behavioral defensive measures may take the form of actual physical avoidance of situations likely to activate dysfunctional/painful schemata.

Although CT has long recognized the importance of a sound therapeutic relationship, the interpersonal processes within CT and the broader array of cognitive-behavioral therapies have received greater emphasis in recent years (Liotti, 1991; Mahoney, 1991; Robins & Hayes, 1993; Safran & Segal, 1990). Interpersonal processes are now seen as important avenues to the exploration and amelioration of dysfunctional interpersonal schemata, which typically receive their strongest developmental influence from early relationships. Due to the early and important influence of interpersonal events in the development of schemata, attachment theory (Bowlby, 1977) has also been incorporated by some cognitive therapists to help clarify the behavioral and cognitive dynamics of the therapeutic relationship (Robins & Hayes, 1993).

Moreover, Safran and Segal (1990) indicate that it is important for a cognitive therapist to attend to his or her own feelings and behaviors elicited by interactions with a patient (although these are not referred to as "countertransference" within the cognitive perspective), and to avoid becoming involved in the patient's dysfunctional interpersonal cycle. They also recommend that the material (thoughts and feelings) uncovered in this type of interaction be thoroughly explored.

This last recommendation highlights on another aspect of cognitive and cognitive-behavioral therapies that may loosely be reflective of their eclectic posture. Namely, these approaches to treatment have been successful with a wide variety of conditions, problems, and disorders. The range of effectiveness attests to the flexibility of the techniques utilized and suggests that these procedures may be used within a prescriptive, strategic framework.

THE RANGE OF EFFECTIVENESS
ASSOCIATED WITH COGNITIVE
AND COGNITIVE-BEHAVIORAL THERAPIES

Historically, the literature in psychology pertaining to comparative outcome studies of psychotherapies for various psychological problems has generally contributed to the conclusion that treatments are broadly equivalent in effectiveness (Shapiro, Barkham, Rees, & Hardy, 1994; Robinson, Berman, & Neimeyer, 1990; Bowers, 1990; Hogg & Deffenbacher, 1988). However, in contrast to those who maintain that research reveals equivalent outcomes among therapies, disciples of cognitive and cognitive-behavioral therapy methods have asserted that their treatments are more effective than others, across a variety of conditions and disorders (Brown, 1997; Blackburn et al., 1986).

The efficacy of cognitive therapy for the treatment of depression is well known, and has been demonstrated in a large number of clinical trials (Dobson, 1989). Studies have illustrated that cognitive therapy has been effective in treating various types of depression, such as unipolar, major, minor, and acute depression (Gitlin, 1995; Billings & Moos, 1984). Positive findings have also been obtained with samples of patients with endogenous depression—a subtype often thought to be refractory to psychotherapy (Simons & Thase, 1992). Whether group or individual, cognitive therapy appears to be effective in reducing symptoms of depression and anxiety and increasing assertiveness (Scogin, Hamblin, & Beutler, 1987; Steuer et al., 1984; Shaffer, Shapiro, Sark, & Coghlan, 1981). A study conducted by Ogles, Sawyer, and Lambert (1995) for the National Institute of Mental Health found that a substantial number of clients completing cognitive treatments for depression showed reliable change on all measures of outcome. In addition, Brown and Barlow (1995) found that cognitive-behavioral therapy evoked significant reductions in somatic depressive symptoms and depressed and anxious mood for patients suffering from alcoholism. In addition to these studies, Scogin et al. (1987) found that cognitive bibliotherapy was more effective in reducing depression than were a delayed-treatment control group and an attention-placebo bibliotherapy condition.

Although this latter finding has not uniformly been supported (Scogin, Bowman, Jamison, Beutler, & Machado, 1994), even failures to replicate have found that patients who score relatively high on measures of cognitive dysfunction tend to have lower scores on posttreatment depression severity measures than those with low levels of cognitive impairment. These findings strongly implicate cognitive functions as important aspects of the change processes related to improvement, regardless of the model of treatment used to address them. If cognitive therapy procedures can change cognitions, therefore, they hold promise for treating these conditions.

Cognitive therapy also does well in comparisons to pharmacotherapy. Historically, research has compared cognitive therapy to pharmacotherapy, and most of the published trials have found cognitive therapy to be at least equal and sometimes superior (Blackburn et al., 1986; Blackburn, Jones, & Lewin, 1986). Specifically, findings have revealed that CT is as efficacious as or more efficacious than standard antidepressant medication (Beck et al., 1985), and it also tends to have lower rates of relapse (Hollon, 1996).

Rush and colleagues (Rush, Beck, Kovacs, & Hollon, 1977; Rush, Beck, Kovacs, Weissenburger, & Hollon, 1982) and Murphy, Simons, Wetzel, and Lustman (1984) found that cognitive therapy was associated with more improvement and less attrition than pharmacotherapy treatment. In fact, patients had a higher rate of dropout when pharmacotherapy alone was compared to cognitive therapy. In addition, the results from these studies also revealed that cognitive therapy exceeded pharmacotherapy in improving the depressive symptatomology dimensions of hopelessness and low self-concept. Even when cognitive therapy is combined with pharmacotherapy, patients tend to report significantly fewer depressive symptoms and negative cognitions at discharge than do patients receiving pharmacotherapy alone (Bowers, 1990). Based upon these studies, it appears that cognitive therapy has a significant impact on the cognitive and vegetative symptoms associated with moderate and severe depression, as well as on the symptoms of mild and transitory depressive states.

Cognitive therapy has also been found to be more effective than behavioral and interpersonal therapies (Shapiro et al., 1994; Wilson, Goldin, & Charbouneau-Powis, 1983). Gaffan, Tsaousis, and Kemp-Wheeler (1995) replicated a study by Dobson (1989) comparing cognitive therapy with other forms of treatment. Although their study focused primarily on allegiance effects, results also yielded evidence that cognitive therapy was superior to other forms of treatment, including behavior therapy. Addis and Jacobson (1996) also found that clients who endorsed characterological and existential reasons for depression responded better to cognitive-behavioral therapy than they did to purely behavioral interventions.

Given these various findings, it seems reasonable to conclude that there is strong support for the value of cognitive or cognitive-behavioral therapy in treating patients with depression, but that the mechanisms through which this effect takes place are still uncertain (Jacobson & Hollon, 1996).

Cognitive therapy also appears to be effective in treating other types of disorders that cause emotional maladjustment. Thus cognitive therapy is effective in treating specific fears and phobias, as well as a host of other anxiety disorders and symptoms. Barlow, O'Brien, and Last (1984) found cognitive therapy to outperform behavioral therapies in the treatment of patients experiencing anxiety. Cognitive-behavioral therapy has also proven to be effective in fostering overall abstinence, both at the end of treatment and during follow-up periods, among patients suffering from alcoholism (Brown & Barlow, 1995). In addition, studies have suggested that cognitive-behavioral therapy is effective in treating patients with eating disorders (Hollon & Beck, 1986). A study (Fairburn, Jones, Peveler, Hope, & O'Connor, 1993) of cognitive-behavioral therapy as a form of treatment for patients with bulimia nervosa found that the treatment effects were substantial, were reflected in all aspects of functioning, and were well maintained. Moreover, Arntz and van den Hout (1996) found that among patients with panic disorder and a secondary diagnosis of either social phobia or mood disorder, cognitive therapy produced superior outcomes in comparison to applied relaxation by reducing the frequency of panic attacks. Cognitive therapy has also been found to be effective in treating patients who experienced problems because of lack of self-assertion (Safran, Alden, & Davison, 1980), problems related to anger and aggression (Schlicter & Horan, 1981), and addictive disorders (Woody et al., 1984).

In addition to studies examining the effects of cognitive therapy on a variety of patient problems and characteristics, an increasing number of studies in the literature have attested to the ability of cognitive therapy interventions to produce meaningful reductions in problem-generated difficulties over a long period of time. A 1-year follow-up study by Kovacs, Rush, Beck, and Hollon (1981), for example, revealed that self-rated depressive symptomatology was significantly lower for those who, 1 year earlier, had completed cognitive therapy than for those who had been treated with pharmacotherapy. Similarly, a 2-year follow-up study of patients who had previously been treated with either cognitive therapy, pharmacotherapy, or both indicated that cognitive therapy was associated with lower relapse rates (Blackburn, Eunson, & Bishop, 1986). Moreover, patients in the pharmacotherapy-only group had a relapse rate that was significantly highest during the 2-year follow-up period.

Clinical research has thus firmly established the efficacy of cognitive and cognitive-behavioral therapy in the treatment of depression, anxiety, and myriad other psychological impairments. Even though it remains unclear what aspects of such therapy are responsible for producing improvement in these various patient groups, it is certain that this treatment is effective and often more effective than other forms of treatment.

Cognitive therapy has certain advantages over many other models by virtue of the variety of conditions for which it is effective, and in this sense has the makings of a flexible and eclectic intervention model. This is not to say, however, that cognitive therapy as traditionally practiced is equally effective for all individuals. Research (e.g., Beutler, Mohr, Grawe, Engle, & MacDonald, 1991) reveals that the efficacy of cognitive therapy is differentially influenced by a variety of qualities that are characteristic of the patient and problem. Such qualities as patient coping styles, complexity, and severity of problems, among others, may influence the way cognitive therapy is applied.

One patient characteristic that has proven to be predictive of patients' response to cognitive therapy is coping style. "Coping style" is defined as a trait-like pattern that is used to minimize negative effects of anxiety. A person's characteristic style of coping is the method that the person usually adopts in interactions with others during anxiety-provoking situations. Cognitive therapy has consistently been found to be most effective among patients who exhibit an inhibited, controlled, inner-directed, and internalizing coping style. For example, Kadden, Cooney, and Getter (1989) evaluated patients suffering from alcoholism and implemented cognitive-based social skills training, a procedure that focused on preventing relapse by remediating behavioral deficits in coping with interpersonal and intrapersonal antecedents to drinking. Although cognitive therapy was approximately as effective as other treatments on the average, their particular form of cognitive therapy was more effective than other approaches among patients who were relatively high on measures of sociopathy or impulsivity. This type of aptitude × treatment interaction was also found in other studies in which patient impulsivity was studied as a treatment moderator. Beutler, Engle, et al. (1991) found that depressed patients who scored high on Minnesota Multiphasic Personality Inventory (MMPI) measures of externalization and impulsivity responded better to a cognitive therapy than to insight-oriented therapies. Beutler and Mitchell (1981) and Beutler, Mohr, et al. (1991) found results consistent with the foregoing among both inpatients and outpatients with depressive symptoms. Likewise, Barber and Muenz (1996) found cognitive therapy to be more effective than other treatment interventions for patients who tended to avoid their problems through a method of externalizing blame.

In addition, most of these studies have found that insight- or awareness-based treatments do better than cognitive therapy among those who do not have strongly impulsive, externalizing traits. For example, Beutler, Mohr, et al. (1991) and Beutler, Engle, et al. (1991) found that cognitive therapy exerted substantially stronger effects among patients with externalizing coping styles than did a client-centered therapy or a supportive, self-directed therapy, respectively. On the other hand, these latter internalizing patients did better with client-centered and self-directed therapy than they did with cognitive therapy.

Similarly, in these latter studies, patient resistance traits and tendencies differentiated the level of benefit achieved from the therapist-guided procedures of cognitive therapy and various patient-led or nondirective procedures. A study by Tasca, Russell, and Busby (1994) examined patient characteristics such as defensive style and psychological-mindedness as mediators of patient preferences for cognitive therapy. Those patients who were expressive and tended to externalize their anger by using projection and turning anger against others tended to choose activity-oriented therapy.

Thus it appears from the literature cited above that cognitive therapy is very effective for clients who avoid their problems, because this treatment intervention tends to prompt clients to confront anxiety-provoking situations through homework and specific behavioral interventions and techniques.

Evidence within the literature also supports the advantages of cognitive treatments among patients whose problems are more complex and severe in nature. Complexity or severity may be associated with such factors as comorbidity, enduring personality disturbances, and chronicity of the condition. As a result, patients who are characterized as having long-standing personality disturbances, or whose problems and symptoms tend to recur and persist over a long period of time, tend to have specific needs pertaining to treatment. Thus the literature has stated that initial severity of depression is another factor that may moderate the efficacy of treatment (Robinson et al., 1990). Nevertheless, cognitive therapy appears to be effective with patients exhibiting symptom characteristics that vary in complexity and severity. Woody et al. (1994) found that among opiate addictions, low- and moderate-severity patients made equal or greater progress with cognitive therapy than with the other treatments. A study by Knight-Law, Sugerman, and Pettinati (1988) found that the effectiveness of behavioral-symptom-focused interventions such as cognitive therapy was highest among those patients whose MMPIs revealed that their problems were reactional and situational and more complex in nature. Similar patterns of interaction were also evident in a study by Beutler, Sandowicz, Fisher, and Albanese (1996), in which CT was most effective among those patients with low levels of distress (acute indicators), when compared with emotionally focused treatments.

Brown and Barlow (1995) examined long-term effects of cognitive-behavioral therapy for patients with panic disorder. Although the results did not support the notion that cognitive therapy has long-term effects on reducing symptomatology, they did suggest that patients with more severe symptomatology were responsive to treatment in the short term. Moreover, patients were neither less able to maintain these treatment gains nor more apt to experience marked fluctuations in symptoms over the longer term.

This latter finding suggests that the long-term effects of cognitive or cognitive-behavioral therapy may partially be a function of interactional matches between type of treatment and patient characteristics. Such a conclusion is supported by other research as well. For instance, Beutler, Mohr, et al. (1991) and Beutler, Engle, et al. (1991) found that patients whose personal characteristics (i.e., internalizing and resistant to direction) indicated that they were poor candidates for cognitive therapy had poorer long-term effects than those who were better matched to the treatment demands. Patients who were well matched to treatment procedures were likely to maintain treatment gains and even to improve during the follow-up period. These findings underline the potential importance of an external coping style and low resistance as indicators for cognitive therapy. In addition, evidence from other sources indicates that situation-specific problems are more responsive to cognitive-behavioral treatments than are chronic and recurrent problems. This has been found to be true among individuals with chemical dependency (Sheppard, Smith, & Rosenbaum, 1988), somatic symptoms (LaCroix, Clarke, Bock, & Doxey, 1986), and chronic back pain (Tref & Yuan, 1983).

From this latter research, it appears that change in cognitive therapy is facilitated are explored and tested in a climate that fosters affective arousal. To address this observation, affect-enhancing techniques have been integrated into cognitive therapy by many therapists as a means of inducing affect among those with low levels of arousal. Robins and Hayes (1993) identified several affective arousal techniques advocated by cognitive therapists, including shame-attacking exercises, imagery dialogues, the use of dreams, repetition and exaggeration of key phrases, and focusing on physical cues/ bodily sensations associated with currently experienced feelings.

Although cognitive therapy has traditionally been conceptualized as present-focused, recent modifications have sought to make it more amenable to explorations of historical contributions to patients' problems (Arnkoff, 1983; Robins & Hayes, 1993; Young, 1990). The examination of cognition within a developmental framework may help induce affective arousal, and thereby enhance the opportunity for a patient and therapist to identify and challenge maladaptive expectations and evaluate faulty assumptions associated with recalled events.

MAKING COGNITIVE THERAPY FIT HUMAN COMPLEXITY

The major impetus for interest in psychotherapy integration comes from the research-generated conclusion that no school of psychotherapy has demonstrated consistent superiority over the others. That is, efforts to define specific methods of psychotherapy that are effective for a specific problem like drug abuse or with a specific symptom like depression have largely concluded that all approaches produce similar mean effects (e.g., Lambert, Shapiro, & Bergin, 1986; Beutler, Crago, & Arizmendi, 1986; Smith, Glass,

& Miller, 1980). Unfortunately, the nonsignificance of treatment main effects often draws more attention than the growing body of research demonstrating that there are meaningful differences in the types of patients for whom different aspects of treatment are effective.

For example, among patients with symptoms of anxiety and depression, research indicates that (1) experiential therapies are more effective than cognitive and dynamic therapies when initial distress about one's condition is insufficient to support movement (Beutler & Mitchell, 1981; Orlinsky & Howard, 1986); (2) nondirective and paradoxical interventions are more effective than directive ones among patients with high levels of pretherapy resistance (i.e., "resistance potential"; Beutler, Mohr, et al., 1991; Beutler, Engle, et al., 1991; Shoham-Salomon & Hannah, 1991; Forsyth & Forsyth, 1982); and (3) therapies that target cognitive and behavior changes through contingency management (e.g., Higgins, Budney, & Bickel, 1994) are more effective among impulsive or externalizing patients than are those that attempt to facilitate insight—an effect that is reversed among patients with less externalizing coping styles (Beutler, Mohr, et al., 1991; Beutler, Engle, et al., 1991; Calvert, Beutler, & Crago, 1988; Sloane, Staples, Cristol, Yorkston, & Whipple, 1975).

Cognitive therapy may be adapted to meet the manifold needs and characteristics of patients suffering from a wide array of problems and diagnoses. In a study now underway in our Psychotherapy Research Lab at the University of California at Santa Barbara, we are utilizing several guiding principles and strategies that inform the systematic application of tactics and techniques drawn from numerous theoretical perspectives. For illustrative purposes, this section addresses some of the techniques and strategies that guide the application of Beck's CT techniques for the internalizing or externalizing patient, for the resistant patient, and for management of arousal level. The techniques of CT may be used with virtually any patient; however, the techniques should be focused or employed differentially, depending on various patient dimensions such as coping style/type of problem, and level of resistance. Although we address this topic in this chapter, some readers may want more detail. For those who are interested in a thorough discussion on identifying various patient–treatment matching dimensions (resistance/reactance level, styles of coping, severity of subjective distress, and functional impairment) and an in-depth treatment of guiding principles, strategies, and technique selection, please refer to Beutler and Harwood (2000) or Beutler and Clarkin (1990).

Unless managed skillfully, patient resistance typically bodes poorly for treatment effectiveness. In a similar vein, relative placement on measures of internalization and externalization (coping traits) require a differential selection of treatment procedures on the part of the therapist, as applied to both in-session and extrasession therapeutic strategies and techniques. It is generally assumed that some patients are likely to resist therapeutic procedures more than others are. "Resistance" has been used both to describe a transitory state and a trait-like quality in psychotherapy. That is, resistance may be characterized as both a dispositional trait and an in-therapy state of oppositional (e.g., angry, irritable, and suspicious) behaviors. Resistance involves both intrapsychic (image of self, safety, and psychological integrity) and interpersonal (loss of interpersonal freedom or power imposed by another) factors (Beutler et al., 1996). Reactance is an extreme example of resistance and is manifested by oppositional and uncooperative behaviors.

A patient's level of resistance or reactance potential is determined by three hypothesized factors (Beutler et al., 1996). The first factor involves the subjective value that is placed on the particular freedom perceived to be threatened. For example, one patient may value highly the freedom afforded by the absence of any fixed schedule of time commitments, while another patient may be relatively comfortable with an imposed schedule or routine. The second factor involves the proportion of freedoms perceived to be threatened or eliminated. Introducing an element in treatment that eliminates or reduces a variety of freedoms (e.g., a homework assignment that proscribes substance use and requires social interaction at an event for a particular amount of time) is likely to generate a high level of reactance among individuals who are resistance-prone, substance-abusing, and socially withdrawn. The third and final factor involves the magnitude of authority and power ascribed to the threatening force or individual. The resistance generated in the case of this third factor arises from a patient's preconceived notions and differential assignment of authority to various professional occupations (e.g., clinicians, those in law enforcement, etc.). In addition, actual interactions with a mental health professional may operate to reduce or exaggerate these notions.

Resistance is easily identifiable, and differential treatment plans for high- and low-resistance patients are easily crafted; however, implementation of these plans is often quite a different matter. Actually overcoming a patient's resistance to the clinician's efforts to help is difficult; it requires the therapist to set aside his or her own resistance and recognize that the patient's oppositional behavior may actually be iatrogenic. Binder and Strupp (1997) found that none of the experienced and highly trained therapists in the Vanderbilt study of psychodynamic psychotherapy were able to work effectively with patient resistance. They observed that therapists were likely to react to patient resistance by becoming angry, critical, and rejecting, all of which reactions reduced the willingness of patients to explore problems.

In general, therapists should do their best to avoid disagreement with highly resistant patients. The collaborative relationship of CT is extremely important for resistant patients, and this treatment component is one that should be emphasized from the initiation of therapy. Socratic questioning (i.e., guided discovery), which is one of the most fundamental techniques of CT, must be handled carefully to avoid any arousal of resistance tendencies. Clinicians should be sure to introduce this technique as a collaborative effort, and they may elicit feedback regarding their patients' willingness to participate; direction and suggestions for exploration may be elicited from the patients as well.

Information regarding a patient's level of resistance potential may be gathered from the patient's history and behavior during recent stressful experiences, or during the process of treatment itself. Examples of behaviors associated with high levels of either *trait* or *state* resistance potential are indicated by the patient behaviors listed in Table 5.1.

Research (Shoham-Solomon, Avner, & Neeman, 1989; Shoham-Salomon & Rosenthal, 1987; Horvath, 1989; Seltzer, 1986) suggests that nondirective, paradoxical, and self-directed procedures produce better outcomes among patients exhibiting high-resistance behaviors. Patient-generated behavioral contracts and "suggested" homework assignments that are self-directed are examples of nondirective therapeutic interventions for managing resistant patients. For patients with extreme and persistent resistance, a paradoxical intervention in which a symptom is prescribed or in which the patients are encouraged to avoid changing for a brief period of time might be considered. Simply put, paradoxical interventions induce

TABLE 5.1. Behaviors Characteristic of Patient Resistance

High *trait* resistance potential	High *state* resistance potential
1. Frequently expresses resentment of others.	1. Has trouble understanding or following instructions.
2. Seems to expect that others will take advantage of him or her.	2. Is stubborn about accepting something that is obvious to the therapist.
3. Tends to be controlling and demanding in intimate relationships.	3. Seems closed to new experiences.
4. Is distrustful and suspicious of others' motives.	4. Responds to suggestions in a passive–aggressive way.
5. Expresses resentment over not having the advantages/opportunities of others.	5. Begins coming late or avoiding appointments.
6. Often has broken the "rules."	6. Expresses fear that the therapist is trying to take advantage of him or her.
7. Enjoys competition.	7. Begins to tenaciously hold a point of view and can't be argued out of a position once it is set.
8. Does the opposite when others try to control him or her.	8. Holds a grudge.
9. Resents those who make the rules.	9. Becomes overtly angry at the therapist.
10. Is happiest when in charge.	

change by discouraging it (Seltzer, 1986). A nondirective, paradoxical intervention could involve suggesting that a patient continue or exaggerate a symptom/behavior. A classic example of a paradoxical intervention involves prescribing wakefulness for a patient complaining of insomnia. An acceptable rationale (e.g., "Your circadian rhythm is not properly set, and staying awake will help you reset your sleep cycle") should typically be provided for this type of intervention. Nonresistant or low-resistance behaviors indicate that patients are generally open to external direction (directive interventions such as assigned homework) and guidance from the therapist. Table 5.2 summarizes some general guidelines for treating high- and low-resistance patients.

An illustration of how CT can be adapted to patient characteristics may be provided by briefly describing how one procedure can be applied to both high-resistance and low-resistance patients. Homework is one extremely helpful element of CT that can be adapted to patient characteristics (Beutler & Harwood, 2000). Three guidelines distinguish the use of homework with high-resistance patients from how homework is assigned and utilized with low-resistance patients. First, homework for resistant patients should be of a self-directed nature (e.g., bibliotherapy selected by the patients from a predetermined list and accompanied by self-help workbooks). The second guideline involves the patients' self-monitoring their own success (e.g., recording self-control procedures or mood ratings in control of drug use and/or depression). The third guideline indicates that there should be relatively little effort on the part of the therapist to check or collect homework assignments. On the other hand, homework for the nonresistant patient may be highly structured and can include assigned readings and exercises designed specifically to alter social behaviors and drug use patterns.

TABLE 5.2. General Guidelines for Treating High- and Low-Resistance Patients

High resistance	Low resistance
1. Provide opportunities for self-directed improvement.	1. Increase relative reliance on procedures that invoke the therapist's authority.
2. Increase reliance on nondirective interventions.	2. May provide direct guidance.
3. Consider using paradoxical interventions.	3. May provide suggestions and interpretation (these are typically well received).
4. Deemphasize the use of confrontive procedures.	4. May assign therapist-guided homework.
5. Deemphasize the use of procedures that invoke the therapist's authority.	5. Use behavioral strategies that structure and monitor therapeutic activities.

In this instance, homework should always be reviewed/checked, and progress should be monitored on a weekly basis.

Another example of how to adapt CT to fit resistance levels involves therapist directiveness. Nondirective therapeutic interventions have been found to be effective with resistant patients; therefore, high levels of recurrent resistance (trait or state) indicate the need for a treatment strategy that ordinarily emphasizes low therapist directiveness, a nonauthoritarian stance, and a nonconfrontive relationship. Nondirective interventions include reflection (including acknowledgment of unhappy and resistant feelings), clarification, questions, support, paradoxical interventions, and an approach–retreat method (in which difficult topics are introduced, followed by the therapist's withdrawal into relative silence). For patients manifesting few indices of resistance, therapists can typically provide guidance and make interpretations, direct suggestions, and assignments. Research suggests that low-resistance patients may in fact do better with authoritative and directive roles than with nondirective ones (Beutler, Engle, et al., 1991).

It is important to remember that resistance states are a function of the particular constraints imposed by the therapeutic environment (resistance *traits* are manifested across situations); therefore, therapists must remain vigilant to in-session levels of manifest state resistance. A summary of directive and nondirective cognitive interventions is provided in Table 5.3.

Internalization and externalization represent opposite poles on a dimension of patients' coping styles; they are conceptualized as trait-like. Both coping styles may be used to reduce uncomfortable experience (i.e., to provide escape or avoidance) whenever it arises. Some patients cope by activating behaviors that allow either direct escape from or avoidance of the feared environment. These are examples of externalization. Others prefer behaviors that control internal experience (i.e., self-blame, compartmentalization, sensitization), such as anxiety. These represent internalization

TABLE 5.3. Examples of Directive and Nondirective Interventions

Directive interventions	Nondirective interventions
1. Asking closed questions.	1. Asking open-ended questions.
2. Providing interpretations.	2. Reflection.
3. Confrontation.	3. Passive acceptance of feelings/ thoughts.
4. Interrupting speech or behavior.	4. Self-monitored homework.
5. Providing information or instructions.	5. Self-directed therapy work.
6. Structured homework.	6. Paradoxical work.
7. Analysis of antecedent–behavior– consequence relationships.	7. Low percentage of occasions when the therapist introduces topics.
8. Activity scheduling.	

styles. However, some patients have complex styles that include coping behaviors characteristic of both internalizers and externalizers.

Internalizing patients are typically characterized by low impulsivity and overcontrol of impulses, whereas externalizers generally exhibit highly impulsive or exaggerated behaviors. In addition, internalizers tend to be more insightful and self-reflective, typically inhibit feelings, tolerate emotional distress better than externalizers, and frequently attribute encountered difficulties to themselves. On the other hand, externalizers tend to deny personal responsibility for either the cause or solution of their problems, experience negative emotions as intolerable, and tend to seek external stimulation. Examples of patient characteristics corresponding to internalizing and externalizing coping styles are provided in Table 5.4.

In the case of an excessively impulsive (externalizing) patient—who, for example, may be a stimulation seeker (i.e., avoiding lack of stimulation), or who may respond avoidantly to the anticipated consequences of social contact—the preferred treatment would be learning to tolerate bland and nonstimulating environments (e.g., via imagery and *in vivo* exposure). Therapeutic procedures designed to facilitate reattribution of responsibility (Beck, Wright, Newman, & Liese, 1993) may also help in the treatment of externalizers who tend to blame others or take a fatalistic view of problems that are under their control. Daily thought records (DTRs or DRDTs as described in Chapter 10, this volume) may help identify impulsive behaviors and reactions (cognitions and affects). Activity schedules can be used to supplement the DTRs by identifying how the patients spend their time (e.g., are the activities characteristic of high stimulation?). Activity schedules also provide a tool for gauging behavioral change. For impulsive individuals re-

TABLE 5.4. Characteristics of Externalizing and Internalizing Patients

Internalizers typically:	Externalizers typically:
1. Are more likely to feel hurt than anger.	1. Are gregarious and outgoing.
2. Are quiet in social gatherings.	2. Seek to impress others.
3. Worry and ruminate a lot before taking action.	3. Seek social status.
4. Feel more than passing guilt, remorse, or shame about minor things.	4. Avoid boredom by seeking novelty, activity, or stimulation.
5. Lack self-confidence.	5. Are insensitive to others' feelings.
6. Like to be alone.	6. Have an inflated sense of importance.
7. Are timid.	7. Are impulsive.
8. Are reluctant to express anger directly.	8. React to frustration with overt anger.
9. Are introverted.	9. Become easily frustrated.
10. Do not go to parties often.	10. Deny responsibility for problems that occur.
11. Do not let feelings show.	11. Have little empathy for others.

covering from substance abuse problems and other problems generated by their impulsive behaviors, stimulus control strategies (e.g., identifying high-risk situations—primarily external for externalizers—and developing adaptive coping responses) may be particularly useful.

For internalizing individuals (e.g., those who may be avoiding uncomfortable feelings, intimacy, or environmental stimulation and activity), treatment may focus on teaching the patients to allow the experience of emotional intensity or to accept the expression of love and intimacy. Although the principles of treatment are the same as for externalizers, the treatment of internalizing individuals is more complex. An internalizing individual's treatment cues are embedded within his or her unique history of conflict and feeling development; therefore, using DTRs and examining the cognitive–affective–behavioral patterns elicited thereby may be a particularly helpful and efficient method for uncovering cues that are indirectly associated with overt symptoms. That is, the DTRs may help the patient and therapist to build bridges from avoided knowledge to insight, or from feelings to awareness. The "downward arrow" technique (Beck et al., 1993) may also be beneficial for internalizers by eliciting "hot" cognitions leading to insight and bringing feelings into focus. Thus a focus on schematic thoughts rather than automatic thoughts may be indicated.

Cognitive skills and restructuring may be enhanced by uncovering the historical origins of the patient's dysfunctional negative schemata and relating them to present functioning. Activity schedules may be useful in identifying withdrawal/lack of social contact or other deficiencies in the range of typical activity, and this information may be used to help identify social schemata.

The patient's level of subjective distress is another dimension that may help guide the differential use of cognitive techniques. A moderate level of emotional intensity or distress is motivating and not debilitating; however, a high level of distress can interfere with therapy, and a low level of emotional intensity fails to motivate the patient to change. Therefore, the management of the patient's subjective distress is an important aspect of most therapeutic endeavors (Orlinsky, Grawe, & Park, 1994; Frank & Frank, 1991). Employing the downward arrow technique in the pursuit of hot cognitions is one way to increase emotional intensity. The downward arrow technique involves the therapist's employing variations on "What does that mean to you?" as applied to the patient's cognitions. This type of questioning technique brings the patient to successively deeper levels of meaning and emotional intensity. For example, Table 5.5 illustrates how a patient may have completed a DTR and the therapy excerpt that may have ensued.

The last statement from the patient in Table 5.5 contains hot cognitions characteristic of the commonly encountered core schema "I'm unlovable," and emotional arousal will accompany the elicitation and explo-

TABLE 5.5. Example of "Downward Arrow" Technique

Situation: At home on a Saturday afternoon.
Emotions: Depressed (80%), anxious (60%).
Automatic thought: I should have a date on Saturday night.

THERAPIST: What does it mean if you don't have a date on Saturday night?
PATIENT: It means that I'll be home by myself on Saturday night.
THERAPIST: What does being home alone on a Saturday night mean?
PATIENT: It means that I'm not out having fun like everybody else.
THERAPIST: And what does that mean to you?
PATIENT: That I'm a loser, nobody loves me, and I'll always be alone.

---

ration of this theme. Following the identification of hot cognitions or core schemata, the structured analysis of dysfunctional thoughts/cognitive errors may be utilized to reduce interfering levels of high emotional intensity. Direct relaxation (i.e., focusing on breathing and muscle relaxation), followed by suggestions for thought insertion such as "I am relaxed and comfortable" or "I can control how I feel," can be particularly helpful for reducing arousal levels.

Similarly, the patient's level of impairment may index the need for longer-term and more intensive therapies. Beutler, Clarkin, and Bongar (2000) found that among 284 patients with depression, anxiety, alcohol misuse, and mixed diagnoses, the level of impairment was a significant indicator for the use of intensive treatments, including adjunctive medication, individual therapy, and alterations in the length and spacing of treatment. Therapists employing CT, like therapists employing any other treatment model, are capable of adapting the frequency and spacing of sessions in order to adapt to the differential needs presented by patients with high levels of social and interpersonal impairment. Several reports suggest that even psychotic patients may benefit from cognitive interventions (Haddock & Slade, 1996; Kingdon & Turkington, 1994). Patients with low social support, low social functioning, and comorbidity may be the best candidates for long-term interventions, frequent sessions, and concomitant pharmacotherapies. Those patients with adequate levels of social support, low impairment, and no Axis II morbidity, on the other hand, may be successfully treated by a time-limited course of cognitive intervention.

The final area of discussion in this section on adjusting treatment elements to fit patient characteristics involves the dimensions of sociotropy and autonomy. Developed specifically to assess these personality dimensions, the Sociotropy–Autonomy Scale (SAS; Beck, Epstein, Harrison, & Emery, 1983) is a 60-item self-report measure that utilizes a 5-point scale format. The personality characteristic of sociotropy has been shown to have stability over time (Blackburn, 1998) and the validity of the SAS Sociotropy scale has been demonstrated (Clark & Beck, 1991); however, the conceptual validity of autonomy has not been consistently demonstrated as applied to differential treatment decisions (Blackburn, 1998). The SAS Autonomy scale is in the process of revision for further validation studies (Clark, Steer, Beck, & Ross, 1995).

Individuals who are highly autonomous present themselves as extremely invested in maintaining independence and freedom from external control. In addition, autonomous individuals value mobility, superior levels of achievement, and choice. These individuals are predicted to be vulnerable to externally imposed constraints or personal limitations that result in a failure to attain goals (Moore & Blackburn, 1996). Individuals who are highly sociotropic are extremely dependent on relationships with others for interpersonal needs. Sociotropic individuals place a high value on acceptance, intimacy, support, and guidance (Blackburn, 1998).

Low-resistance potential is characterized by avoidance of confrontation with others and acceptance of direction from those in authority, similar to the sociotropic individual's need for acceptance, support, and guidance from others (Allen, Horne, & Trinder, 1996). In addition, autonomous individuals appear to share similarities with those scoring high on measures of resistance. Opposition to attempted (or perceived) control from others and a need to be in charge characterize high resistance. These characteristics seem to parallel the autonomous individual's need for independence and mobility. If these patient dimensions are correlated and if this is demonstrated empirically, therapeutic interventions can be selected according to the aforementioned guidelines for the dimension of resistance. That is, nondirective and patient self-monitored interventions should be most likely to produce a positive outcome for autonomous/high-resistance patients. On the other hand, sociotropic/low-resistance patients should be most likely to respond best to directive interventions, frequent interpretations, and direct guidance from the therapist.

SUMMARY

Recent years have seen a proliferation of eclectic viewpoints. Haphazard eclecticism is the most widely practiced but least systematic approach to eclecticism. Theoretical integrationism is widely practiced, but may be too abstract to provide clear and practical guidance for implementing treatments. Systematic eclecticism may suffer from being too narrow and atheoretical. However, in this chapter we have argued that the theoretical and practical foundations of cognitive and cognitive-behavioral therapies (particularly Beck's CT) provide a framework and platform by which to develop strategic eclectic interventions.

The tradition of adhering to empirical guidelines, the foundation in sound measurement methods, and the absence of confounding theoretical constructs provide a suitable environment in which to extend the use of cognitive interventions and to apply them more discriminatingly than is typically done. We see in the wide diversity of problems for which cognitive or cognitive-behavioral therapy is applicable, and in the level of effects associated with its procedures, the opportunity to increase the specificity of the procedures. This integration can be accomplished by adapting procedures to such dimensions as the patient's level of impairment, resistance, coping style, and level of distress. Adapting recommendations for treatment frequency and length (associated with patient functional impairment), degree of directiveness (associated with patient resistance), focus on symptoms or schematic thoughts (associated with patient coping style), and attention to hot cognitions (associated with level of patient distress) may make it possible to further increase the already powerful effects of cognitive therapy. In the last part of this chapter, we have outlined some general guidelines and patient dimensions that may assist the practitioner to adapt the procedures of Beck's CT to the unique needs of each patient.

REFERENCES

Addis, M. E., & Jacobson, N. S. (1996). Reasons for depression and the process and outcome of cognitive-behavioral psychotherapies. *Journal of Consulting and Clinical Psychology, 64*(6), 1417–1424.

Allen, N. B., Horne, D. J. L., & Trinder, J. (1996). Sociotropy, autonomy, and dysphoric emotional responses to specific classes of stress: A psychophysiological evaluation. *Journal of Abnormal Psychology, 105,* 25–33.

Andrews, J. D. W., Norcross, J. C., & Halgin, R. P. (1992). Training in psychotherapy integration. In J. C. Norcross & M. R. Goldfried (Eds.), *Handbook of psychotherapy integration* (pp. 563–592). New York: Basic Books.

Arkowitz, H. (1995). Common factors or processes of change in psychotherapy? *American Psychological Association, 2*(1), 94–100.

Arkowitz, H., & Messer, S. B. (1984). *Psychoanalytic therapy and behavior therapy: Is integration possible?* New York: Plenum Press.

Arnkoff, D. B. (1983). Common and specific factors in cognitive therapy. In M. J. Lambert (Ed.), *Psychotherapy and patient relationships* (pp. 85–125). Homewood, IL: Dorsey Press.

Arntz, A., & van den Hout, M. (1996). Psychological treatments of panic disorder without agoraphobia: Cognitive therapy vs. applied relaxation. *Behaviour Research and Therapy, 34,* 113–121.

Barber, J. P., & Muenz, L. R. (1996). The role of avoidance and obsessiveness in matching patients to cognitive and interpersonal psychotherapy: Empirical findings from the treatment for Depression Collaborative Research Program. *Journal of Consulting and Clinical Psychology, 64*(5), 951–958.

Barlow, D. H., O'Brien, G. T., & Last, C. G. (1984). Couples treatment of agoraphobia. *Behavior Therapy, 18*, 441–448.

Beck, A. T. (1991). Cognitive therapy as *the* integrative therapy. *Journal of Psychotherapy Integration, 3*, 191–198.

Beck, A. T. (1993). Cognitive therapy: Nature and relation to behavior therapy. *Journal of Psychotherapy Practice and Research, 2*, 345–356.

Beck, A. T., et al. (1989). Treatment of depression with cognitive therapy and amitriptyline. *Archives of General Psychiatry, 42*(2), 142–148.

Beck, A. T., Epstein, N., Harrison, R. P., & Emery, G. (1983). *Development of the Sociotropy–Autonomy Scale: A measure of personality factors in psychopathology.* Unpublished manuscript, University of Pennsylvania.

Beck, A. T., & Weishaar, M. E. (1989). Cognitive therapy. In R. J. Corsini & D. Wedding (Eds.), *Current psychotherapies* (4th ed., pp. 285–320). Itasca, IL: Peacock.

Beck, A. T., Wright, F. D., Newman, C. F., & Liese, B. S. (1993*). Cognitive therapy for substance abuse.* New York: Guilford Press.

Beutler, L. E. (1983). *Eclectic psychotherapy: A systematic approach.* New York: Pergamon Press.

Beutler, L. E., & Clarkin, J. E. (1990). *Systematic treatment selection: Toward targeted therapeutic interventions.* New York: Brunner/Mazel.

Beutler, L. E., Clarkin, J. E., & Bongar, B. (2000). *Guidelines for the systematic treatment of the depressed patient.* New York: Oxford University Press.

Beutler, L. E., Crago, M., & Arizmendi, T. G. (1986). Therapist variables in psychotherapy process and outcome. In S. L. Garfield & A. E. Bergin (Eds.), *Handbook of psychotherapy and behavior change* (3rd ed., pp. 257–310). New York: Wiley.

Beutler, L. E., Engle, D., Mohr, D., Daldrup, R. J., Bergan, J., Meredith, K., & Merry, W. (1991). Predictors of differential and self-directed psychotherapeutic procedures. *Journal of Consulting and Clinical Psychology, 59*, 333–340.

Beutler, L. E., & Harwood, T. M. (2000). *Prescriptive therapy: Systematic treatment selection with special emphasis on treating co-morbid depression and substance abuse.* New York: Oxford University Press.

Beutler, L. E., & Mitchell, R. (1981). Psychotherapy outcome in depressed and impulsive patients as a function of analytic and experiential treatment procedures. *Psychiatry, 44*, 297–306.

Beutler, L. E., Mohr, D. C., Grawe, K., Engle, D., & MacDonald, R. (1991). Looking for differential effects: Cross-cultural predictors of differential psychotherapy efficacy. *Journal of Psychotherapy Integration, 1*, 121–142.

Beutler, L. E., Sandowicz, M., Fisher, D., & Albanese, A. L. (1996). Resistance in psychotherapy: What conclusions are supported by research. *In Session: Psychotherapy in Practice, 2*, 77–86.

Beutler, L. E., Williams, R. E., & Wakefield, P. J. (1993). Obstacles to disseminating applied psychological science. *Journal of Applied and Preventive Psychology,* 2, 38–53.

Beutler, L. E., Williams, R. E., Wakefield, P. J., & Entwistle, S. R. (1995). Bridging scientist and practitioner perspectives in clinical psychology. *American Psychologist, 50,* 984–994.

Billings, A. B., & Moos, R. H. (1984). Coping, stress, and social resources among adults with unipolar depression. *Journal of Personality and Social Psychology, 46,* 877–891.

Binder, J. L., & Strupp, H. H. (1997). Negative process: A recurrently discovered and underestimated facet of therapeutic process and outcome in the individual psychotherapy of adults. *Clinical Psychology: Science and Practice, 4,* 121–139.

Blackburn, I. M. (1998). Cognitive therapy. In A. S. Bellack & M. Hersen (Eds.), *Comprehensive clinical psychology* (Vol. 1, pp. 51–84). New York: Pergamon.

Blackburn, I. M., Eunson, K. M., & Bishop, S. (1986). A two-year naturalistic follow-up of depressed patients treated with cognitive therapy, pharmacotherapy, and a combination of both. *Journal of Affective Disorders, 10,* 67–75.

Blackburn, I. M., Jones, S., & Lewin, R. J. (1986). A two year naturalistic follow-up of depressed patients treated with cognitive therapy, pharmacotherapy, and combination of both. *Journal of Affective Disorders, 10,* 67–75.

Bowers, W. A. (1990). Treatment of depressed in-patients: Cognitive therapy plus medication, relaxation plus medication, and medication alone. *British Journal of Psychiatry, 156,* 73–78.

Bowlby, J. (1977). The making and breaking of affectional bonds: II. Some principles of psychotherapy. *British Journal of Psychiatry, 130,* 421–431.

Brown, G. W. (1997). A psychosocial perspective and the aetiology of depression. In A. Honig & H. M. van Praag (Eds.), *Depression: Neurological, psychopathological, and therapeutic advances* (pp. 343–362). Chichester, England: Wiley.

Brown, T. A., & Barlow, D. H. (1995). Long-term outcome in cognitive-behavioral treatment of panic disorder: Clinical predictors and alternative strategies for assessment. *Journal of Consulting and Clinical Psychology, 63,* 754–765.

Calvert, S. J., Beutler, L. E., & Crago, M. (1988). Psychotherapy outcome as a function of therapist–patient matching on selected variables. *Journal of Social and Clinical Psychology, 6,* 104–117.

Clark, D. A., & Beck, A. T. (1991). Personality factor in dysphoria: A psychometric refinement of Beck's Sociotropy–Autonomy scale. *Journal of Psychopathology and Behavioral Assessment, 13,* 369–388.

Clark, D. A., Steer, R. A., Beck, A. T., & Ross, L. (1995). Psychometric characteristics of revised sociotropy and autonomy scales in college students. *Behavior Research and Therapy, 33,* 325–334.

Dobson, K. S. (1989). A meta-analysis of the efficacy of cognitive therapy for depression. *Journal of Consulting and Clinical Psychology, 57*(3), 414–419.

Fairburn, C. G., Jones, R., Peveler, R. C., Hope, R. A., & O'Connor, M. (1993). Psychotherapy and bulimia nervosa: Longer-term effects of interpersonal psychotherapy, behavior therapy, and cognitive behavior therapy. *Archives of General Psychiatry, 50,* 419–428.

Fava, G. A. (1986). Psychotherapy research: Clinical trials versus clinical reality. *Psychotherapy and Psychosomatics, 46,* 6–12.

Forsyth, N. L., & Forsyth, D. R. (1982). Internality, controllability, and the effectiveness of attributional interpretation in counseling. *Journal of Counseling Psychology, 29,* 140–150.

Frank, J. D., & Frank, J. B. (1991). *Persuasion and healing: A comparative study of psychotherapy* (3rd ed.). Baltimore: University Press.

Freedheim, D. K., Freudenberger, H. J., Kessler, J. W., & Messer, S. B. (1992). *History of psychotherapy: A century of change.* Washington, DC: American Psychological Association.

Gaffan, E. A., Tsaousis, J., & Kemp-Wheeler, S. M. (1995). Researcher allegiance and meta-analysis: The case of cognitive therapy for depression. *Journal of Consulting and Clinical Psychology, 63,* 966–980.

Garfield, S. L. (1981). Evaluating the psychotherapies. *Behavior Therapy, 12,* 295–307.

Gitlin, M. J. (1995). Effects of depression and antidepressants on sexual functioning. *Bulletin of the Menninger Clinic, 59,* 232–248.

Goldfried, M. R. (1995). *From cognitive-behavior therapy to psychotherapy integration.* New York: Springer.

Goldfried, M. R., & Padawar, W. (1982). Current status and future direction in psychotherapy. In M. R. Goldfried (Ed.), *Converging themes in psychotherapy* (pp. 3–52). New York: Springer.

Goldstein, A. P., & Stein, N. (1976). *Prescriptive psychotherapy.* New York: Pergamon.

Haddock, G., & Slade, P. D. (Eds.). (1996). *Cognitive behavioural interventions with psychotic disorders.* New York: Routledge.

Heppner, P. P., & Anderson, W. P. (1985). On the perceived non-utility of research in counseling. *Journal of Counseling and Development, 63,* 545–547.

Higgins, S. T., Budney, A. J., & Bickel, W. K. (1994). Applying behavioral concepts and principles to the treatment of cocaine dependence. *Drug and Alcohol Dependence, 34,* 87–97.

Hogg, J. A., & Deffenbacher, J. L. (1988). A comparison of cognitive and interpersonal-process group therapies in the treatment of depression among college students. *Journal of Counseling Psychology, 35*(3), 304–310.

Hollon, S. D. (1996). The efficacy and effectiveness of psychotherapy relative to medications. *American Psychologist, 51*(10), 1025–1030.

Hollon, S. D., & Beck, A. T. (1986). Cognitive and cognitive-behavioral therapies. In S. L. Garfield & A. E. Bergin (Eds.), *Handbook of psychotherapy and behavior change* (3rd ed., pp. 443–482). New York: Wiley.

Horvath, A. (1989, June). *There are no main effects, only interactions.* Paper presented at the annual meeting of the Society for Psychotherapy Research, Toronto.

Jacobson, N. S., & Hollon, S. D. (1996). Cognitive-behavioral therapy versus pharmacotherapy: Now that the jury's returned its verdict, it's time to present the rest of the evidence. *Journal of Consulting and Clinical Psychology, 64,* 74–80.

Kadden, R. M., Cooney, N. L., & Getter, H. (1989). Matching alcoholics to coping skills or interactional therapy: Posttreatment results. *Journal of Consulting and Clinical Psychology, 56*(1), 48–55.

Kingdon, D., & Turkington, D. (1994). *Cognitive-behavioral therapy of schizophrenia.* New York: Guilford Press.

Knight-Law, A., Sugerman, A., & Pettinati, H. (1988). An application of an MMPI classification system for predicting outcome in a small clinical sample of alcoholics. *American Journal of Drug and Alcohol Abuse, 14*(3), 325–334.

Kovacs, M., Rush, A. J., Beck, A. T., & Hollon, S. D. (1981). Depressed outpatients treated with cognitive therapy or pharmacotherapy: A one-year follow-up. *Archives of General Psychiatry, 38,* 33–39.

LaCroix, M., Clarke, M., Bock, C., & Doxey, N. (1986). Physiological changes after biofeedback and relaxation training for multiple-pain tension-headache patients. *Perceptual and Motor Skills, 63*(1), 139–153.

Lazarus, A. (1996). The utility and futility of combining treatments in psychotherapy. *Clinical Psychology: Science and Practice, 3,* 59–68.

Lambert, M. J., Shapiro, D. A., & Bergin, A. E. (1986). The effectiveness of psychotherapy. In S. L. Garfield & A. E. Bergin (Eds.), *Handbook of psychotherapy and behavior change* (3rd ed., pp. 157–211). New York: Wiley.

Liotti, G. (1991). Patterns of attachment and the assessment of interpersonal schemata: Understanding and changing difficult patient–therapist relationships in cognitive psychotherapy. *Journal of Cognitive Psychotherapy, 5,* 105–114.

Mahoney, M. J. (1991). *Human change processes.* New York: Basic Books.

Moore, R. G., & Blackburn, I. M. (1996). The stability of sociotropy and autonomy in depressed patients undergoing treatment. *Cognitive Therapy and Research, 20,* 69–80.

Morrow-Bradley, C., & Elliott, R. (1986). Utilization of psychotherapy research by practicing psychotherapists. *American Psychologist, 41*(2), 188–197.

Murphy, G. E., Simons, A. D., Wetzel, R. D., & Lustman, P. J. (1984). Cognitive therapy and pharmacotherapy: Singly and together in the treatment of depression. *Archives of General Psychiatry, 41,* 33–41.

Norcross, J. C. (1987). *Casebook of eclectic psychotherapy.* New York: Brunner/Mazel.

Norcross, J. C., Martin, J. R., Omer, H., & Pinsof, W. M. (1996). When and how does psychotherapy integration improve clinical effectiveness?: A roundtable. *Journal of Psychotherapy Integration, 6,* 295–332.

Ogles, B. M., Sawyer, J. D., & Lambert, M. J. (1995). Clinical significance of the National Institute of Mental Health Treatment of Depression Collaborative Research Program data. *Journal of Consulting and Clinical Psychology, 63*(2), 321–326.

Orlinsky, D. E., Grawe, K., & Parks, B. K. (1994). *Process and outcome in psychotherapy: Noch einmal.* In A. E. Bergin & S. L. Garfield (Ed.), *Handbook of psychotherapy and behavior change* (4th ed., pp. 270–376). New York: Wiley.

Orlinsky, D. E., & Howard, K. I. (1986). Process and outcome in psychotherapy. In S. L. Garfield & A. E. Bergin (Eds.), *Handbook of psychotherapy and behavior change* (3rd ed., pp. 311–384). New York: Wiley.

Robins, C. J., & Hayes, A. M. (1993). An appraisal of cognitive therapy. *Journal of Consulting and Clinical Psychology, 61,* 1–10.

Robinson, L. A., Berman, J. S., & Neimeyer, R. A. (1990). Psychotherapy for the treatment of depression: A comprehensive review of controlled outcome research. *Psychological Bulletin, 108,* 30–49.

Rush, A. J., Beck, A. T., Kovacs, M., & Hollon, S. D. (1977). Comparative efficacy of cognitive therapy and pharmacotherapy in the treatment of depressed outpatients. *Cognitive Therapy and Research, 1*(1), 17–37.

Rush, A. J., Beck, A. T., Kovacs, M., Weissenburger, J., & Hollon, S. T. (1982). Comparison of the effects of cognitive therapy and pharmacotherapy on hopelessness and self-concept. *American Journal of Psychiatry, 139,* 862–866.

Safran, J., Alden, L., & Davison, P. (1980). Client anxiety level as a moderator variable in assertion training. *Cognitive Therapy and Research, 4*(2), 189–200.

Safran, J., & Messer, S. (1997). Psychotherapy integration: A postmodern critique. *American Psychologist, 4,* 140–152.

Safran, J., & Segal, Z. V. (1990). *Interpersonal process in cognitive therapy.* New York: Basic Books.

Schlicter, K. J., & Horan, J. J. (1981). Effects of stress inoculation on the anger and aggression management skills of institutionalized juvenile delinquents. *Cognitive Therapy and Research, 5,* 359–365.

Scogin, F., Bowman, D., Jamison, C., Beutler, L. E., & Machado, P. P. (1994). Effects of initial severity of dysfunctional thinking on the outcome of cognitive therapy. *Clinical Psychology and Psychotherapy, 1*(3), 179–184.

Scogin, F., Hamblin, D., & Beutler, L. E. (1987). Bibliotherapy for depressed older adults: A self-help alternative. *Gerontologist, 27,* 383–387.

Seltzer, L. F. (1986). *Paradoxical strategies in psychotherapy: A comprehensive overview and guidebook.* New York: Wiley.

Shaffer, C. S., Shapiro, J., Sark, L. I., & Coghlan, D. J. (1981). Positive changes in depression, anxiety, and assertion following individual and group cognitive behavior therapy intervention. *Cognitive Therapy and Research, 5,* 149–157.

Shapiro, D. A., Barkham, M., Rees, A., & Hardy, G. E. (1994). Effects of treatment duration and severity of depression on the effectiveness of cognitive-behavioral and psychodynamic–interpersonal psychotherapy. *Journal of Consulting and Clinical Psychology, 62,* 522–534.

Sheppard, D., Smith, G. T., & Rosenbaum, G. (1988). Use of MMPI subtypes in predicting completion of a residential alcoholism treatment program. *Journal of Consulting and Clinical Psychology, 56,* 590–596.

Shoham-Salomon, V., Avner, R., & Neeman, R. (1989). You are changed if you do and changed if you don't: Mechanisms underlying paradoxical interventions. *Journal of Consulting and Clinical Psychology, 57,* 590–598.

Shoham-Soloman, V., & Hannah, M. T. (1991). Client–treatment interactions in the study of differential change process. *Journal of Consulting and Clinical Psychology, 59,* 217–225.

Shoham-Salomon, V., & Rosenthal, R. (1987). Paradoxical interventions: A meta-analysis. *Journal of Consulting and Clinical Psychology, 55,* 22–27.

Simons, A. D., & Thase, M. E. (1992). Biological markers, treatment outcome, and 1-year follow-up in endogenous depression: Electroencephalographic sleep studies and response to cognitive therapy. *Journal of Consulting and Clinical Psychology, 60,* 392–401.

Sloane, R. B., Staples, F. R., Cristol, A. H., Yorkston, N. J., & Whipple, K. (1975). *Psychotherapy versus behavior change.* Cambridge, MA: Harvard University Press.

Smith, M. L., Glass, G., & Miller, T. I. (1980). *The benefits of psychotherapy.* Baltimore: Johns Hopkins University Press.

Steuer, J. L., Mintz, J., Hammen, C. L., Hill, M. A., Jarvik, L. F., McCarley, T., Motoike, P., & Rosen, R. (1984). Cognitive-behavioral and psychodynamic group psychotherapy in the treatment of geriatric depression. *Journal of Consulting and Clinical Psychology, 52,* 180–189.

Stricker, G., & Gold, J. (1996). Psychotherapy integration: An assimilative, psychodynamic approach. *Clinical Psychology: Science and Practice, 3*(1), 47–58.

Tasca, G. A., Russell, V., & Busby, K. (1994). Characteristics of patients who choose between two types of group psychotherapy. *International Journal of Group Psychotherapy, 44*(4), 499–508.

Thorne, F. C. (1962). Self-consistency theory and psychotherapy. *Annals of the New York Academy of Sciences, 96,* 877–888.

Tref, D. M., & Yuan, H. A. (1983). The use of the MMPI in a chronic back pain rehabilitation program. *Journal of Clinical Psychology, 39*(1), 46–53.

Wachtel, P. L. (1978). On some complexities in the application of conflict theory to psychotherapy. *Journal of Nervous and Mental Disease, 166,* 457–471.

Wilson, G. T. (1989). Behavior therapy. In R. J. Corsini & D. Wedding (Eds.), *Current psychotherapies* (4th ed., pp. 241–282). Itasca, IL: Peacock.

Wilson, P. H., Goldin, J. C., & Charbouneau-Powis, M. (1983). Comparative efficacy of behavioural and cognitive treatments of depression. *Cognitive Therapy and Research, 7,* 111–124.

Woody, G. E., McClellan, A. T., Luborsky, L., & O'Brien, C. P. (1985). Sociopathy and psychotherapy outcome. *Archives of General Psychiatry, 42,* 1081–1086.

Young, J. E. (1990). *Cognitive therapy for personality disorders: A schema-focused approach.* Sarasota, FL: Professional Resource Exchange.

PART TWO

THE THERAPIES

6

Self-Management Therapies

PAUL D. ROKKE
LYNN P. REHM

Self-management approaches to psychological treatment encompass a variety of techniques, strategies, and models. The term "self-management" has developed a somewhat differentiated use from the similar terms in behavioral psychology of "self-regulation" and "self-control." "Self-regulation" tends to be used more often as a generic term referring to a variety of processes and techniques involving the voluntary control of psychological, behavioral, and physiological processes. It is used to describe biofeedback procedures, for example, as well as cognitive-behavioral procedures. The terms "self-control" and "self-management" have been used more consistently to refer to tactics and procedures of control over cognitive and behavioral processes. The term "self-control" has lost favor in the literature because of its connotations of willpower and containment of the expression of emotions. "Self-management," in contrast to "self-control," is a semantically less loaded term. It is also applied in different ways within cognitive-behavioral theory and practice. First, "self-management" refers to certain natural processes by which individuals direct and control their own behavior. The observable consequences of these processes may be assessed—for example, the ability to delay gratification or tolerate pain. Many therapy strategies and theories of self-management attempt to model these natural processes. Second, the term "self-management" refers to specific methods within cognitive-behavioral approaches to therapy. Often the term is used to refer to methods that are adjuncts to in-office therapy procedures. They are intended to extend the newly acquired behaviors to home and daily life. These generalization strategies depend upon a person's being able to administer a program that may involve practicing new behaviors or manipulating antecedents and consequences of behaviors. Third, "self-management" can refer to specific theoretical models of processes by which people direct and control their behavior. Models may be abstractions of natural processes or may involve translations of learning principles into operations performed by an individual to control his or her own behavior. These models offer procedures and processes by which individuals acquire generalized skills for behavioral adaptation and change. This chapter focuses on models of self-management and their application as therapy methods or techniques.

Although specific definitions of self-management may vary with the individual models, the models themselves share certain common assumptions and features. To begin with, there is an underlying assumption that individuals can behave essentially as if they were two persons—a controlled person, who is acting in an environment and responding to a variety of internal and external cues and consequences; and a controlling person, who is capable of manipulating internal and external cues and consequences for the purposes of achieving some long-range goals. It is assumed that such processes normally and naturally operate within every individual, and that thinking in terms of such processes is therefore useful for purposes of intervention and treatment. Intervention is seen as intervention on the controlling processes. Self-management therapies involve teaching new controlling processes derived from psychological concepts or behavior modification principles. Self-management therapy procedures can be typically characterized not as applying learning principles to individuals, but as teaching the principles to those individuals so that they can apply them to themselves. Therapy thus involves procedures for teaching controlling strategies to the individual.

Self-management models stress the notion of the person in the person × situation interaction. The therapeutic skills represent individual differences that are relatively consistent across time and place. They are generalized skills that the person may apply as the strategy to similar situations. Generalized application to actual life situations is the central focus of self-management therapy procedures. Such therapies attempt to sample situations from real life, bring them into the therapy office for practice, and then send the individual out to apply the strategies in real life.

Self-management therapy procedures focus on methods for the individual to achieve long-term goals. Models and techniques have typically focused on problems of self-control in which behavior directed toward delayed reinforcers is not supported by immediate reinforcers. Traditional self-control or self-management problems include persistence—that is, maintaining behavior toward a delayed positive reinforcement despite immediate punishments, as in the cases of jogging or sticking to a diet. Optimal long-term adjustment requires effort, persistence, and resistance to temptation.

In order to model the behavior required for achieving long-range goals, most self-management theories assume some sort of internal, unobservable processes. They assume that in one form or another, individuals make inferences or abstractions about external contingencies and consequences, and that response strategies are based on these internal representations. These models fall within the social learning or cognitive-behavioral models in clinical psychology. The nature of the assumptions made, however, varies among self-management theories. Some theoretical models of self-management avoid such internal constructs. For example, within a radical behavioral paradigm, Skinner (1953) suggested a number of strategies whereby individuals manipulate their environment in order to influence their own future behavior and obtain future rewards. This chapter focuses on three prominent models within the cognitive-behavioral literature: (1) Albert Bandura's (1977a, 1977b, 1997) self-efficacy model, (2) Donald Meichenbaum's self-instruction strategies (e.g., Meichenbaum & Cameron, 1973), and (3) Frederick Kanfer's self-control model (Kanfer, 1970; Kanfer & Karoly, 1972a, 1972b). Though other models might have been included in this chapter, including Carver and Scheier's (1982) information-processing model, Eric Klinger's (1982) model of cognitive plans and concerns, or Richard Lazarus's (1974) work on coping strategies under stress, the models we have chosen to write about are representative, and each has generated extensive research and a variety of clinical applications.

MODELS OF SELF-MANAGEMENT

Bandura's Model

Bandura (1969, 1977a, 1977b, 1997) has written extensively about social-cognitive factors that influence human learning and behavior change. A construct that has been given a primary role in his conceptual scheme is "self-efficacy." The following discussion focuses on defining self-efficacy, on the role self-efficacy may play in behavioral performance, and on the implications this concept may have for self-management approaches to therapy.

Bandura (1977a) distinguishes between "efficacy expectancies" and "outcome expectancies." An "outcome expectancy" can be defined as a person's judgment about whether the performance of a given behavior will produce a particular outcome. An "efficacy expectancy," on the other hand, refers to the individual's estimate about whether he or she can successfully execute that behavior.

Bandura (1980) suggests that perceived self-efficacy is a major determinant in whether or not a behavior is initiated, in the amount of effort expended, and in how long a person will persist in the face of adverse circumstances. For example, people participate frequently in activities in which they feel competent and avoid those in which they feel less competent. Of course, a person can feel very competent at performing a particular behavior and still not perform it because there is no incentive for doing so. It also follows that those people who are more confident in their abilities will persist longer in the face of obstacles and adverse conditions than those who are not confident. An individual is more willing and more likely to expend effort on a task he or she is sure of being able to do than on a task he or she is unsure of being able to do. Performance and persistence are dependent on the interaction of the strength of the person's evaluation of his or her abilities and the relative value of the anticipated outcome goal.

According to Bandura (1997), efficacy expectations are formed through information derived from four primary sources. Listed in order of their hypothesized power in influencing efficacy expectations, these sources are (1) actual performance accomplishments, (2) vicarious experience, (3) verbal persuasion, and (4) physiological and affective states. Note that these sources are also listed in order of the relative amounts of behavior- and situation-specific information available from them.

Direct experience with the behavior and situation of interest is the most important source of information on which self-efficacy expectations can be based. Repeated successes in a particular situation may raise efficacy expectations, while failures may serve to lower them. The manner in which success or failure experiences influence efficacy and future performance, however, depends on the attributions of causation that the individual makes for the quality of the performance and the outcome (Weiner et al., 1971). Whether an individual makes internal or external and stable or unstable attributions about the cause of the outcome may influence both the individual's sense of efficacy and his or her expectancies of favorable outcomes.

The observation of another person performing a behavior of interest can also influence an individual's efficacy expectations. This occurs primarily through a process of social comparison. The degree of influence that observation will have on efficacy expectancies depends in part on the perceived personal relevance of the information obtained. Efficacy expectancies will be tempered by a number of factors, including the model's characteristics, the similarity of these characteristics to those of the observer, and the nature of the behavior × situation interaction (i.e., whether the model exhibits mastery of the behavior or some initial failures followed by persistence and subsequent success).

Verbal persuasion is a valuable tool in changing a person's efficacy expectations, largely because of its relative convenience in terms of availability and ease of implementation. Initial expectations may be raised in varying degrees, depending on whether the content of the persuasive message is consistent with the individual's prior experience. The likelihood of acting on a persuasive message depends on how well the advice matches with one's previous understanding and beliefs about the causal relationships between the particular behaviors and outcomes involved. The effects of verbal persuasion, however, may be weak and temporary because they are not founded on experience. Furthermore, they may be quickly dismissed in the face of experiential disconfirmation.

The final source of information relevant to judgments of personal efficacy is the perception of physiological arousal and affective states. These states are frequently relied on at the moment in which situational demands are placed on a person. Physiological arousal may interfere with performance and also signal vulnerability, thus serving as a negative influence on judgments of efficacy. The presence of physiological states associated with perceptions of relaxation and calm may be associated with feelings of confidence and expected success. Affective states can influence efficacy judgments both directly by their informative value and indirectly through their effects on cognitive processes. In making a judgment, one's emotional reaction may play as important a role as any other information that may be available. Mood may also influence evaluative judgments because it serves to direct attention and may introduce biases in the recall of relevant information. Positive mood can serve to increase judgments of efficacy and negative mood can lower such judgments, whether one is concerned with achievement situations (Forgas, Bower, & Moylan, 1990) or health behavior (Salovey & Birnbaum, 1989).

In light of the discussion above, certain characteristics of self-efficacy can be noted. Self-efficacy is seen as central to adequate functioning and a sense of competency. Self-efficacy, however, is not a single-dimensional, overarching trait. Self-efficacy represents a system of beliefs, each of which is specific to a particular area of functioning. These beliefs can refer to behavioral as well as cognitive skills. Because they are founded on the basis of experience and are situation- and behavior-specific, they are also expected to vary across individuals, to vary within individuals across situations, and to change over time.

Several studies have been conducted by Bandura and his colleagues to validate the construct of self-efficacy. A strong association has been demonstrated between an individual's level of perceived self-efficacy and his or her subsequent level of performance accomplishments, regardless of the method used for enhancing self-efficacy (Bandura, 1982). The concept of self-efficacy has been applied to a variety of areas of human functioning, including gender development (Bussey & Bandura, 1992), managerial performance (Wood, Bandura, & Bailey, 1990), pain (Bandura, O'Leary, Taylor, Gauthier, & Gossard, 1987), academic attainment (Zimmerman, Bandura, & Martinez-Pons, 1992), anxiety (Bandura, 1988), and athletic or motor skills (Carroll & Bandura, 1985). It has also been suggested that self-efficacy theory explains the rate of change during the course of treatment (Bandura & Adams, 1977).

Bandura (1977a) argues that effective psychological treatments, of any form, are successful in part because they alter people's expectations of personal efficacy. Self-management approaches to therapy that focus specifically on instigating the development of skills that people can implement on their own may be especially well suited to enhancing self-efficacy. Although the causal role of perceived self-efficacy in effecting positive treatment outcomes has yet to be unequivocally demonstrated, the concept has many implications for clinical practice. Treatments that can maximally influence self-efficacy provide graduated success experiences in performance-based procedures, consider and utilize self-attributional processes and self-evaluative information, encourage individuals to develop their own abilities, and allow individuals personal choice and responsibility for the management of their behavior. Procedures that can maximally influence perceived self-efficacy will maximize treatment effectiveness.

Meichenbaum's Model

Self-instructional training was an outgrowth of ideas in the developmental literature (Meichenbaum, 1977). Luria (1961, cited in Meichenbaum, 1977), among others, suggested that self-control over the initiation and inhibition of voluntary motor behaviors in children develops through predictable stages. Control over a child's behavior, initially directed by parental speech, is gradually shifted to the child's own overt speech, and finally becomes internalized as the child's covert speech (thoughts, internal dialogue) assumes a self-directive role. Meichenbaum (1977) proposed a form of treatment that makes this process explicit.

Self-instructional training is a form of self-management that focuses on the importance of a person's self-instructions. An explicit assumption is that an individual's self-instructions mediate behavior and behavior change. In many cases maladaptive self-statements may contribute to a person's problems. The learning and application of more adaptive self-instructions are the goals of self-instructional training. Since cognitive strategies are not situation bound and can be "carried with" the individual, it may be expected that training in the systematic use of self-instructional techniques can enhance treatment effectiveness and generalization.

Self-instructions can play two primary roles in governing desired behaviors. In the acquisition of new skills, self-instructions can serve as useful cues for the recall of appropriate behavior sequences or for redirecting and correcting behavior errors. In the correction of maladaptive behavior, self-instructions can interrupt automatic behavioral or cognitive chains and can prompt the use of more adaptive responses. Self-instructional skills will probably not be effective in the absence of requisite behavioral skills, but may be very useful in the learning of new skills and in enhancing the performance of adaptive responses.

Meichenbaum (1977) has described three phases of self-instructional training that outline his general approach to therapy. The first phase consists primarily of information gathering, which allows an accurate conceptualization of the problem. This process involves a cooperative venture between the client and the therapist, each contributing experience and expertise in such a way that the therapist can clearly understand the nature of the presenting problem and the client can feel that he or she has had direct input into the therapeutic process and has been understood.

In addition to assessing the nature, extent, and duration of the presenting problem, the therapist will begin to assess the role of maladaptive cognitions. Cognitive processes occurring in problem situations may be quite automatic and initially difficult for the client to identify clearly. Formal assessment strategies may be useful to evaluate the role of maladaptive cognitions and to teach the client to pay attention to his or her covert language activity during problem situations. Common strategies for assessment include in-session imaginal techniques and extrasession self-monitoring assignments. A therapist can ask a client to imagine a problem situation and describe his or her probable internal dialogue to the therapist. Discussion of the quality of these statements, and of their relationship to affect and behavior, is a useful assessment and instructional procedure. Self-monitoring, whether done in more formal written records or simply by having the client begin to listen to him- or herself with a "third ear," can also be very useful. Homework assignments contribute to the gathering of information about the frequency, intensity, and duration of problems, as well as to the ability to make meaningful situational analyses and to understand the role cognitions play in maintaining the problem. Conducting initial sessions in this manner allows the client and therapist to develop a common conceptualization of the problem and sets the stage for the presentation of a treatment rationale that will be credible and acceptable to the client. This process should lead to the formulation of an initial treatment plan.

The second phase of self-instructional training has been described as a process of "trying on" the conceptualization of the problem. Discussion of the rationale and treatment plan, in the context of ongoing observation of the problem, allows the client the opportunity to test the logic of the rationale and to see whether it "fits." The rationale of self-instructional training focuses on helping the client develop skills that will allow him or her to change the problem behavior or cope in problem situations, and especially on learning more adaptive self-statements, which can be substituted for the negative self-statements that are currently contributing to the problem.

Whereas the first two stages of therapy are primarily concerned with preparing the client for change, the third stage is directed toward promoting change. This promotion occurs through active attempts to change the client's self-statements to modify behavior. Several authors have discussed a variety of techniques for modifying self-statements (e.g., Coleman & Beck, 1981; Ellis, 1962).

Meichenbaum and Goodman (1971) originally outlined their procedures for training impulsive children in self-instructional techniques. They used a five-step process. First, an adult model performed a task while talking to him- or herself out loud. The important self-statements were thus modeled for the child. The child then performed the same task under direction of the therapist's instructions (i.e., using the same or similar statements that the therapist had made to him- or herself). The child then performed the task while instructing him- or herself aloud. The overt nature of the self-instructions was gradually faded so that the child repeated the task while whispering the self-instructions, and finally while guiding his or her performance solely by private (covert) speech. Meichenbaum and Goodman (1971) found that self-instructional procedures, in comparison to placebo and assessment control conditions, resulted in significantly improved performance for impulsive children on the Porteus Maze, on the Performance IQ of the Wechsler Intelligence Scale for Children, and on a measure of cognitive impulsivity.

These procedures have been adapted for use with adults with a variety of problems—for example, stroke or dementia (Brown, Gouvier, & Blanchard-Fields, 1990), schizophrenia (Meichenbaum & Cameron, 1973), anger, anxiety, and pain (DiGiuseppe, McGowan, Simon, & Gardner, 1990; Heimberg & Barlow, 1988; Meichenbaum & Turk, 1976). Generally, the important features of self-instructional training include education about the particular problem and the modeling and rehearsal of relevant behavioral and cognitive skills. These skills may include problem-solving strategies, focusing attention, response guidance, self-evaluation, and self-reinforcement skills, all of which can serve to enhance coping and self-correcting skills. There should be opportunities for the client to develop self-instructional strategies that best fit personal needs and desires. The rehearsal of these strategies, under imaginal or *in vivo* conditions with input, modeling, and feedback from the therapist, should also be planned. Many cognitive-behavioral therapies can be expanded and perhaps enhanced by the inclusion of self-instructional strategies. Strategies such as relaxation training, systematic desensitization, and assertion training can all include a self-instructional component.

Kanfer's Model

Kanfer (1970; Kanfer & Karoly, 1972a, 1972b) has proposed a feedback-loop model of self-management and has elaborated on the components of this process. He views self-control as a series of processes in which an individual engages to alter the probability of a response in the relative absence of immediate external supports. Self-control processes are engaged when the person perceives that ongoing behavior is not producing the desired consequences. For example, a person may perceive a problem in eating behavior upon finding that last summer's clothes now fit too tightly, or a problem in smoking behavior upon discovering that a pack of cigarettes that was bought just a few hours earlier is empty. The same processes may be engaged if, during a conversation at a party, an individual perceives that the other person seems irritated or uninterested. In each of these instances, the person begins to employ a three-stage feedback loop involving self-monitoring, self-evaluation, and self-reinforcement processes.

In the self-monitoring stage of the loop, the person observes his or her own behavior. This may involve the observation of either the behavior itself or the behavior along with its antecedents and consequences, and the inter-relationships among these elements. Self-monitoring may also involve attending to internal events, such as thoughts and emotions. Self-monitoring implies a conscious attention to some specific category of behavior. It may be accomplished in many ways. It may be done in a very informal, unsystematic fashion; for instance, one may have a general impression that a particular meal is consistent with long-range weight goals or not. On the other hand, self-monitoring can be very systematic—for example, recording calorie counts for each item consumed. Monitoring behavior involves awareness of and attention to certain classes of events, an ability to make accurate discriminations among them, and an awareness of the importance of relationships among events. Self-monitoring skills may be acquired in a variety of ways, and this acquisition may be an important aspect of childhood social development. Individual differences in the use, skill, and effectiveness of self-monitoring exist among persons. One may speak of individuals' developing certain self-monitoring styles or of behavior problems' involving specific self-monitoring deficits. Certain styles of self-monitoring may be considered maladaptive.

The second stage in Kanfer's model is self-evaluation. "Self-evaluation" refers to a comparison between one's performance and a criterion or standard. The index of performance is derived from self-monitoring; the index may therefore be a relatively informal abstraction or a systematic measurement of the behavior. Criteria or standards may be derived from a variety of sources. Many generalized standards are internalized in the course of development and come in the form of internalized rules (e.g., "I should always do the best I can"). They may derive from experiences relative to other people (e.g., "I should be in the top 5% of anything I do academically") or from external sources of expertise (e.g., "For my sex and height, I should eat no more than 2,000 calories per day"). Criteria may vary on many dimensions. They may be relatively specific and differentiated or general and undifferentiated. They may or may not be realistic or appropriate. Inappropriate standard setting may be another potential form of maladaptive self-control.

On the basis of the comparison to a standard, the individual makes a judgment that the behavior did or did not meet the standard. This judgment is evaluative and involves a determination of whether a behavior was good or bad, a success or a failure. Such evaluative judgments may therefore involve an affective component, depending upon the importance of the behavior involved. Negative affect about oneself and low self-esteem may derive from repeated judgments that one has not met internalized standards in the self-evaluation process.

The third stage in the self-control loop is self-reinforcement. This model assumes that individuals control their own behavior through the administration of contingent rewards and punishments, just as one person might control the behavior of another. Self-reinforcement supplements external reinforcement in controlling behavior. Self-reinforcements may be covert or overt. People may reward themselves covertly with self-congratulation or an internal sense of accomplishment or pride (patting themselves on the back). People may overtly reward behavior by allowing themselves a pleasurable experience—for example, going to a movie contingent on a week of following a diet. Of course, individuals may self-administer both covert and overt rewards and may do so for the same behavior. Self-reinforcement is the mechanism whereby individuals strengthen and maintain behavior in the face of contradictory external reinforcement. Persistence and resistance to temptation are accomplished by self-administered reinforcement for attaining the behavior and self-punishment for lapses or giving in to temptations. Self-reinforcement functions to maintain consistency in behavior and to bridge situations in which desirable external reinforcers are delayed and immediate reinforcers for less desirable alternative behavior are readily available. Self-reward and self-punishment habits and skills may vary from one individual to another. Some individuals may use reward more consistently or more effectively than others. Self-reward skills may vary independently of self-punishment skills.

In general, the self-control feedback loop consists of the behavior by which people exert control over and modify their own behavior. Self-monitoring, self-evaluation, and self-reinforcement processes can be involved in developing a jogging program, in losing weight, or in quitting smoking. These processes may also be involved when changing the topic of a conversation to maintain a positive relationship with another person at a party. The model assumes that these are processes that people engage in naturally, but also implies that the processes can be made explicit and externalized for therapeutic purposes. Individuals can be taught specific new self-monitoring, self-evaluation, and self-reinforcement skills and procedures.

Two other concepts deserve comment for a full explication of Kanfer's model: commitment and attributions. Kanfer and his colleagues have emphasized the importance of commitment to engaging in self-correcting behavior. After perceiving the desirability of change, a client must make a commitment to continue engaging in the self-control process to accomplish such a change. Commitment is an important issue, since in many instances self-modification programs involve considerable effort, and both positive and negative consequences accrue from making the change. Commitment may be made easier by discomfort, by fear of social disapproval over inaction, by the presence of others making similar commitments, or by the encouragement and support of relevant others. Commitment may be more difficult if the goal is difficult and distant, or if the behavior is not publicly observable and not supported by others in the environment (see Kanfer, 1977). Attention to issues involved in making commitments is very important for therapy procedures using self-management concepts.

The second important concept to add to the self-control model is that of attribution of causality. The various stages of the self-control process imply that the person believes that the behavior involved is under personal control. If the behavior or consequence is partly or entirely under the control of another person, or perceived as being under the control of another, then efforts at self-control can be futile. Rehm (1977) has suggested that attributional processes are particularly important in the self-evaluation stage of the model. Attributions of causality must be internal before a behavior can be judged as good or bad, or as a success or a failure. A person may perceive him- or herself as being accurate and successful at a child's task, but may not evaluate this performance as commendable in any way because doing well is attributed to the easy nature of the task. Similarly, a person may perceive him- or herself as failing at a task outside the person's own area of expertise and thus may not condemn him- or herself for it. Attribution theory, developed by Weiner and his colleagues (e.g., Weiner et al., 1971), is generally applicable to these considerations. They suggest that attributions of causality in real life can generally be classified according to two primary dimensions: (1) internal versus external, and (2) stable versus unstable over time. Kanfer and Hagerman (1981) have developed an elaborated form of the self-control model in which attributional processes are involved at each of the three major stages. This model has not been as applied as extensively as the former model.

APPLICATIONS

Treatment of Anxiety

Several authors have suggested that perceived inefficacy may be related to fearful behavior, cognitions, and affect. Sarason (1975), for example, equated anxiety with a type of self-preoccupation that can be characterized by a heightened concern over one's inadequacies. Thus, if one were presented with a situation that demanded a decision or some type of active response, doubts about one's ability to cope with the situation would be associated with increased anxiety and would interfere with one's ability to attend to and carry out the task at hand. Beck, Emery, and Greenberg (1985), following the work of Lazarus (1966), identify the importance of secondary appraisal processes in the experience of anxiety. If a person perceives threat, it is the judgment of available resources and of the person's ability to use them that determines the emotional and behavioral responses. Others also postulate that self-doubt and the misattribution of cause away from the self are central mechanisms in problems of anxiety and stress (e.g., Abramson, Seligman, & Teasdale, 1978; Alloy, Kelly, Mineka, & Clements, 1990; Lazarus, 1981).

Bandura (1997) focuses on the importance of an individual's perceived inability to cope with a potentially aversive situation as a primary mechanism in the development of anxiety and fear. To the extent that a particular therapy instills a sense of controllability or predictability—that is, to the extent that the individual comes to believe that he or she is able to prevent, change, avoid, or generally cope with the aversive situation—anxiety and fear will be reduced. From this point of view, low self-efficacy expectations are identified as the primary problems, and improvements in self-efficacy during therapy are seen as the critical mechanisms of change. It is hypothesized that treatments that are effective in enhancing perceptions of self-efficacy should therefore be more effective in changing behavior.

Research conducted by Bandura and his colleagues has not focused on developing a treatment approach consistent with self-efficacy theory. Rather, they have utilized a variety of current behavioral and cognitive treatments in efforts to validate the concept of self-efficacy and to demonstrate its causal role in therapeutic change. Many of these treatments have utilized skills approaches that include *in vivo* and covert modeling, shaping, rehearsal, and feedback. A strong association has in fact been demonstrated between an individual's level of perceived self-efficacy and his or her subsequent level of performance accomplishments, regardless of the method used for enhancing self-efficacy (Bandura, 1982). Performance-based treatment strategies have been hypothesized to serve as the major source of efficacy information. These strategies have been demonstrated to increase levels of perceived self-efficacy (Bandura, 1982), to be effective in the treatment of agoraphobia (Bandura, Adams, Hardy, & Howells, 1980), and to be more effective than vicarious modes of therapy for snake phobia (Bandura, Adams, & Beyer, 1977).

Stress inoculation training is a variant of self-instructional training that consists of a multicomponent coping skills package with particular applicability to anxiety. Initial tests of this approach were successful with anxious and phobic subjects (Meichenbaum, 1972; Meichenbaum & Turk, 1976). Meichenbaum (1977) has described this approach as a behavioral analogue to the immunization model in medicine. When a person is inoculated, he or she is given an opportunity to deal with a low dose of the stress-related stimulus in a controlled environment. The experience of learning to cope with small and manageable units of the problematic stimuli will help the person develop skills to cope with larger concerns in other settings. There are three operational phases in stress inoculation training: education, rehearsal, and application. Each of these phases is discussed in turn.

The first phase of stress inoculation training is educational in nature. The presentation of one or two current theoretical approaches to stress reactions can serve to provide the client with a conceptual framework for understanding his or her own responses. It is important that the theories used are credible, are easily adapted to the client's own experiences, and lead logically to the implementation of the particular coping strategies that will be recommended. Although the scientific merit of any theory used is ultimately important, it is important to recognize the practicality of being able to present the theory in a manner that is understandable and believable to the client.

Meichenbaum and Turk (1976) have suggested the use of Schachter's (1966) theory of emotion with anxious or phobic clients. Following Schachter's theory, they explain to a client that fear reactions appear to involve two major components—heightened physiological arousal and cognitive events (images and self-statements)—which may in fact create more anxiety. From this perspective, then, treatment can be focused on reducing physiological arousal and substituting more positive self-statements for the habitual anxiety-producing self-statements. Various forms of relaxation training and cognitive coping techniques can be employed to enable the client to address these two components of anxiety-related responses.

The second component of stress inoculation training is the rehearsal phase. During this period of treatment, various coping techniques are presented and discussed with the client. These may include active behavioral responses as well as cognitive coping strategies. Clients may learn as much as they can about the phobic object or an upcoming stressful event, in order to be able to realistically assess the risks involved and to provide for more realistic expectations. They can explore escape and response alternatives to expected decision points in the stressful experience. They can also develop relaxation skills. Cognitive strategies may include changing negative self-statements to more positive and adaptive ones, and using imaginal strategies to influence attentional and affective aspects of the setting (e.g., imagining a pleasant scene, or imagining successfully completing a sequence of coping behaviors). Having a "menu" of options for clients to choose from will allow them to try out and pick those strategies that they are most comfortable with and that they feel they can use most effectively. The availability of a range of options from which to choose may also enhance the clients' sense of control in the situation and contribute to the credibility of the treatment. Three or four different coping strategies can be generated and developed for use by a particular client. The client can rehearse these strategies in imagination and in role-playing situations with the therapist, always with the goal of refining them and becoming more proficient in their use.

The third phase of stress inoculation training consists of the application of the coping strategies in a series of graduated stressful situations. It is generally recommended that a client begin with situations that are mildly stressful, with the application of the strategies to the final target being held off until the client has successfully used the strategies in other situations and is well prepared to handle the final stressor. The therapist can expose the client to a variety of stressors in the office, including imaginal and *in vivo* stressors, in order to give the client practice in a controlled yet still stressful situation. It is suggested that clients begin to test out their skills in other mildly stressful situations as they go through their daily routines.

Throughout treatment a self-instructional approach is used, so that clients learn to observe their responses and to use appropriate self-statements to guide them through the coping strategies. This process includes preparing for a stressor by reminding oneself of the strategy to be used and the behaviors involved in carrying out the strategy; confronting the stressful situation and encouraging oneself to meet the challenge; engaging in the coping strategies themselves; and finally rewarding oneself for a successful performance, either by covertly commenting on the good performance or by providing for some other positive consequence. The particular self-statements that a client uses can be tailored to his or her particular needs and situation. A number of statements should be generated as examples, however, to encourage variety and to enable the client to recognize differences among situations. Variety can also be used to demonstrate the problem-solving, coping, and self-regulatory nature of covert dialogues.

Several studies have included self-instructional training as an independent treatment or in conjunction with exposure for social phobia and agoraphobia (Hoffart, 1993). The early studies tended to focus primarily on changing the self-talk associated with anxiety states. In these studies, self-instructional training by itself was shown to reduce symptomatology, but evidenced poorer outcomes than exposure alone and rarely added additional benefits to exposure (Emmelkamp, Brilman, Kuiper, & Mersch, 1986; Emmelkamp & Mersch, 1982; Emmelkamp, Mersch, Vissia, & Van der Helm, 1985). More recently the broader stress inoculation package has been applied to a variety of problems (Meichenbaum & Deffenbacher, 1988), including posttraumatic stress disorder (PTSD) (Meichenbaum, 1994). Though few studies have examined the full package with anxiety disorders among adults, there is considerable support for its use with children and adolescents (Maag & Kotlash, 1994; Ollendick & King, 1998).

Treatment of Pain

Current conceptualizations of acute and chronic pain recognize that pain is a complex phenomenon that is influenced as much by psychological and social variables as it is by sensory and physiological variables (Karoly & Jensen, 1987; Litt, 1996; Turk, Meichenbaum, & Genest, 1983). In particular, self-efficacy and perceived control seem to be important contributors to coping with pain. In both laboratory (Baker & Kirsch, 1991; Bandura, Cioffi, Taylor, & Brouillard, 1988; Litt, 1988) and clinical (Council, Ahern, Follick, & Kline, 1988; Jensen, Turner, & Romano, 1991; Litt, Nye, & Shafer, 1995; Manning & Wright, 1983) studies, self-efficacy has been found to be a significant predictor of coping effort and pain. In addition, early studies showed that predictability and control can serve to reduce stress and pain (Averill, 1973; Bowers, 1968; Miller, 1979; Staub, Tursky, & Schwartz, 1971). Subsequent studies have demonstrated that these factors interact. Bandura et al. (1988) and his colleagues showed that high levels of self-efficacy to manage a taxing cognitive task were associated with lower stress and no activation of endogenous opioids during exposure to pain. In contrast, perceived inefficacy led to increased stress and opioid activation. Cognitive coping interventions can serve to increase self-efficacy (Bandura, 1997), as can experiential manipulations (Gattuso, Litt, & Fitzgerald, 1992; Litt, 1988). When an individual is faced with a stressful medical or dental procedure in which the aversive stimulus is not necessarily controllable, some degree of perceived control may be introduced by offering the individual a choice of coping strategies (Rokke & al'Absi, 1992; Rokke & Lall, 1992), though choice may only be beneficial to the extent that the individual perceives him- or herself to be efficacious in coping (Litt, 1988; Rokke, Al Absi, Lall, & Oswald, 1991).

Self-instructional strategies and the stress inoculation program have also been applied to pain-related problems (e.g., Genest & Turk, 1979; Horan, Hackett, Buchanan, Stone, & Demchik-Stone, 1977; Klepac, Hauge, Dowling, & McDonald, 1981). As a further example of this form of self-management therapy, each of the three phases of stress inoculation is presented here as it is applied to coping with pain. Though the predictability of events associated with stressful medical and dental procedures makes the stress inoculation package and its emphasis on preparatory practice especially useful for situations involving acute pain, it can also be applied to problems associated with chronic pain.

One conceptualization of pain that appears to fit well in the educational phase of stress inoculation is Melzack and Wall's (1965) gate control theory of pain. The gate control theory postulates that pain is a complex phenomenon consisting not only of the physiological and sensory–discriminative aspects that are often so readily apparent, but also of motivational–affective and cognitive–evaluative components. Although Melzack and Wall (1965) presented a physiological basis for this theory, it is more important for the client simply to understand that there is a scientific basis for these hypothesized components of pain than it is for him or her to know the physiological details. It should be emphasized that sensory, affective, and motivational components are recognized as important aspects of the pain experience.

Commonly observed experiences can serve as useful analogies to this model and may help the client to accept the notion that influencing psychological parameters can affect his or her experience of pain. The physiological component can be illustrated easily by the expected reaction to accidentally putting one's hand on a hot stove top. There is an immediate reflexive motor reaction that removes the hand from the stove, which is followed by sensations described as pain. Often in these situations, not only does one have the intense noxious physical stimulus that is perceived as pain-inducing, but there are also some automatic, self-protective, physiological responses, including increased muscle tension. This response can be related to chronic or acute pain situations, in which habitual muscle tension may serve to exacerbate the perception of anxiety and pain.

Situations analogous to the motivational and affective components may include the following: a football player or other athlete who is injured during competition but, because he is in a particular motivational state, continues in the competition without experiencing undue pain; a person with a pounding headache who goes to answer the telephone and doesn't realize that he or she has a headache again until several minutes later, when he or she hangs up and his or her attention is no longer distracted by the conversation; personal experiences demonstrating that on days when one is "down," tired, or irritable, the pain of a stubbed toe or bumped knee is worse than when one is feeling good and ambitious.

Finally, the cognitive–evaluative component of this pain theory can be illustrated to the client by pointing out that it is a natural tendency for people to evaluate their behaviors and their experiences. Usually the kind of evaluation one makes (i.e., good or bad) is based on one's prior experiences in similar situations. Thus one's experience of pain may be influenced by one's evaluation of the pain. For example, an evaluation like "This headache is terrible; it's the worst one I've ever had," not only may indicate the severity of the pain, but may heighten the concern of the individual and thus exacerbate the headache. In contrast, if a person were able to say, "Well, this headache isn't too bad; I can remember much worse," he or she may be able to continue with the tasks at hand and positively influence the experience of pain by reducing the adverse effects of negative evaluations. This conceptualization leads very nicely to the introduction of cognitive-behavioral techniques that can serve to influence attentional, motivational, emotional, and physical aspects of pain.

Skills taught during the second phase of treatment are very similar to those used with anxiety. Various coping techniques are presented, and the client may choose and practice those that he or she and the therapist agree may be most useful. The client may learn as much as he or she can about the stressor (e.g., upcoming surgery), in order to develop realistic expectations and a plan for dealing with predictable stressors. Relaxation skills and cognitive coping skills may also be developed. A variety of cognitive coping strategies can be used as diversions and as ways to address affective and evaluative components of the pain. These may include imagining a pleasant scene, imagining that one is a secret agent resisting torture, describing the painful stimulus in terms other than "painful" (e.g., while having a tooth drilled, a person may describe the sensations as "warm," "cool," "vibrating," or "massaging"), counting backward by multiples of seven, examining artwork in the room, and listening to music. Any cognitive activity that the client would like to do, and that can hold his or her attention and positively influence his or her mood under adverse conditions, may be tried as a potentially useful strategy for coping with pain. Three to four particular strategies should be clearly defined and developed in enough detail that they can be efficiently rehearsed and implemented.

The final phase of stress inoculation involves applying the developed strategies to painful situations. Some investigators have utilized laboratory methods of inducing pain (e.g., cold pressor, arm shock, and electrical stimulation of tooth pulp), in order to help clients practice their skills under controlled conditions and thus help improve their pain tolerance (Horan et al., 1977; Klepac et al., 1981). It should be noted that both Horan et al. and Klepac et al. tested for generalization of treatment effects and found that improvements made on one training stimulus were not evidenced on a second stimulus that was not targeted during treatment. Efforts should be made during treatment to enhance the generalization and maintenance of effects to the desired target objectives.

Treatment of Depression

Neither the Bandura self-efficacy model nor the Meichenbaum self-instructional model has been applied extensively to the treatment of depression. The Bandura model is theoretically quite applicable to depressive phenomena, however. Depression may be characterized by a generalized low sense of self-efficacy. The model is related to Seligman's learned helplessness model of depression (Abramson et al., 1978; Seligman, 1975, 1981). In the revised helplessness model, a factor contributing to vulnerability to depression is a negative attributional style. On the basis of attribution theory (Weiner et al., 1971), it is hypothesized that persons prone to depression attribute the causes of negative events to internal, stable, and global factors and attribute the causes of positive events to external, unstable, and specific causes. This tendency produces helpless attributions, in that such persons feel constantly responsible for negative events and incapable of producing positive events. Bandura (1977a) has agreed that causal attributional processes may be important in developing efficacy expectations. The Seligman model suggests that a depressive attributional style should interact with an aversive major life event to produce a generalized helpless belief and thus depression. Seligman (1981) differentiates between "personal" helplessness (i.e., a belief that one is individually incapable of producing certain responses) and "universal" helplessness (i.e., the belief that desirable consequences are not under anyone's personal control). This distinction corresponds to Bandura's differentiation between conceptions of efficacy and outcome expectations. Efficacy is personal, whereas outcome expectations refer to contingencies in the external world.

Seligman (1981) suggests that four general therapy strategies should be useful in modifying helplessness: (1) environmental enrichment, which involves placing the person in an environment that is relatively undemanding and that provides a variety of success and efficacy experiences; (2) personal control training, in which the individual is taught specific skills to give him or her greater control in certain pertinent domains; (3) resignation training, in which the individual is helped to accept his or her helplessness in certain domains in ways that should either reduce the aversiveness of the helplessness or reduce the desirability of the unattainable goal; and (4) attribution retraining, in which the individual is taught to attribute failures and successes in a more positive and realistic fashion.

Meichenbaum's self-instructional approach is also related to certain ideas about the nature of depression. Various experts have identified negative thoughts or negative self-statements typical of depression (e.g., Beck, 1976; Ellis, 1962). There is empirical evidence that depressed individuals are more likely to make covert negative self-statements (e.g., Missel & Sommer, 1983; Vestre, 1984). Vasta and Brockner (1979) had subjects actually monitor their positive and negative self-evaluative thoughts, and found that the frequency of negative self-statements correlated with self-esteem. Craighead and Craighead (1980) have argued that negative self-statements may be typical of a number of psychological disorders and that modifying such self-statements is an important target of psychotherapy. They further argue that methods from attitude research that produce persuasive modification of self-statements should be applicable to psychotherapy. Meichenbaum's methodologies can be considered effective teaching methods relative to modifying self-statements. Self-statement change has been the target of some cognitive-behavioral therapy interventions for depression. Mahoney (1971) had a depressed patient practice positive self-evaluative thoughts by pairing them with frequent daily events. Zeiss, Lewinsohn, and Munoz (1979) and Rehm, Kaslow, and Rabin (1987) have described therapy programs specifically targeting changes in self-statements. Applications of Meichenbaum's specific techniques to depression would be consistent with these efforts and could be a fruitful line of future research.

Extensive work on the treatment of depression has been derived from the Kanfer self-control model. Several authors have suggested the applicability of self-control concepts to depression (Bandura, 1971; Marston, 1968; Mathews, 1977), and self-control procedures have been applied in various case studies (e.g., Jackson, 1972). The most extensive work has been derived from the self-control or self-management model of depression proposed by Rehm (1977). This model suggests that depression can be thought of as a set of one or more deficits in self-management behavior. Six deficits are postulated: (1) Depressed individuals attend selectively to negative events in their environment to the exclusion of positive events; (2) depressed persons attend selectively to the immediate as opposed to the long-range outcomes of their behavior; (3) depressed individuals tend to set stringent self-evaluative standards for their behavior; (4) depressed individuals make negative attributions for their behavior, such that they attribute positive outcomes to external factors and negative outcomes to internal factors; (5) as a result of one or more of the preceding deficits, depressed individuals administer insufficient positive reinforcement to themselves; and (6) depressed individuals administer excessive self-punishment to themselves. The first two deficits involve self-monitoring behavior; the second two involve self-evaluation behavior (it is assumed that self-attribution acts as a modifier on self-evaluation); and the final two involve self-reinforcement behavior. Fuchs and Rehm (1977) developed a psychotherapy program based on this model to modify these deficits. The program has been expanded and revised in a series of therapy outcome studies (see Rehm, 1984). The program is a highly structured group therapy, the format of which is defined in a detailed therapist's manual. The program involves didactic presentations of self-management concepts, exercises that help participants to acquire and use the concepts, discussion of the applicability of the concepts to individual participants, and homework assignments enabling participants to practice nondepressive self-management skills between sessions.

The therapy program begins by presenting the general argument that mood is related to activity and to self-statements about activities. It is suggested that depressed individuals tend to focus in a distorted fashion on negative activities and to make resulting negative self-statements. A homework assignment is given in which participants are required to keep a daily log, self-monitoring positive activities and self-statements. Daily mood is also recorded, and an exercise in the second session plots daily mood and a daily number of events to point out the association between the two. An immediate- versus delayed-outcome exercise helps participants attend to positive delayed outcomes of behavior, and self-monitoring homework assignments continue the focus on activities with naturally occurring positive delayed outcomes.

In the self-evaluation phase of the therapy program, goal-setting worksheets are filled out by participants, helping them to define goals in positive, realistic, attainable ways and to break these goals down into subgoal activities. The self-monitoring assignment continues with special emphasis on monitoring subgoal behaviors. Attributional concepts are taught in sessions focusing on positive and negative events. Participants practice writing nondepressed attributions as positive self-statements for positive and negative events during the week.

In the self-reinforcement phase of the program, participants are taught principles of self-reinforcement and develop both overt and covert self-reinforcement strategies. Overt self-reinforcement involves the use of easy and accessible positive activities, to be engaged in contingently following more difficult subgoal activities. Covert reinforcement involves using positive self-statements as contingent rewards following difficult positive activities or subgoal activities. As the program is currently used, basic concepts are taught in the first 7 weekly sessions of a 10-session program. The final 3 sessions are used for continued practice and consolidation of the use of the principles involved.

The therapy program has been evaluated in six outcome studies by Rehm and his colleagues. The first two studies involved validation of the program in contrast to traditional control conditions. Using symptomatic depressed women who were volunteers from the local community, Fuchs and Rehm (1977) compared self-management therapy to a nonspecific group therapy condition and a waiting-list control condition. On standard self-report measures of depression, participants in the self-management therapy condition improved significantly more than those in nonspecific group therapy condition, who in turn improved significantly more than participants in the waiting-list control condition. Rehm, Fuchs, Roth, Kornblith, and Romano (1979) compared the self-management program to a social skills assertiveness training program. Self-management participants showed greater improvement on target measures of self-management behavior, and social skills participants showed greater improvement on target measures of assertiveness. Both groups improved significantly in depression, but the self-management condition was significantly superior. The 1-year follow-up of participants in these two studies (Romano & Rehm, 1979) found that participants in both self-management and control (nonspecific and assertion) therapy conditions remained improved relative to pretest. However, the self-management participants reported fewer and less intense episodes of depression during the year, as well as fewer instances of having obtained additional therapy. This finding, which has been replicated in 1-year follow-up studies of the subsequent four studies in this series, suggests that individuals who have been through the self-management program have acquired skills that allow them to deal more effectively with episodes of depression and to do so without additional therapy intervention.

The second two studies in the series attempted to dismantle the major components of the self-management program. Rehm et al. (1981) compared five therapy conditions: (1) the self-monitoring therapy component alone, (2) self-monitoring plus self-evaluation components, (3) self-monitoring plus self-reinforcement components, (4) self-monitoring plus self-evaluation plus self-reinforcement components (i.e., the full self-management program), and (5) a waiting list control condition. Participants in all of the active treatments did better than those in the waiting-list control condition, but no consistent significant differences were found on a variety of depression outcome measures. Kornblith, Rehm, O'Hara, and Lamparski (1983) compared the following conditions: (1) the full self-management program, (2) self-monitoring and self-evaluation components, (3) the self-management principles without the behavioral homework assignments, and (4) a control treatment consisting of a problem-oriented dynamic group psychotherapy. No significant differences resulted among the therapy conditions, all of which reduced depression to a clinically significant degree. Interpretation of these results is problematic. It may be that the major effects of the full self-control program are incorporated within the self-monitoring phase of the program, and that the later components simply elaborate on those effects. Session-by-session tracking of the improvement in depression suggested that the vast majority of improvement in the program occurs in the first few weeks, so that it may be very difficult to detect the effects due to later program components. The explicitness of the program led many of the subjects in the condition where no explicit homework assignments were given to develop their own homework assignments. Finally, it is also possible that the complete program, as implemented at the time, was simply too complicated. Each time a homework assignment was made, it was added to all of the previous assignments. This structure made the program more difficult to do and may have canceled out the positive effects of the content in the later sessions of the program. As a consequence, the program was revised so that the monitoring log continued throughout the program, but the focal homework assignments were changed for each of the following sections.

The final two studies in the series concerned the specific behavioral and cognitive targets of the self-control program. Separate self-management programs were devised targeting activity increase (behavioral target) versus self-statements (cognitive target), along with a combined-target condition. Rehm (1984) discussed a study in which these versions of the self-management program were compared to a waiting-list control; it was found that participants in all three active therapy conditions improved to a greater extent than those in the waiting-list control, with no differences among the three active therapies. This result validated the idea that each therapy was indeed an active and effective therapy strategy in and of itself. Rehm et al. (1987) compared the same three conditions against one another, with larger numbers of participants in each condition. Various pre- and posttherapy measures were designed to assess specific behavioral and cognitive deficits. Again, all three programs were effective in alleviating depression, with no significant differences among them. Interestingly, each program was effective regardless of the degree of cognitive or behavioral deficits at pretest, and each program was equally effective in producing changes in cognitive and behavioral targets.

The self-management program has also been evaluated in other contexts using the self-management therapy manuals. Fleming and Thornton (1980) compared a cognitive therapy based on that of Shaw (1977) with the self-management program based on the Fuchs and Rehm (1977) manual, and with a nondirective therapy control condition. Participants in all conditions improved significantly at posttest and follow-up, with the greatest improvement on several measures shown by those in the self-management therapy condition. Roth, Bielski, Jones, Parker, and Osborn (1982) compared the self-management therapy to self-management therapy plus a tricyclic antidepressant drug. Although participants in the drug condition responded faster during therapy, at posttest and 3-month follow-up there were no significant differences between the two conditions. Two small studies using the Fuchs and Rehm (1977) manual were reported by Rothblum, Green, and Collins (1979). Both studies compared two versions of the self-management therapy program, one emphasizing client responsibility for selecting behaviors for monitoring and goal setting, and the other stressing the therapist's role in goal setting. Results tended to favor the active role of the therapist, which is more consistent with the original therapy. Tressler and Tucker (1980) compared a version of the self-management program consisting of self-monitoring and self-evaluation with a version consisting of self-monitoring and self-reinforcement. At posttest and 12-week follow-up, the self-monitoring and self-reinforcement condition proved significantly superior.

Other investigators have reported preliminary results with varied populations. Glanz and Dietz (1980) offered the program as part of a community outreach program from a community mental health center. A diverse group of currently depressed persons, previously depressed persons, and spouses or other relatives of depressed persons participated and showed gains on depression inventory scores. Kornblith and Greenwald (1982) gave a preliminary report on applying the self-management program with inpatients. Sulz and Lauter (1983) used a modified self-control program in a clinical trial with inpatients. The program has also been applied to depressed patients in a day treatment center (van den Hout, Arntz, & Kunkels, 1995). A current project involves the application of self-management therapy in a trauma recovery program for veterans with PTSD and major depression (Dunn et al., 1995). Rogers, Kerns, Rehm, Hendler, and Harkness (1982) reported that the program was effective in reducing depression among renal dialysis patients.

Self-management therapy has not been limited to a single age group. Reynolds and Coats (1986), Stark, Reynolds, and Kaslow (1987), and Rehm and Sharp (1996) have all applied self-management therapy to children and adolescents. Rokke and his colleagues have successfully applied the self-management program to older adults. They found that self-management therapy could be helpful to older adults when offered in a group therapy format (Rokke, Tomhave, & Jocic, 2000), and that when offered individually, self-management therapy was effective for targeting either behavioral or cognitive change (Rokke, Tomhave, & Jocic, 1999). The program appears to be an effective treatment for depression with broad therapeutic effects. It is applicable to a variety of depressed patients.

It should also be noted that various self-management strategies and techniques are also incorporated in other major cognitive and behavioral programs for depression. For example, Lewinsohn's activity increase program (Lewinsohn, Antonuccio, Steinmetz, & Teri, 1984) involves extensive self-monitoring of pleasant events, although the self-monitoring is used primarily as an assessment device. Self-reinforcement methods are sometimes used to motivate involvement in pleasant activities. Self-monitoring is also used in Beck's cognitive therapy (Beck, Rush, Shaw, & Emery, 1979). In Beck's program, self-monitoring data are used to challenge irrational and distorted interpretations of events. Future research will be needed to identify the relative contribution of more specific components of the therapy program and to match self-management therapy or its components to specific subtypes of depressed individuals.

ASSESSMENT TECHNIQUES

Self-Monitoring

The assessment methodology most clearly associated with self-management approaches to treatment is self-monitoring. "Self-monitoring" refers to a systematic recording of observations by the client of his or her own behavior. A full discussion of the forms and characteristics of self-monitoring is beyond the scope of this chapter, which focuses on practical applications to anxiety, depression, and pain research. In the typical use of self-monitoring, clients keep logs of events that occur in their lives between therapy sessions. Most often, the occurrence of each event in a class is recorded, but time-sampling formats may also be employed.

Self-monitoring has the advantage of providing real-life data on a client's functioning with regard to a problem behavior on a day-to-day basis. Since the client collects the data, subjective events can also be "observed." For example, the client may record incidences of emotional responses or of thoughts associated with experiences. Frequently the purpose of the self-monitoring is to observe the connection between external events and internal subjective responses.

Self-monitoring requires daily effort on the part of the client, and thus compliance may be a problem. In practice, assignments must be kept simple, concise, and clearly relevant to the problem. The reactivity of self-monitoring is another important consideration. Having people record their own behavior influences the occurrence of the behavior. Ordinarily, undesirable behaviors are decreased by self-monitoring and desirable behaviors are increased. Reactivity is a problem for representative sampling when self-monitoring is used for assessment, but it may be usefully employed when self-monitoring is part of an intervention. Self-monitoring may be used for the purposes of problem assessment, evaluation of progress or outcome, keeping track of completion of homework assignments, or intervention per se.

A typical use of self-monitoring in self-management therapy for anxiety is to record situations in which anxiety arises. This monitoring may be part of problem assessment as a way of discovering common characteristics of anxiety situations, or it may be an evaluation of progress with the expectation of decreased frequency across weeks of therapy. Many aspects of the anxiety response may be monitored. Ratings of intensity of subjective anxiety or of physiological concomitants may be additional ways to assess progress. Monitoring correlated thoughts, self-evaluation, or efficacy ratings may provide useful feedback for therapy planning.

In his depression therapy program, Lewinsohn (Lewinsohn et al., 1984) has participants monitor daily mood and daily pleasant events to identify mood-related events as targets for intervention. He and his colleagues have developed lists of events, pleasant events, unpleasant events, and interpersonal events, for use in selecting items for self-monitoring for different purposes. The Rehm self-management therapy program uses a Positive Activities List to prompt participants with classes of activities that may have occurred, but that may have been overlooked. Activities are recorded at or close to the time they occur, and a summary mood rating is recorded at the end of the day. In recent versions of the program, positive self-evaluations (self-statements) are also recorded throughout the day. Data are used as a means of teaching principles about behavior and emotion, and as progress feedback. The self-monitoring assignment is viewed both as assessment and as a form of intervention on natural styles of self-observation.

Beck (Beck et al., 1979; DeRubeis, Tang, & Beck, Chapter 10, this volume) uses self-monitoring in various ways in his cognitive therapy approach to depression. Among these is a multiple-column technique. When a client becomes aware of an increase in dysphoria, he or she records the date and a brief description of the situation in the first two columns. The emotional reaction itself is recorded in the third column. In the fourth column, the client records the thought that presumably intervened between the situation and the emotional reaction. In the fifth column, a more adaptive, positive interpretation of the situation is recorded. Finally, the client rates his or her degree of confidence in the statements in the fourth and fifth columns—for example, "The boss's brusqueness shows he doesn't like me" (60% confident), and "He's just in a hurry" (50% confident). Depending on the circumstances, the therapist may elect to use only a few of these columns. These data are used to help the client practice disputing distorted interpretations of experiences in a realistic and convincing manner.

Self-monitoring in pain programs again usually involves situational assessments of the occurrence and/or intensity of pain. The patient may attempt various activities and record pain levels, or may employ various pain reduction techniques and record subsequent levels of pain. As with interventions for anxiety and depression, the data provide assessments for directing interventions; they may be part of the interventions per se, and they provide progress feedback to the patient.

Self-Control Questionnaire

The Self-Control Questionnaire (SCQ) was initially developed as a device to assess the teaching effectiveness of the self-management therapy program for depression (Fuchs & Rehm, 1977). Item content is derived from the deficits in self-management behavior that the model posits are contributory causes of depression. The SCQ was intended as an outcome measure to assess the effectiveness of the program in accomplishing the specific proximal purpose of acquisition of these concepts by participants—that is, the modification of these attitudes and beliefs. The SCQ consists of 40 statements of attitudes and beliefs about self-management behaviors and cognitions related to depression. Instructions require the examinee to indicate the degree to which each statement is characteristic of him or her on a 5-point scale from "A = Very characteristic of me, extremely descriptive" to "E = Very uncharacteristic of me, extremely undescriptive." Nineteen items are phrased to reflect positive, nondepressive attitudes, and 21 to reflect negative, depressed attitudes. Sample items include "Planning each step of what I have to do helps me to get things done well," and "It's no use trying to change most of the things that make me miserable."

Internal-consistency alpha coefficients of .82 and .88 have been reported for the SCQ. Test–retest reliability over a 5-week period was reported to be .86 by O'Hara, Rehm, and Campbell (1982). In a sample of 101 clinically depressed community volunteers, the scale correlated .42 with the Rosenbaum Self-Control Schedule (Rosenbaum, 1980a; see below), which is a measure of a broad range of self-control skills. In the same sample, the SCQ correlated .16 with the Beck Depression Inventory (BDI). In a sample of normal women, O'Hara et al. (1982) found a correlation of .31 with the BDI. In a series of outcome studies of the self-management therapy program for depression, the SCQ has consistently shown significant improvement in scores from pre- to posttherapy (see Rehm, 1984). Posttest scores have differentiated self-management patients from patients in waiting-list, traditional therapy, and assertion training conditions. Pretreatment scores have not predicted depression outcome in these studies. O'Hara et al. (1982) did find that the SCQ contributed significantly to the prediction of postpartum depression when included in a battery administered in the second trimester of pregnancy.

The SCQ was originally written on a logical basis to tap the concepts and skills that are targeted by the self-management therapy program for depression. Although the scale has worked relatively well for these purposes, the original scale had little formal psychometric development. An expanded scale with specific subscales for each of the major targets of the program is near completion and will be published in the near future.

Learned Resourcefulness Scale

The Learned Resourcefulness Scale was originally titled the Self-Control Schedule (Rosenbaum, 1980a). The scale consists of 36 statements of self-management behaviors. Respondents indicate on a 6-point Likert scale the degree to which each behavior is characteristic of them. Twelve items refer to the use of cognitions to manage emotional and physiological sensations; 11 items refer to the use of problem-solving strategies; 4 items refer to perceived ability to delay gratification; and 9 items refer to general self-efficacy expectations. Psychometric data from six samples indicated good internal-consistency and test–retest reliability (Rosenbaum, 1980a).

Rosenbaum demonstrated the validity of the Learned Resourcefulness Scale by showing that it was related to successful self-management behavior in several settings. Individuals scoring high on the scale were shown to tolerate pain better on a cold pressor test (Rosenbaum, 1980b) and to cope better with seasickness (Rosenbaum & Rolnick, 1983). The scale was subsequently reconceptualized as measuring the opposite of learned helplessness and was thus renamed the Learned Resourcefulness Scale (Rosenbaum, 1983). Work was reported on the relationship of the scale to coping among epilepsy patients (Rosenbaum & Palmon, 1984). The scale can be seen as a rather broad measure of self-management behaviors, potentially applicable to many situations.

The Frequency of Self-Reinforcement Questionnaire

Heiby (1982) has developed a scale aimed at assessing a much more specific form of self-management behavior—namely, self-reinforcement. The Frequency of Self-Reinforcement Questionnaire consists of 30 true–false items and is intended to assess use of self-reinforcing statements and positive self-attitudes. Validity has been shown by comparing scores to ratings by another person and to self-monitored self-reinforcement records (Heiby, 1982). Depressed individuals score lower on the scale (Heiby, 1981), and low scorers are more likely to respond with depression to low levels of external reinforcement (Heiby, 1983). Training in self-reinforcement was found to increase later self-monitored self-reinforcement behavior (Heiby, Ozaki, & Campos, 1984). This scale has the potential to be a useful scale for assessing a specific component of self-management behavior in various contexts.

Efficacy

The measurement of efficacy expectations, as defined by Bandura, requires behavior- and situation-specific information. There is thus no single measurement instrument available for assessing self-efficacy; different problem areas and situations require different instruments. Bandura has developed his own instruments for the investigation of self-efficacy in the context of fearful situations (e.g., Bandura et al., 1977, 1980; Bandura, Reese, & Adams, 1982). Other investigators have extended the investigation of self-efficacy into areas such as weight reduction (Chambliss & Murray, 1979), assertiveness (Kazdin, 1979; Lee, 1984), cigarette smoking (Condiotte & Lichtenstein, 1981; DiClemente, 1981; McIntyre, Lichtenstein, & Mermelstein, 1983), and pain (Anderson, Dowds, Pelletz, Edwards, & Peeters Asdourian, 1995; Lawson, Reesor, Keefe, & Turner, 1990). In most cases, the assessment of self-efficacy has occurred within the context of a structured research program investigating the role of the self-efficacy construct in behavior change. Very few of these studies have commented on the clinical utility of this construct or on the use of the particular assessment devices in clinical settings.

In general, efficacy expectations can be measured along three primary dimensions: level, strength, and generality. That is, tasks can vary on several dimensions that can usually be ordered in terms of some attribute, such as their level of difficulty, complexity, or stressfulness. The level of an individual's efficacy expectations should correspond to the task level that he or she expects to be able to perform. The individual's degree of conviction about his or her ability to perform this particular task should correspond to the strength dimension. Finally, efficacy expectations may vary in how broadly they are applied across situational and time parameters.

Bandura (1977a, 1982) has proposed a strategy for measuring self-efficacy. Subjects are presented with a list of behavioral tasks that are arranged in a hierarchical fashion, such that easier, less complex tasks appear early in the list, followed by more difficult ones. For each of these tasks, subjects are asked to respond simply whether or not they think they can perform the behavior in question. For each task that they state they could perform, subjects are asked to rate the strength of their self-judged efficacy on a 100-point probability scale. This scale ranges from 0 (high uncertainty) to 100 (complete certainty that the behavior can be performed). The number of items checked "Can Do" represents the level of self-efficacy, whereas the average certainty rating across all items represents the strength of self-efficacy.

Many of the studies of this construct have also included behavioral measures with tasks that correspond directly to the items on the self-efficacy measure. Investigators have thus been able to evaluate the relationship between perceived efficacy and the actual level of performance. Bandura's (1980) "microanalytic" technique calls for calculating the congruence (i.e., percentage of agreement) between efficacy judgments and performance of specific tasks. Others (e.g., Kirsch, 1985) have argued that correlational analyses may best reveal the relationship between self-efficacy and behavior. In noting that the utility of any analysis of self-efficacy will be enhanced to the degree that it is both "fine-grained and interpretable," Lee (1985) suggests that agreement measures such as the chi-square and the phi coefficient may also be good alternatives.

Several assumptions of this assessment model and its problems should be noted. One primary assumption is that individuals have had enough prior experience with the particular behaviors or situations to estimate their abilities adequately. Other assumptions are that the instrument elicits responses indicative of maximal rather than typical levels of performance, and that the items are arranged in hierarchical order. Bandura developed this approach to assessment in the context of simple or specific phobias while trying to understand or predict approach behavior. Items relevant to specific behaviors occurring in specific situations could be readily identified and arranged in hierarchical fashion without too much difficulty. These methods, however, do not lend themselves well to situations in which the problem behaviors involved are very complex or are by nature not clearly hierarchical. Although the concept of self-efficacy may be potentially useful in areas such as depression, pain, and social skills, strategies for measuring self-efficacy expectancies in these circumstances have been less well developed. Moe and Zeiss (1982) attempted to offer some solutions to these problems in the study of social skills by proposing the use of more molar attributes associated with acceptable performance, rather than limiting assessment to molecular behavior. They used 12 attributes (e.g., "warm," "attractive," "friendly," "trusting") that could be rated in each of 12 different social situations. These attributes were not viewed as being hierarchical, yet level or magnitude of self-efficacy could still be assessed by calculating the mean number of attributes checked for the different situations. As research on self-efficacy is conducted in relation to new problem areas, the reliability of measurement must be demonstrated, and the clinical utility of the construct should be addressed.

Self-Instruction

Self-instructional training provides the therapist with a general framework for approaching a variety of problems. Because it is a general approach, there is not a single assessment device or strategy associated with self-instructional training. Any measures that are typically used for a given problem area, (e.g., anxiety, fear, pain) may be incorporated into self-

instructional therapy. Since this is an approach that pays particular attention to self-evaluative cognitions, however, several measures directed specifically to self-statements may be of use. Several authors have attempted to
develop self-report measures to assess cognitive events (i.e., self-statements)
that may be useful in studying depressive phenomena. These include the
Expanded Attributional Style Questionnaire (Peterson & Villanova, 1988),
the Automatic Thoughts Questionnaire (Hollon & Kendall, 1980), the
Dysfunctional Attitude Scale (Weissman & Beck, 1978), and the Hopelessness Scale (Beck, Weissman, Lester, & Trexler, 1974).

CONCLUDING REFLECTIONS

Self-management interventions and assessment methods have been applied
to many populations and problems. This chapter has focused on applications to anxiety, depression, and pain. It should also be clear that a number
of specific models and theories fall under the general heading of self-management. This chapter has focused on those of Bandura, Kanfer, and
Meichenbaum. The common threads among the techniques and models involve the assumption that therapeutic change and progress toward long-
range goals can be brought about by teaching individuals general skills in
managing their own behavior in problematic situations. Generalization and
maintenance of outcome are enhanced by giving responsibility to clients for
carrying out the change strategies in real-life situations. Self-management
approaches will continue to make their contributions to therapy, assessment, and conceptualization of psychopathology independently and in conjunction with other models and methods.

REFERENCES

Abramson, L. Y., Seligman, M. E. P., & Teasdale, J. D. (1978). Learned helplessness
    in humans: Critique and reformulation. *Journal of Abnormal Psychology, 87*,
    49–74.
Alloy, L. B., Kelly, K. A., Mineka, S., & Clements, C. M. (1990). Comorbidity of
    anxiety and depressive disorders: A helplessness–hopelessness perspective. In J.
    D. Maser & C. R. Cloninger (Eds.), *Comorbidity of mood and anxiety disor-
    ders* (pp. 499–543). Washington, DC: American Psychiatric Press.
Anderson, K. O., Dowds, B. N., Pelletz, R. E., Edwards, W. T., & Peeters
    Asdourian, C. (1995). Development and initial validation of a scale to measure
    self-efficacy beliefs in patients with chronic pain. *Pain, 63*(1), 77–84.
Averill, J. R. (1973). Personal control over aversive stimuli and its relationship to
    stress. *Psychological Bulletin, 80*, 286–303.

Baker, S. L., & Kirsch, I. (1991). Cognitive mediators of pain perception and tolerance. *Journal of Personality and Social Psychology, 61,* 504–510.

Bandura, A. (1969). *Principles of behavior modification.* New York: Holt, Rinehart & Winston.

Bandura, A. (1971). Vicarious and self-reinforcement processes. In R. Glaser (Ed.), *The nature of reinforcement* (pp. 228–278). New York: Academic Press.

Bandura, A. (1977a). Self-efficacy: Toward a unifying theory of behavioral change. *Psychological Review, 84,* 191–215.

Bandura, A. (1977b). *Social learning theory.* Englewood Cliffs, NJ: Prentice-Hall.

Bandura, A. (1980). Gauging the relationship between self-efficacy judgment and action. *Cognitive Therapy and Research, 4,* 263–268.

Bandura, A. (1982). Self-efficacy mechanism in human agency. *American Psychologist, 37,* 122–147.

Bandura, A. (1988). Self-efficacy conception of anxiety. *Anxiety Research, 1,* 77–98.

Bandura, A. (1997). *Self-efficacy: The exercise of control.* New York: Freeman.

Bandura, A., & Adams, N. E. (1977). Analysis of self-efficacy theory of behavioral change. *Cognitive Therapy and Research, 1,* 287–308.

Bandura, A., Adams, N. E., & Beyer, J. (1977). Cognitive processes mediating behavioral change. *Journal of Personality and Social Psychology, 35,* 125–139.

Bandura, A., Adams, N. E., Hardy, A. B., & Howells, G. N. (1980). Tests of the generality of self-efficacy theory. *Cognitive Therapy and Research, 4,* 39–66.

Bandura, A., Cioffi, D., Taylor, C. B., & Brouillard, M. E. (1988). Perceived self-efficacy in coping with cognitive stressors and opioid activation. *Journal of Personality and Social Psychology, 55,* 479–488.

Bandura, A., O'Leary, A., Taylor, C. B., Gauthier, J., & Gossard, D. (1987). Perceived self-efficacy and pain control: Opioid and nonopioid mechanisms. *Journal of Personality and Social Psychology, 53,* 563–571.

Bandura, A., Reese, L., & Adams, N. E. (1982). Microanalysis of action and fear arousal as a function of differential levels of perceived self-efficacy. *Journal of Personality and Social Psychology, 43,* 5–21.

Beck, A. T. (1976). *Cognitive therapy and the emotional disorders.* New York: International Universities Press.

Beck, A. T., Emery, G., & Greenberg, R. T. (1985). *Anxiety disorders and phobias.* New York: Basic Books.

Beck, A. T., Rush, A. J., Shaw, B. F., & Emery, G. (1979). *Cognitive therapy of depression.* New York: Guilford Press.

Beck, A. T., Weissman, A., Lester, D., & Trexler, L. (1974). The measurement of pessimism: The Hopelessness Scale. *Journal of Consulting and Clinical Psychology, 42,* 861–865.

Bowers, K. S. (1968). Pain, anxiety, and perceived control. *Journal of Consulting and Clinical Psychology, 32,* 596–602.

Brown, L. M., Gouvier, W. D., & Blanchard-Fields, F. (1990). Cognitive interventions across the life-span. In A. M. Horton, Jr. (Ed.), *Neuropsychology across the life-span: Assessment and treatment* (pp. 133–153). New York: Springer.

Bussey, K., & Bandura, A. (1992). Self-regulatory mechanisms governing gender development. *Child Development, 63,* 1236–1250.

Carroll, W. R., & Bandura, A. (1985). Role of timing of visual monitoring and motor rehearsal in observational learning of action patterns. *Journal of Motor Behavior, 17,* 269–281.

Carver, C. S., & Scheier, M. F. (1982). An information processing perspective on self-management. In P. Karoly & F. H. Kanfer (Eds.), *Self-management and behavior change: From theory to practice* (pp. 93–128). New York: Pergamon Press.

Chambliss, C. A., & Murray, E. J. (1979). Efficacy attribution, locus of control, and weight loss. *Cognitive Therapy and Research, 4,* 349–353.

Coleman, R. E., & Beck, A. T. (1981). Cognitive therapy for depression. In J. F. Clarkin & H. I. Glazer (Eds.), *Depression: Behavioral and directive intervention strategies* (pp. 111–130). New York: Garland Press.

Condiotte, M. M., & Lichtenstein, E. (1981). Self-efficacy and relapse in smoking cessation programs. *Journal of Consulting and Clinical Psychology, 49,* 648–658.

Council, J. R., Ahern, D. K., Follick, M. J., & Kline, C. L. (1988). Expectancies and functional impairment in chronic low back pain. *Pain, 33,* 323–331.

Craighead, L. W., & Craighead, W. E. (1980). Implications of persuasive communication research for the modification of self-statements. *Cognitive Therapy and Research, 4,* 117–135.

DiClemente, C. C. (1981). Self-efficacy and smoking cessation maintenance. *Cognitive Therapy and Research, 5,* 175–187.

DiGiuseppe, R., McGowan, L., Simon, K.-S., & Gardner, F. (1990). A comparative outcome study of four cognitive therapies in the treatment of social anxiety. *Journal of Rational Emotive and Cognitive Behavior Therapy, 8,* 129–146.

Dunn, N. J., Brothers-Braun, G., Rehm, L. P., Hamilton, J. D., de Leon, C., & Kearney, J. (1995, November). *Treatment of depression in patients with PTSD: A challenge in the treatment of trauma.* Poster presented at the annual meeting of the International Society for Traumatic Stress Studies, Boston.

Ellis, A. (1962). *Reason and emotion in psychotherapy.* New York: Stuart.

Emmelkamp, P. M., Brilman, E., Kuiper, H., & Mersch, P. P. (1986). The treatment of agoraphobia: A comparison of self-instructional training, rational emotive therapy, and exposure in vivo. *Behavior Modification, 10,* 37–53.

Emmelkamp, P. M., & Mersch, P. P. (1982). Cognition and exposure in vivo in the treatment of agoraphobia: Short-term and delayed effects. *Cognitive Therapy and Research, 6,* 77–90.

Emmelkamp, P. M., Mersch, P. P., Vissia, E., & Van der Helm, M. (1985). Social phobia: A comparative evaluation of cognitive and behavioral interventions. *Behaviour Research and Therapy, 23,* 365–369.

Fleming, B. M., & Thornton, D. W. (1980). Coping skills training as a component in the shortterm treatment of depression. *Journal of Consulting and Clinical Psychology, 48,* 652–655.

Forgas, J. P., Bower, G. H., & Moylan, S. J. (1990). Praise or blame?: Affective influences on attributions for achievement. *Journal of Personality and Social Psychology, 59,* 809–819.

Fuchs, C. Z., & Rehm, L. P. (1977). A self-control behavior therapy program for depression. *Journal of Consulting and Clinical Psychology, 45,* 206–215.

Gattuso, S. M., Litt, M. D., & Fitzgerald, T. E. (1992). Coping with gastrointestinal endoscopy: Self-efficacy enhancement and coping style. *Journal of Consulting and Clinical Psychology, 60,* 133–139.

Genest, M., & Turk, D. C. (1979). A proposed model for behavioral group therapy with pain patients. In D. Upper & S. M. Ross (Eds.), *Behavioral group therapy, 1979: An annual review.* Champaign, IL: Research Press.

Glanz, L. M., & Dietz, R. E. (1980, August). *Building individual competence: Coping with depression and fear.* Paper presented at the meeting of the American Psychological Association, Montreal.

Heiby, E. M. (1981). Depression and frequency of self-reinforcement. *Behavior Therapy, 12,* 549–555.

Heiby, E. M. (1982). A self-reinforcement questionnaire. *Behaviour Research and Therapy, 20,* 397–401.

Heiby, E. M. (1983). Toward the prediction of mood change. *Behavior Therapy, 14,* 110–115.

Heiby, E. M., Ozaki, M., & Campos, P. E. (1984). The effects of training in self-reinforcement and reward: Implications for depression. *Behavior Therapy, 15,* 544–549.

Heimberg, R. G., & Barlow, D. H. (1988). Psychosocial treatments for social phobia. *Psychosomatics, 29,* 27–37.

Hoffart, A. (1993). Cognitive treatments of agoraphobia: A critical evaluation of theoretical basis and outcome evidence. *Journal of Anxiety Disorders, 7,* 75–91.

Hollon, S. D., & Kendall, P. C. (1980). Cognitive self-statements in depression: Development of an Automatic Thoughts Questionnaire. *Cognitive Therapy and Research, 4,* 383–395.

Horan, J., Hackett, G., Buchanan, J., Stone, C., & Demchik-Stone, D. (1977). Coping with pain: A component analysis. *Cognitive Therapy and Research, 1,* 211–221.

Jackson, B. (1972). Treatment of depression by self-reinforcement. *Behavior Therapy, 3,* 298–307.

Jensen, M. P., Turner, J. A., & Romano, J. M. (1991). Self-efficacy and outcome expectancies: Relationship to chronic pain coping strategies and adjustment. *Pain, 44,* 263–269.

Kanfer, F. H. (1970). Self-regulation: Research, issues, and speculations. In C. Neuringer & J. L. Michael (Eds.), *Behavior modification in clinical psychology* (pp. 178–220). New York: Appleton-Century-Crofts.

Kanfer, F. H. (1977). Self-regulation and self-control. In H. Zeir (Ed.), *The psychology of the 20th century.* Zurich: Kindler Verlag.

Kanfer, F. H., & Hagerman, S. (1981). The role of self-regulation. In L. P. Rehm (Ed.), *Behavior therapy for depression: Present status and future directions* (pp. 143–180). New York: Academic Press.

Kanfer, F. H., & Karoly, P. (1972a). Self-control: A behavioristic excursion into the lion's den. *Behavior Therapy, 2,* 398–416.

Kanfer, F. H., & Karoly, P. (1972b). Self-regulation and its clinical application: Some additional conceptualizations. In R. C. Johnson, P. R. Dokecki, & O. H. Mowrer (Eds.), *Socialization: Development of character and conscience* (pp. 428–437). New York: Holt, Rinehart & Winston.

Karoly, P., & Jensen, M. P. (1987). *Multimethod assessment of chronic pain*. New York: Pergamon Press.

Kazdin, A. E. (1979). Imagery elaboration and self-efficacy in the covert modeling treatment of unassertive behavior. *Journal of Consulting and Clinical Psychology*, 47, 725–733.

Kirsch, I. (1985). Response expectancy as a determinant of experience and behavior. *American Psychologist*, 40, 1189–1202.

Klepac, R. K., Hauge, G., Dowling, J., & McDonald, M. (1981). Direct and generalized effects of three components of stress inoculation for increased pain tolerance. *Behavior Therapy*, 12, 417–424.

Klinger, E. (1982). On the self-management of mood, affect, and attention. In P. Karoly & F. H. Kanfer (Eds.), *Self-management and behavior change: From theory to practice* (pp. 129–164). New York: Pergamon Press.

Kornblith, S. J., & Greenwald, D. (1982, November). *Self-control therapy with depressed inpatients*. Paper presented at the meeting of the Association for Advancement of Behavior Therapy, Los Angeles.

Kornblith, S. J., Rehm, L. P., O'Hara, M. W., & Lamparski, D. M. (1983). The contribution of self-reinforcement training and behavioral assignments to the efficacy of self-control therapy for depression. *Cognitive Therapy and Research*, 7, 499–527.

Lawson, K. C., Reesor, K. A., Keefe, F. J., & Turner, J. A. (1990). Dimensions of pain-related cognitive coping: Cross-validation of the factor structure of the Coping Strategy Questionnaire. *Pain*, 43, 195–204.

Lazarus, A. A. (1981). *The practice of multimodal therapy: Systematic, comprehensive, and effective psychotherapy*. New York: McGraw-Hill.

Lazarus, R. S. (1966). *Psychological stress and the coping process*. New York: McGraw-Hill.

Lazarus, R. S. (1974). Psychological stress and coping in adaptation and illness. *International Journal of Psychiatry in Medicine*, 5, 321–333.

Lee, C. (1984). Accuracy of efficacy and outcome expectations in predicting performance in a simulated assertiveness task. *Cognitive Therapy and Research*, 8, 37–48.

Lee, C. (1985). Efficacy expectations as predictors of performance: Meaningful measures of microanalytic match. *Cognitive Therapy and Research*, 9, 367–370.

Lewinsohn, P. M., Antonuccio, D. O., Steinmetz, J. L., & Teri, L. (1984). *The Coping with Depression course*. Eugene, OR: Castalia.

Litt, M. D. (1988). Self-efficacy and perceived control: Cognitive mediators of pain tolerance. *Journal of Personality and Social Psychology*, 54, 149–160.

Litt, M. D. (1996). A model of pain and anxiety associated with acute stressors: Distress in dental procedures. *Behaviour Research and Therapy*, 34, 459–476.

Litt, M. D., Nye, C., & Shafer, D. (1995). Preparation for oral surgery: Evaluating elements of coping. *Journal of Behavioral Medicine*, 18, 435–459.

Maag, J. W., & Kotlash, J. (1994). Review of stress inoculation training with children and adolescents: Issues and recommendations. *Behavior Modification*, 18, 443–469.

Mahoney, M. J. (1971). The self-management of covert behavior: A case study. *Behavior Therapy, 2,* 575–578.

Manning, M. M., & Wright, T. L. (1983). Self-efficacy expectancies, outcome expectancies, and the persistence of pain control in childbirth. *Journal of Personality and Social Psychology, 45,* 421–431.

Marston, A. R. (1968). Dealing with low self-confidence. *Educational Research, 10,* 134–138.

Mathews, C. O. (1977). A review of behavioral theories of depression and a self-regulation model for depression. *Psychotherapy: Theory, Research and Practice, 14,* 79–86.

McIntyre, K. O., Lichtenstein, E., & Mermelstein, R. J. (1983). Self-efficacy and relapse in smoking cessation: A replication and extension. *Journal of Consulting and Clinical Psychology, 51,* 632–633.

Meichenbaum, D. H. (1972). Cognitive modification of test anxious college students. *Journal of Consulting and Clinical Psychology, 39,* 370–380.

Meichenbaum, D. H. (1977). *Cognitive-behavior modification: An integrative approach.* New York: Plenum Press.

Meichenbaum, D. H. (1994). *A clinical handbook/practical therapist manual for assessing and treating adults with post-traumatic stress disorder (PTSD).* Waterloo, Ontario, Canada: Institute Press.

Meichenbaum, D. H., & Cameron, R. (1973). Training schizophrenics to talk to themselves: A means of developing attentional controls. *Behavior Therapy, 4,* 515–534.

Meichenbaum, D. H., & Deffenbacher, J. L. (1988). Stress inoculation training. *Counseling Psychologist, 16,* 69–90.

Meichenbaum, D. H., & Goodman, J. (1971). Training impulsive children to talk to themselves: A means of developing self-control. *Journal of Abnormal Psychology, 77,* 115–126.

Meichenbaum, D. H., & Turk, D. (1976). The cognitive-behavioral management of anxiety, anger, and pain. In P. O. Davidson (Ed.), *The behavioral management of anxiety, depression and pain* (pp. 1–34). New York: Brunner/Mazel.

Melzack, R., & Wall, P. (1965). Pain mechanisms: A new theory. *Science, 150,* 971–979.

Miller, S. M. (1979). Controllability and human stress: Method, evidence and theory. *Behaviour Research and Therapy, 17,* 287–304.

Missel, P., & Sommer, G. (1983). Depression and self-verbalization. *Cognitive Therapy and Research, 7,* 141–148.

Moe, K. O., & Zeiss, A. M. (1982). Measuring self-efficacy expectations for social skills: A methodological inquiry. *Cognitive Therapy and Research, 6,* 191–205.

O'Hara, M. W., Rehm, L. P., & Campbell, S. B. (1982). Predicting depressive symptomatology: Cognitive-behavioral models and postpartum depression. *Journal of Abnormal Psychology, 91,* 457–461.

Ollendick, T. H., & King, N. J. (1998). Empirically supported treatments for children with phobic and anxiety disorders: Current status. *Journal of Clinical Child Psychology, 27,* 156–167.

Peterson, C., & Villanova, P. (1988). An Expanded Attributional Style Questionnaire. *Journal of Abnormal Psychology, 97*, 87–89.

Rehm, L. P. (1977). A self-control model of depression. *Behavior Therapy, 8*, 787–804.

Rehm, L. P. (1984). Self-management therapy for depression. *Advances in Behaviour Research and Therapy, 6*, 83–98.

Rehm, L. P., Fuchs, C. Z., Roth, D. M., Kornblith, S. J., & Romano, J. M. (1979). A comparison of self-control and assertion skills treatments of depression. *Behavior Therapy, 10*, 429–442.

Rehm, L. P., Kaslow, N. J., & Rabin, A. S. (1987). Cognitive and behavioral targets in a self-control therapy program for depression. *Journal of Consulting and Clinical Psychology, 55*, 60–67.

Rehm, L. P., Kornblith, S. J., O'Hara, M. W., Lamparski, D. M., Romano, J. M., & Volkin, J. (1981). An evaluation of major components in a self-control behavior therapy program for depression. *Behavior Modification, 5*, 459–490.

Rehm, L. P., & Sharp, R. N. (1996). Strategies in the treatment of childhood depression. In M. A. Reinecke, F. M. Dattilio, & A. Freeman (Eds.), *Cognitive therapy with children and adolescents: A casebook for clinical practice* (pp. 103–123). New York: Guilford Press.

Reynolds, W. M., & Coats, K. I. (1986). A comparison of cognitive-behavioral therapy and relaxation training for the treatment of depression in adolescents. *Journal of Consulting and Clinical Psychology, 54*, 653–660.

Rogers, P. A., Kerns, R., Rehm, L. P., Hendler, E. D., & Harkness, L. (1982, August). *Depression mitigation in hemo-dialysands: A function of self-control training.* Paper presented at the meeting of the American Psychological Association, Washington, DC.

Rokke, P. D., & al'Absi, M. (1992). Matching pain coping strategies to the individual: A prospective validation of the Cognitive Coping Strategy Inventory. *Journal of Behavioral Medicine, 15*, 611–625.

Rokke, P. D., Al Absi, M., Lall, R., & Oswald, K. (1991). When does a choice of coping strategies help?: The interaction of choice and locus of control. *Journal of Behavioral Medicine, 14*, 491–504.

Rokke, P. D., & Lall, R. (1992). The role of choice in enhancing tolerance to acute pain. *Cognitive Therapy and Research, 16*, 53–65.

Rokke, P. D., Tomhave, J. A., & Jocic, Z. (1999). The role of client choice and target selection in self-management therapy for depression in older adults. *Psychology and Aging, 14*, 155–169.

Rokke, P. D., Tomhave, J. A., & Jocic, Z. (2000). Self-management therapy and educational group therapy for depressed elders. *Cognitive Therapy and Research, 24*, 99–119.

Romano, J. M., & Rehm, L. P. (1979, April). Self-control treatment of depression: One-year follow-up. In A. T. Beck (Chair), *Factors affecting the outcome and maintenance of cognitive therapy.* Symposium presented at the meeting of the Eastern Psychological Association, Philadelphia.

Rosenbaum, M. (1980a). A schedule for assessing self-control behaviors: Preliminary findings. *Behavior Therapy, 11*, 109–121.

Rosenbaum, M. (1980b). Individual differences in self-control behaviors and tolerance of painful stimulation. *Journal of Abnormal Psychology, 89,* 581–590.

Rosenbaum, M. (1983). Learned resourcefulness as a behavioral repertoire for the
self-regulation of internal events: Issues and speculations. In M. Rosenbaum,
C. M. Franks, & Y. Jaffe (Eds.), *Perspectives on behavior therapy in the eighties* (pp. 55–73). New York: Springer.

Rosenbaum, M., & Palmon, N. (1984). Helplessness and resourcefulness in coping
with epilepsy. *Journal of Consulting and Clinical Psychology, 52,* 244–253.

Rosenbaum, M., & Rolnick, A. (1983). Self-control behaviors and coping with seasickness. *Cognitive Therapy and Research, 7,* 93–98.

Roth, D., Bielski, R., Jones, M., Parker, W., & Osborn, G. (1982). A comparison of
self-control therapy and combined self-control therapy and antidepressant
medication in the treatment of depression. *Behavior Therapy, 13,* 133–144.

Rothblum, E., Green, L., & Collins, R. L. (1979, April). *A comparison of self-control and therapist control in the treatment of depression.* Paper presented at
the meeting of the Eastern Psychological Association, Philadelphia.

Salovey, P., & Birnbaum, D. (1989). Influence of mood on health-relevant cognitions. *Journal of Personality and Social Psychology, 57,* 539–551.

Sarason, I. G. (1975). Anxiety and self-preoccupation. In I. G. Sarason & C. D.
Spielberger (Eds.), *Stress and anxiety* (Vol. 2, pp. 27–44). Washington, DC:
Hemisphere.

Schachter, S. (1966). The interaction of cognitive and physiological determinants of
emotional state. In C. Spielberger (Ed.), *Anxiety and behavior.* New York: Academic Press.

Seligman, M. E. P. (1975). *Helplessness: On depression, development, and death.*
San Francisco: Freeman.

Seligman, M. E. P. (1981). A learned helplessness point of view. In L. P. Rehm (Ed.),
Behavior therapy for depression: Present status and future directions (pp.
123–142). New York: Academic Press.

Shaw, B. F. (1977). Comparison of cognitive therapy and behavior therapy in the
treatment of depression. *Journal of Consulting and Clinical Psychology, 45,*
543–551.

Skinner, B. F. (1953). *Science and human behavior.* New York: Free Press.

Stark, K. D., Reynolds, W. M., & Kaslow, N. J. (1987). A comparison of the relative efficacy of self-control therapy and a behavioral problem-solving therapy
for depression in children. *Journal of Abnormal Child Psychology, 15,* 91–
113.

Staub, E., Tursky, B., & Schwartz, G. E. (1971). Self-control and predictability:
Their effects on reactions to aversive stimulation. *Journal of Personality and
Social Psychology, 18,* 157–162.

Sulz, K. D., & Lauter, H. (1983). Stationaire Verhaltens therapie der Depression:
Ein multimodaler Ansatz in der klinischen Praxis [Inpatient behavior therapy
of depression: Multimodal approach in clinical practice]. *Psychiatric Praxis,
10,* 33–40.

Tressler, D. P., & Tucker, R. D. (1980, November). *The comparative effects of self-
evaluation and self-reinforcement training in the treatment of depression.* Pa-

per presented at the meeting of the Association for Advancement of Behavior Therapy, New York.

Turk, D. C., Meichenbaum, D., & Genest, M. (1983). *Pain and behavioral medicine: A cognitive-behavioral perspective.* New York: Guilford Press.

van den Hout, J. H., Arntz, A., & Kunkels, F. H. (1995). Efficacy of a self-control therapy program in a psychiatric day-treatment center. *Acta Psychiatrica Scandinavica, 92,* 25–29.

Vasta, R., & Brockner, J. (1979). Self-esteem and self-evaluative covert statements. *Journal of Consulting and Clinical Psychology, 47,* 776–777.

Vestre, N. D. (1984). Irrational beliefs and self-reported depressed mood. *Journal of Abnormal Psychology, 93,* 239–241.

Weiner, B., Frieze, I., Kukla, A., Reed, L., Rest, S., & Rosenbaum, R. M. (1971). *Perceiving the causes of success and failure.* New York: General Learning Press.

Weissman, A. N., & Beck, A. T. (1978, November). *Development and validation of the Dysfunctional Attitude Scale.* Paper presented at the meeting of the Association for Advancement of Behavior Therapy, Chicago.

Wood, R., Bandura, A., & Bailey, T. (1990). Mechanisms governing organizational performance in complex decision-making environments. *Organizational Behavior and Human Decision Processes, 46,* 181–201.

Zeiss, A. M., Lewinsohn, P. M., & Munoz, R. (1979). Nonspecific improvement effects in depression using interpersonal, cognitive, and pleasant events focused treatment. *Journal of Consulting and Clinical Psychology, 47,* 427–439.

Zimmerman, B. J., Bandura, A., & Martinez-Pons, M. (1992). Self-motivation for academic attainment: The role of self-efficacy beliefs and personal goal setting. *American Educational Research Journal, 29,* 663–676.

7

Problem-Solving Therapies

THOMAS J. D'ZURILLA
ARTHUR M. NEZU

Problem-solving therapy, or the clinical application of problem-solving training (PST),[1] began in the late 1960s and early 1970s as part of the cognitive-behavioral movement in the field of behavior modification (Kendall & Hollon, 1979). At a symposium on the role of cognitive factors in behavior modification at the 1968 American Psychological Association convention, D'Zurilla and Goldfried presented a paper arguing that social skills training programs should include training in problem-solving skills to facilitate generalized improvements in social competence. This paper was later expanded and published in 1971 under the title "Problem Solving and Behavior Modification." In 1976, Spivack, Platt, and Shure published their influential book *The Problem-Solving Approach to Adjustment*, which presented evidence on the relationship between social problem-solving ability and psychopathology; it also described several early studies on PST with children, adolescents, and adults.

Since the early 1970s, rapidly growing numbers of PST programs have been reported in the clinical, counseling, and health psychology literature. Focusing on children, adolescents, and adults, PST has been employed as a treatment method (alone or part of a treatment package), a maintenance strategy, and a prevention program. These interventions have been applied within a variety of clinical settings, including individual, group, marital/couple, and family therapy and counseling. In addition, there have been preventive applications in nonclinical settings such as workshops, academic courses, and seminars. Participants have presented with a wide range of problems and disorders, including schizophrenia, depression, stress and anxiety disorders, suicidal ideation and behavior, substance abuse, weight problems, relationship problems, mental retardation, cancer, and other health problems.

The present chapter focuses on PST for adolescents and adults. First we describe the theoretical and empirical foundations of PST, and then we discuss the clinical applications of PST. The latter discussion includes a description of a generic PST program and a discussion of the current empirical status of PST.

THEORETICAL AND EMPIRICAL FOUNDATIONS

Definitions of Major Concepts

Any adequate theory of social problem solving must clearly define three major concepts: (1) "problem solving", (2) "problem", and (3) "solution." It is also important for theory, research, and practice to distinguish between the concepts of "problem solving" and "solution implementation." The definitions presented below are based on concepts previously discussed by Davis (1966), D'Zurilla and Goldfried (1971), D'Zurilla and Nezu (1982, 1999), and Skinner (1953).

As it occurs in the natural environment, "problem solving" may be defined as the self-directed cognitive-behavioral process by which a person attempts to identify or discover effective or adaptive solutions for specific problems encountered in everyday living. As this definition implies, problem solving is conceived here as a conscious, rational, effortful, and purposeful activity. In the fields of clinical, counseling, and health psychology, "social problem solving" has become the most popular term for this phenomenon (D'Zurilla & Nezu, 1982). The adjective "social" is not meant to limit the study of problem solving to any particular type of problem; it is used only to highlight the fact that the focus of study is on problem solving that occurs within the natural social environment. Thus theory and research on social problem solving and PST deal with all kinds of problems in living, including impersonal problems (e.g., finances, property), personal/intrapersonal problems (cognitive, emotional, behavioral, health), interpersonal problems (e.g., marital/couple and family conflicts), and community and societal problems (e.g., crime, public services).

A "problem" (or "problematic situation") is defined as any life situation or task (present or anticipated) that demands a response for adaptive functioning, but for which no effective response is immediately apparent or available to the person, due to the presence of some obstacle or obstacles. The demands in a problematic situation may originate in the environment (e.g., objective task demands) or within the person (e.g., a personal goal, need, or commitment). The obstacles may include novelty, ambiguity, unpredictability, conflicting stimulus demands, performance skill deficits, or lack of resources. A specific problem may be a single time-limited event (e.g., missing a train to work, an acute illness), a series of similar or related events (e.g., repeated unreasonable demands from one's boss, repeated violations of curfew by one's adolescent daughter), or a chronic, ongoing situation (e.g., continuous pain, boredom, or feelings of loneliness).

A "solution" is a situation-specific coping response or response pattern (cognitive and/or behavioral), which is the product or outcome of the problem-solving process when it is applied to a specific problematic situation. An *effective* solution is one that achieves the problem-solving goal (i.e., changing the situation and/or one's emotional reactions to it so that it is no longer perceived as a problem), while at the same time maximizing other positive consequences and minimizing negative consequences. The relevant consequences include effects on others as well as oneself, and long-term outcomes as well as short-term effects.

As noted above, a theory of social problem solving should also distinguish between the concepts of "problem solving" and "solution implementation." These two processes are conceptually different and require different sets of skills. "Problem solving" refers to the process of *finding* solutions to specific problems, whereas "solution implementation" refers to the process of *carrying out* those solutions in the actual problematic situations. Problem-solving skills are assumed to be general, whereas solution implementation skills are expected to vary across situations depending on the type of problem and solution. Because they are different, problem-solving skills and solution-implementation skills are not always correlated. Hence, some clients may possess poor problem-solving skills but good solution implementation skills, or vice versa. Because both sets of skills are required for effective functioning or social competence, it is often necessary to combine PST with training in other social and behavioral skills in order to maximize positive outcomes (McFall, 1982).

A Prescriptive Model of Social Problem Solving

The great majority of PST programs reported in the literature have been based on a prescriptive model of social problem solving originally described by D'Zurilla and Goldfried (1971) and later expanded and refined by D'Zurilla and Nezu (1982, 1990, 1999). This model assumes that problem-solving outcomes in the real world are largely determined by two major, partially independent processes: (1) problem orientation and (2) problem-solving proper. "Problem orientation" is the motivational part of the problem-solving process, whereas "problem solving proper" is the process by which a person attempts to find an effective or adaptive solution to a particular problem through the rational application of problem-solving strategies and techniques.

PROBLEM ORIENTATION

Problem orientation consists of an attentional set to recognize problems when they occur during the course of everyday living, together with a set of relatively stable cognitive–emotional schemata describing how a person typically thinks and feels about problems in living and his or her own general problem-solving ability. A positive or constructive problem orientation produces positive emotions and approach tendencies; sets the occasion for problem-solving behavior; keeps attention focused on constructive problem-solving activities; and maximizes effort, persistence, and tolerance for frustration and uncertainty. In contrast, a negative or dysfunctional problem orientation generates negative emotions and avoidance tendencies; increases destructive worrying; and reduces effort, persistence, and tolerance for frustration and uncertainty. In the present model, the major problem orientation variables are (1) problem perception, (2) problem attribution, (3) problem appraisal, (4) perceived control, and (5) time/effort commitment.

"Problem perception" refers to the general tendency or readiness to recognize problems when they occur during the course of daily living, rather than ignoring or denying them. Problem perception is important because it activates the other problem orientation schemata and sets the occasion for problem solving proper. "Problem attribution" refers to a person's causal beliefs concerning problems in living. A positive or facilitative problem attribution involves the general readiness or tendency to perceive problems as normal and inevitable life events for everyone, rather than attributing them to some personal and stable defect or deficiency. Problem attribution is likely to influence "problem appraisal," which refers to a person's evaluation of the significance or relevance of a problem for personal and/or social well-being. A positive problem appraisal is the general tendency to perceive a problem as a challenge or potential benefit, rather than viewing it only as a harmful or threatening situation. "Perceived control" has two components: (1) generalized problem-solving self-efficacy, or the general belief that one is capable of solving problems and implementing solutions effectively; and (2) generalized positive problem-solving outcome expectancy, or the general belief that problems in living are "solvable." "Time/effort commitment" also has two components: (1) the likelihood that an individual will estimate accurately the time it will take to solve a particular problem successfully, and (2) the likelihood that the individual will be willing to devote the necessary time and effort to problem solving.

PROBLEM SOLVING PROPER

In the present model, problem solving proper involves the application of four major problem-solving skills that are designed to maximize the probability of finding the "best" or most effective solution for a particular problem: (1) problem definition and formulation, (2) generation of alternative solutions, (3) decision making, and (4) solution implementation and verification. These four skills may be viewed as a set of specific goal-directed tasks enabling a person to solve a particular problem successfully. Each task has its own unique purpose or function in the problem-solving process.

In the real-life setting, problem solving usually begins with a problem that is "messy" or ill defined (i.e., vague, ambiguous, or irrelevant cues, inaccurate or distorted information, unclear goals). Hence the purposes of "problem definition and formulation" are to (1) gather as much relevant, factual information about the problem as possible; (2) clarify the nature of the problem; (3) set realistic problem-solving goals; and (4) reappraise the significance of the problem for personal and/or social well-being. This important problem-solving skill also includes the ability to recognize and correct irrational beliefs and other cognitive distortions that often contribute to ill-defined problems and pseudoproblems (Beck, Rush, Shaw, & Emery, 1979; Ellis & Dryden, 1997). The function of "generation of alternative solutions" is to make available as many solution alternatives as possible, in such a way as to maximize the likelihood that the "best" (most preferred) solution will be among them. Based on Osborn's (1963) method of "brainstorming," this problem-solving skill emphasizes three basic principles: (1) quantity (the more solution alternatives that are produced, the more good-quality ideas will be made available), (2) deferment of judgment (more good-quality solution ideas will be generated when the person suspends evaluation of ideas until later in the problem-solving process), and (3) variety (the greater the range or variety of solution ideas, the more good quality ideas will be discovered).

The purposes of the third problem-solving skill, "decision making," are to evaluate (compare and judge) the available solution alternatives and to select the "best" one(s) for implementation in the problematic situation. The present decision-making model is based primarily on expected-utility theory, where choice behavior is based on a rational benefit–cost analysis (Beach & Mitchell, 1978; Edwards, 1961). The functions of the fourth problem-solving skill, "solution implementation and verification," are to assess the solution outcome and verify the "effectiveness" of the chosen solution strategy in the real-life problematic situation. This task involves four steps: (1) performance of the solution behavior; (2) self-monitoring of the consequences or effects of the solution on the person and the environment; (3) self-evaluation (comparing the actual outcome to the predicted outcome); and, depending on satisfaction with the solution outcome, either (4a) self-reinforcement if the problem is solved or (4b) troubleshooting and recycling if the problem remains (i.e., returning to the problem-solving process in an attempt to find a better solution).

The order in which the above-described problem-solving skills are presented represents a logical and useful sequence for training and systematic, efficient application. However, in actual practice effective problem solving usually involves movement back and forth from one task to another before the process is finally terminated with the discovery of a satisfactory solution. For example, questions are often raised about the problem during the generation of alternative solutions and decision-making tasks that lead to a better understanding of the problem or a reevaluation of problem-solving goals. Likewise, evaluation of solution alternatives during decision making often suggests modifications or improvements that make available more good-quality solution alternatives. Most importantly, information obtained during solution implementation and verification, which involve the evaluation of solution outcome in the actual problematic situation, often indicates that the chosen solution is ineffective, requiring the problem solver to go back to one or more of the previous stages in an attempt to identify a better solution. The problem solver exits from the process only when a satisfactory solution is found.

A number of experimental studies have found support for the efficacy of individual model components and/or different combinations of components by providing training in the particular component(s) and observing the effects on some measure of problem-solving performance or adaptive coping (e.g., D'Zurilla & Nezu, 1980; Cormier, Otani, & Cormier, 1986; Nezu & D'Zurilla, 1979, 1981a, 1981b; Nezu & Ronan, 1987). For a full description of these studies, the reader is referred to D'Zurilla and Nezu (1999).

The Interpersonal Cognitive Problem-Solving Model

After the D'Zurilla, Goldfried, and Nezu model, the next most frequently used social problem-solving model in PST is the interpersonal cognitive problem-solving (ICPS) model described by Spivack et al. (1976). Although these two models were developed independently, they are very similar. According to the ICPS model, interpersonal problem-solving competence depends on six major subskills: (1) "sensitivity to interpersonal problems" (ability to recognize the range of interpersonal problems that an individual might encounter in normal living), (2) "causal thinking" (ability to understand that thoughts, actions, and feelings are responses to prior events in the interpersonal sphere), (3) "consequential thinking" (awareness that social acts have an impact on oneself and others), (4) "alternative thinking" (capacity to produce alternative solutions to common interpersonal problems), (5) "means–ends thinking" (ability to think through, step by step, the actions that will be required to achieve a given social goal), and (6) "perspective taking" (capacity to consider the feelings, thoughts, and motives of others). One of the major applications of ICPS training has been in the area of substance abuse (Platt, Taube, Metzger, & Duome, 1988; Platt, Husband, Hermalin, Cater, & Metzger, 1993).

Measures of Social Problem Solving

In both research and clinical practice involving PST, it is important to assess not only a person's general level of social problem-solving ability, but also his or her strengths and weaknesses across the different components of social problem-solving ability (e.g., problem orientation, generation of alternative solutions, decision making). Hence it is useful to distinguish between two general types of social problem-solving measures: (1) process measures and (2) outcome measures.

"Process measures" directly assess the general cognitive and behavioral activities (e.g., attitudes, skills) that facilitate or inhibit the discovery of effective or adaptive solutions for specific problems, whereas "outcome measures" assess the quality of those specific solutions. Hence process measures are used to assess specific strengths and deficits in social problem-solving ability, whereas outcome measures are used to evaluate problem-solving performance, or the ability of a person to apply his or her skills effectively to specific problems. An outcome measure can be viewed as an global indicator of social problem-solving ability, but, unlike a process measure, it does not provide any information about the specific components of social problem-solving ability.

Process measures can be subdivided into inventories and process performance tests. As the term is used here, a "problem-solving inventory" is a broad survey of a person's problem-solving attitudes, strategies, and techniques, both positive (facilitative) and negative (inhibitive). Some inventories also estimate the extent to which the person actually uses the problem-solving skills that he or she possesses, as well as the manner in which these techniques are typically applied (e.g., efficiently, systematically, impulsively, carelessly, etc.). Most problem-solving inventories are pencil-and-paper questionnaires that employ Likert-type items, but other formats can be used for this purpose as well, such as structured interviews, audiotape procedures, and computer-assisted methods.

The "performance test" format presents the person with a task that requires him or her to use a specific problem-solving skill (e.g., problem recognition, problem definition and formulation, generation of alternative solutions, decision making). The individual's task performance is then judged or evaluated, and this measure is viewed as an indicator of his or her level of ability in that particular skill area (see D'Zurilla & Nezu, 1980; Nezu & D'Zurilla, 1979, 1981a, 1981b; Spivack et al., 1976).

All outcome measures are performance tests. However, instead of testing one particular skill or component of the problem-solving process, outcome measures assess overall problem-solving performance by presenting the person with a problem and asking him or her to solve it, after which the quality of the solution is evaluated. Most outcome measures employ hypothetical test problems, but subjects' solutions for their real current problems have also been assessed (e.g., Marx, Williams, & Claridge, 1992; Schotte & Clum, 1987). When real problems are used, subjects may be asked to report their solutions verbally (either before or after they implement their solutions), or solution implementation may be directly observed (either in the natural environment or in some simulated or role-played problem-solving situation).

Published studies on social problem solving and PST have used many different process and outcome measures. Unfortunately, a number of these measures have been presented without sufficient test construction information and/or psychometric data to permit an evaluation of their reliability and validity. Here, we consider only measures that have adequate published test information and data. The major process measures are the Social Problem-Solving Inventory (SPSI; D'Zurilla & Nezu, 1990), the SPSI—Revised (SPSI-R; D'Zurilla, Nezu, & Maydeu-Olivares, in press; Maydeu-Olivares & D'Zurilla, 1996), the SPSI for Adolescents (SPSI-A; Frauenknecht & Black, 1995), the Problem-Solving Inventory (PSI; Heppner, 1988; Heppner & Petersen, 1982), the Problem-Solving Self-Efficacy and Problem-Solving Skills scales of the modified PSI (Maydeu-Olivares & D'Zurilla, 1997), and the Rational Processing scale of the Perceived Modes of Processing Inventory (Burns & D'Zurilla, 1999).

The major outcome measures are the Means–Ends Problem-Solving procedure (Platt & Spivack, 1975; Spivack, Shure, & Platt, 1985), the Interpersonal Problem-Solving Assessment Technique (Getter & Nowinski, 1981), the Adolescent Problems Inventory (Freedman, Rosenthal, Donahoe, Schlundt, & McFall, 1978), and the Inventory of Decisions, Evaluations, and Actions (Goddard & McFall, 1992). For a more thorough description and critical evaluation of these measures, as well as a description of additional social problem-solving measures, the reader is directed to D'Zurilla and Maydeu-Olivares (1995), D'Zurilla and Nezu (1999), Spivack et al. (1976), and Platt et al. (1988).

A Relational/Problem-Solving Model of Stress

The major assumption underlying the use of PST is that much of what we view as "psychopathology" can be understood as ineffective or maladaptive coping behavior and its consequences. That is, a person is unable to resolve certain stressful problems in his or her life, and the person's inadequate attempts to do so are having negative effects, such as anxiety, depression, anger, physical symptoms, and the creation of new problems (D'Zurilla & Goldfried, 1971). Given this assumption, the theory of PST is best conceptualized within a relational/problem-solving model of stress, in which the concept of social problem solving is given a central role as a general coping strategy that increases adaptive situational coping, general competence, and psychological and physical wellness—which in turn reduce and prevent the negative effects of daily stress on psychological and physical well-being (D'Zurilla, 1990; D'Zurilla & Nezu, 1999; Nezu & D'Zurilla, 1989). This model integrates Richard Lazarus's relational model of stress (Lazarus, 1999; Lazarus & Folkman, 1984) with the social problem-solving model presented here.

Lazarus defines "stress" as a particular type of person–environment relationship or transaction in which demands are appraised by the person as taxing or exceeding coping resources and endangering well-being (Lazarus & Folkman, 1984). Earlier, we have defined a "problem" as a life situation that demands a response for adaptive functioning, but for which no effective response is immediately available to the person. From a comparison of these two relational definitions, it can be concluded that a problematic situation is a stress situation if it is at all difficult and significant for well-being. According to Lazarus's model, a person in a stress situation significantly influences both the quality and intensity of stress responses through two major processes: (1) cognitive appraisal and (2) coping.

"Cognitive appraisal" is the process by which a person determines the "meaning" or personal significance of a specific stressful encounter with the environment. Two important kinds of cognitive appraisal are primary and secondary appraisal. "Primary appraisal" refers to the person's evaluation of the relevance of the encounter for physical, social, or psychological well-being. "Secondary appraisal" involves the person's evaluation of his or her coping resources and options with respect to the particular stressful encounter. The term "coping" refers to the various cognitive and behavioral activities by which the person attempts to manage stressful situational demands, as well as the emotions that they generate. Two major types of coping are problem-focused and emotion-focused coping. "Problem-focused coping" is directed at changing the stressful situation for the better (i.e., meeting, changing, or controlling situational demands). "Emotion-focused coping," on the other hand, is aimed at managing the emotions that are generated by the stressful situation. Research has shown that in general, problem-focused coping predominates when stressful conditions are appraised as changeable or controllable, whereas emotion-focused coping predominates when these conditions are appraised as unchangeable or uncontrollable (see Lazarus, 1999). Although neither strategy is universally effective, problem-focused coping is generally considered to be the more useful and adaptive form of coping. In Lazarus's model, "problem solving" is defined as a form of problem-focused coping, which means that problem-solving goals are equated with mastery goals or control of the environment. In this view, problem solving is futile and maladaptive when stressful conditions are unchangeable.

The relational/problem-solving model retains the basic assumptions and essential features of Lazarus's relational model of stress. However, these features are cast within a general social problem-solving framework, and problem solving is given an expanded and more important role as a general coping strategy. Within this model, stress is viewed as a function of the reciprocal relations among three major variables: (1) stressful life events, (2) emotional stress responses, and (3) problem-solving coping.

"Stressful life events" are life experiences that present a person with strong demands for personal, social, or biological readjustment (Bloom, 1985). Two important types of stressful life events that affect most people are major negative life events and daily problems. A "major negative life event" is a large event or happening, such as a major negative life change, that calls for sweeping readjustments in a person's life (e.g., divorce, death of a loved one, job loss, major illness or injury). A "daily problem" (or "daily problematic situation") is a more narrow and specific life event characterized by a perceived discrepancy between adaptive demands and available coping responses. In the stress literature, these specific stressful events are also called "daily hassles" (Kanner, Coyne, Schaefer, & Lazarus, 1981). Although daily problems are less dramatic than major negative life events, research suggests that the frequency of these stressors may have a greater impact on psychological and physical well-being than the number of major negative life events may have (Burks & Martin, 1985; Kanner et al., 1981; Nezu, 1986a; Nezu & Ronan, 1985; Weinberger, Hiner, & Tierney, 1987).

The concept of "emotional stress" refers to the immediate emotional responses of a person to a stressful life event, as modified or transformed by appraisal and coping processes (Lazarus, 1999). Although emotional stress responses are often negative, including such feelings as anxiety, anger, disappointment, and depression, they can also be positive in nature (e.g., hope, relief, exhilaration). Negative emotions are likely to predominate when a person (1) appraises a problem as harmful or threatening to well-being, (2) doubts his or her ability to cope with the situation effectively, and/or (3) makes ineffective or maladaptive coping responses. On the other hand, positive emotions may be experienced when the person (1) appraises the stress situation as a challenge or opportunity for benefit, (2) believes that he or she is capable of coping with the situation effectively, and (3) makes coping responses that are effective in reducing harmful or threatening conditions and/or the negative emotions generated by them.

The most important concept in the relational/problem-solving model is "problem-solving coping". This is a unifying concept that integrates all cognitive appraisal and coping activities within a general social problem-solving framework. Problem-solving coping is conceived as a general coping process by which a person generates and selects specific coping responses for specific problematic stress situations. A person who uses the problem-solving coping strategy identifies a stress situation; perceives it as a problem to be solved; carefully attempts to identify, discover, or invent a solution (effective or adaptive coping responses); implements the chosen solution; and then carefully observes and evaluates the outcome. In contrast with Lazarus's view of problem solving as a form of problem-focused coping, problem solving is conceived within this model as a broader, more versatile coping strategy, in that problem-solving goals are not limited to mastery goals. The goals may include problem-focused goals, emotion-focused goals, or both, depending on the nature of the particular problematic situation and how it is defined and appraised. When the situation or major aspects of it are appraised as changeable or controllable, then problem-focused goals are emphasized, although the person may also set an emotion-focused goal if emotional distress is extremely high. On the other hand, if the situation is largely unchangeable or uncontrollable, then emotion-focused goals are emphasized.

The relational/problem-solving model provides a cognitive-behavioral framework for assessing clinical problems, as well as a theoretical rationale for PST. To assess clinical problems, the problem-solving therapist identifies and pinpoints major negative life events, current daily problems, emotional stress responses, problem orientation deficits and distortions, problem-solving skills deficits, and other coping skills deficits. Based on this assessment, PST is then applied to improve problem orientation and problem-solving skills. This is expected to increase adaptive situational coping, general competence, and psychological and physical wellness—which in turn are expected to reduce, moderate, or prevent the negative effects of stress on psychological and physical well-being.

Over the past two decades, numerous studies have provided support for the major assumptions of the relational/problem-solving model (see review by D'Zurilla & Nezu, 1999). These studies have examined the relations between social problem solving and a wide range of adaptational outcomes, including measures of situational coping; behavioral competence (e.g., social performance, academic performance, caregiving effectiveness); positive psychological well-being (e.g., positive affectivity, self-esteem, life satisfaction); psychological distress and symptomatology (e.g., depression, anxiety, suicidal ideation); and health-related behaviors, symptoms, and adjustment. The subject populations in these studies have included high school students, college students, middle-aged adults, elderly adults, depressed college students, emotionally disturbed adolescents, suicidal adolescents, clinically depressed adults, suicidal adults, adults with agoraphobia, adults with alcoholism or other drug addictions, other adult psychiatric patients, abusive and neglectful mothers, pregnant women, patients with cancer, physically disabled individuals, and caregivers of people with serious illness and disabilities. The strongest support for the relational/problem-solving model is provided by studies demonstrating that problem solving moderates or mediates the negative effects of stressful life events on emotions (e.g., Folkman & Lazarus, 1988; Nezu, 1986b; Nezu, Nezu, Faddis, DelliCarpini, & Houts, 1995; Nezu, Nezu, Saraydarian, Kalmar, & Ronan, 1986; Nezu & Ronan, 1985, 1988; Kant, D'Zurilla, & Maydeu-Olivares, 1997).

CLINICAL APPLICATIONS

PST Procedures

Based on a thorough cognitive-behavioral assessment, a clinician decides whether PST may be a useful intervention strategy for a given client and, if so, how it may be used most effectively. PST is potentially useful in the treatment of any disorder in which a client is experiencing multiple daily problems and stresses and is not coping effectively with them. PST is particularly appropriate when the assessment suggests that the client's ineffective coping may be related to deficits in problem orientation and/or problem-solving skills. Then, depending on the nature of the disorder and other treatment requirements, PST may be used as the sole treatment, as part of a broader treatment package, or as a posttreatment maintenance strategy. Although deficits in problem-solving ability are used to identify the most appropriate cases for PST, the problem-solving approach is concerned with higher-level functioning and not merely the correction of "deficiencies." Hence we would argue that *most* clients are likely to benefit from some PST aimed at maximizing problem-solving ability in order to prevent the development of new clinical problems.

The goal of PST is to help clients identify and resolve current life problems that are antecedents of maladaptive responses, while at the same time teaching general skills that will enable them to deal more effectively and independently with future problems. In addition to solving these antecedent problems, PST can have a direct impact on maladaptive responses, such as anxiety, depression, pain, overeating, or problem drinking, if they are viewed conceptually as "problems to be solved." For example, a problem formulation for depression may be the following: "My girlfriend has just informed me that she is ending our relationship because she no longer loves me. I am feeling extremely depressed and inadequate. What can I do to make myself feel better?" For tension-induced pain, a problem statement may be this: "I am sitting at my desk trying to complete a difficult report that is due tomorrow, but I cannot concentrate because I have a terrible headache. I have already taken aspirin, but it has not worked. What can I do to relieve my headache pain?" An example of a problem statement for overeating is this: "I am sitting at home alone watching TV, and I have a strong urge to go out and buy some ice cream, but I know that I have already reached my calorie limit for the day. What can I do to keep myself from giving in to the urge to go out and get some ice cream?"

Although it is often useful to treat maladaptive responses as problems to be solved, the emphasis in PST should always be on the identification and resolution of the current antecedent problems that are causally related to these responses, because this approach is more likely to produce durable and generalized reductions in maladaptive behavior. However, in cases where antecedent problematic situations are difficult to identify, define, and/or change, a problem-solving strategy that focuses on changing maladaptive responses to the problem (e.g., emotional distress) may be the most effective or adaptive coping strategy (D'Zurilla & Nezu, 1999; Nezu, 1987).

When PST is used in conjunction with other treatment methods, it should not be applied apart from these approaches as a separate, distinct treatment procedure. Instead, we believe that therapy is best conducted within an overall PST framework, in which the other treatment methods are applied at the appropriate points in training, as needed either to facilitate problem-solving performance or to deal directly with some serious problematic situation or maladaptive response. For example, cognitive restructuring techniques may be needed to correct cognitive distortions when treatment is focusing on the identification and definition of current life problems related to depression (Nezu, Nezu, & Perri, 1989); anxiety reduction techniques may be required when a person's anxiety is disrupting problem-solving thinking or when fear or anxiety is seriously inhibiting effective solution performance; and social skills training techniques may also be necessary to facilitate effective solution implementation.

In addition to its application within a conventional, open-ended therapy framework, PST may also be applied as a structured, time-limited, psychotherapy/skills training program designed to be completed in approximately 8 to 16 weekly sessions lasting 1 1/2 to 2 hours, depending on the needs of the particular target population (in most published outcome studies on PST, the number of sessions varies from 8 to 12). These training programs may be used as a treatment, maintenance, or prevention strategy. They may be adapted to an individual setting, a small-group setting with six to eight group members, or larger-group settings such as a course or workshop structure. The advantages of individual training are privacy, more individual attention, and greater flexibility to tailor the program to a particular individual's needs. The advantages of a group program are the motivating effects of group discussion, the sharing of ideas and experiences, modeling, social support, and the efficient use of trained therapists or instructors. Groups may be conducted by one group leader or two coleaders, preferably a male–female team (see Nezu, Nezu, Friedman, Faddis, & Houts, 1998, for a compendium of PST-related "group therapy tips").

PST employs several methods of training, including the Socratic method, which emphasizes the use of questions and discussions that guide and encourage clients to formulate their own conclusions, as well as didactic instruction, coaching, modeling, rehearsal, performance feedback, positive reinforcement, and shaping. Didactic instruction is used to explain the rationale and course of treatment and to provide an initial description of effective problem-solving principles and techniques. Modeling includes written and verbal examples to demonstrate various problem-solving operations and tasks, using both hypothetical and real-life problems presented by the therapist. Rehearsal involves actual practice in problem solving, using various in-session problem-solving exercises as well as homework assignments. Performance feedback is provided by the therapist during the problem-solving exercises and through self-monitoring and self-evaluation in the natural environment. Positive reinforcement includes the therapist's praise and the natural reinforcement of successful verbal problem solving in session, as well as successful problem-solving performance in the real-life setting. Shaping involves specific training in the problem-solving process in progressive steps, with each new step being contingent on successful performance in the previous step.

The remainder of this section contains a global description of training in the major components of the social problem-solving model described earlier: problem orientation and problem solving proper (i.e., the effective application of problem definition and formulation, generation of alternative solutions, decision making, and solution implementation and verification). This description is generic in its focus regarding the client or patient population. Because of space limitations, we can only present an outline of the actual training manual. A more complete generic manual is available in D'Zurilla and Nezu (1999). For additional treatment manuals targeted for specific populations, the reader is directed to Nezu et al. (1989) for patients with clinical depression, and to Nezu et al. (1998) for patients with cancer. In addition, a PST manual designed for patients with alcoholism or other drug addictions is available in Platt et al. (1988). This manual is based on the ICPS model described by Spivack et al. (1976).

It is important to note that although the training framework presented below is sequentially delineated, actual training is more flexible and fluid. Rather than implementing PST in a static, sequential manner, clinicians should highlight the dynamic interplay among the various components. For example, the use of brainstorming principles can be used throughout training to generate a wide variety of problem-solving goals or a comprehensive list of anticipated consequences, instead of during the generation-of-alternatives procedure only.

PROBLEM ORIENTATION

The first problem-solving process reflects a general response set involved in understanding and reacting to stressful problems. This orientation can have either a generalized facilitative or inhibiting effect on the remaining problem-solving tasks. Therefore, actual training in this process is geared toward helping individuals adopt a positive or adaptive problem orientation, which includes the following:

- The ability to recognize a problem accurately when it occurs.
- The belief that problems are a normal and inevitable part of life.
- The ability to identify or attribute the "cause" of the problem accurately.
- The tendency to appraise new problems as "challenges," rather than as "catastrophes" or situations to be avoided.
- The belief in one's ability to cope effectively with stressful problems.
- The knowledge that complex problems may require substantial time and effort to resolve them.
- The desire to solve problems in a timely manner.
- The ability to inhibit the tendency to be impulsive when solving stressful problems.

To facilitate adopting such an orientation, we recommend the "reverse-advocacy role-play strategy." According to this technique, the therapist pretends to adopt a particular belief about problems reflective of a *negative* orientation, and asks the patient to provide reasons why that belief is irrational, illogical, incorrect, or maladaptive. Such beliefs may include the following statements: "Problems are not common to everyone; if I have a problem, that means that I am crazy!", "All my problems are caused by me", "There is always a perfect solution to any problem", or "People are not able to change; this is the way that I will always be." At times, when the client has difficulty generating arguments against such a position, the therapist then adopts a more *extreme* form of the belief, such as "No matter how long it takes, I will continue to try and find the perfect solution to my problem."

If prior clinical assessment indicates that the patient has generalized distortions in information processing, such as a negative attributional style, negative appraisals, cognitive distortions, and/or irrational beliefs, then treatment should also be geared to change them. Cognitive restructuring strategies, such as those of Beck's cognitive therapy, are recommended in such cases as adjunctive strategies (e.g., Beck et al., 1979).

A second important part of this problem-solving process involves teaching patients to recognize and label problems accurately when they occur. To facilitate this process, therapists can use various problem checklists (e.g., Mooney & Gordon, 1950) to help sensitize patients to the array of problems that may occur across a range of areas of life. In addition, patients should also be asked to discuss personal problems that they have experienced or may experience across these areas, such as marriage, work, friendships, religion, career, finance, relationships, and so on.

Clients are also taught to use feelings or emotions as "cues" or "signals" that a problem exists. We have found it helpful to use visual images of either a traffic stoplight that is flashing red or a waving red flag as signals to "STOP AND THINK." Essentially, it is important to teach patients to recognize various situations as problems and to label them as such. Accurately labeling a situation as a problem serves to help people confront the situation instead of avoiding it, and to inhibit the tendency to respond impulsively or automatically to the situation.

As part of this training, patients are helped to identify the specific ways they experience emotions in general. This process includes physiological arousal and somatic changes, such as fatigue, pain, mood changes, and thoughts such as "I believe that nothing is going to change." A client is taught to *reframe* these reactions from an "overwhelming emotional state of being" to a signal that "something is wrong," just as the image of the red traffic light signals the client to "STOP AND THINK." Attention is then redirected to the problem the individual is experiencing, with the immediate goal of continuing to engage in the remaining problem-solving tasks.

Clinical Example. The following is a clinical example, adapted from Nezu, Nezu, Rothenberg, and D'Zurilla (1996),[2] of a dialogue between a patient and a PST therapist demonstrating how to engage in the reverse-advocacy role-play exercise. The client was a 40-year-old salesman, Steve, who abused alcohol and suffered from depression. He entered treatment several months after he and his wife had separated; he was experiencing feelings of hopelessness and suicidal ideation.

THERAPIST: Steve, it seems at times that the way you think may have an impact on your feelings. I would like to try a role-play exercise in which I'll take the part of an old friend of yours that you haven't seen in a few months. Just go along with me for now, even if you find yourself agreeing with what I say, because I'd like to make a certain point. Your job during this exercise is to try your best to make a case against any statements I make that sound irrational or illogical to you, okay?

STEVE: Okay, I'll give it a try.

THERAPIST: (*Beginning the role play*) I know I seem real down lately. I've been a really terrible friend, and I wouldn't blame you if you never wanted to talk to me again.

STEVE: What's going on with you? What's wrong?

THERAPIST:What's going on? Everything! Absolutely everything! I can't even think of one thing that's going right. My girlfriend has been acting strange lately, and I think that she is going to end things with me. Also, my boss reminded me that I have to be evaluated for a raise in the next few weeks. I know for sure that I won't get a raise, and then I'll have to find another job to pay the rent. Forget it! There's no hope for me.

STEVE: Why give up? You have worked hard at your job. You don't know about your girlfriend—what's she doing that's so strange?

THERAPIST: I don't know. None of my work has paid off. My efforts are pointless. It's all coming down to this . . . a disaster!

STEVE: Your efforts are not pointless. A lot of people have rough times at work, and you don't know about your girlfriend. Why don't you talk to her? I know how you feel.

THERAPIST: No, you don't! Not like this! Don't you know what this means? I definitely won't get the raise. I will have to move out of my apartment. Losing my job and apartment will just make my girlfriend dump me.

STEVE: Look, you don't even know if you're not getting the raise. You don't even have any evidence to say why your girlfriend is leaving you. You don't even sound like you're willing to talk to her. You seem like you're having a rough time right now, but every one has problems like this from time to time. You have to be willing to try to do something about it.

THERAPIST: I don't know. This seems worse than anything I have ever seen or heard before.

STEVE: You have to look at this a little differently. First, you need more information about this stuff. You can't come to these conclusions based on what you have told me so far. Anyway, if these things do happen, you'll find a way to get on with your life. Everyone has problems. You are not expected to be perfect.

THERAPIST: I feel like I should be perfect and make my boss and my girlfriend happy.

STEVE: It's impossible to be perfect and to never have any problems.

THERAPIST: Are you sure about that?

STEVE: Of course I am sure. You have to be realistic. I'm sure that there are some things you can do to help.

Note that in this example the therapist presented both a problem that was relevant to the patient's own life experience, and a situation that the patient could objectively appraise. The therapist's aim was to strengthen the rational and adaptive attitude that this individual already held concerning failing in interpersonal relationships. A patient should not perceive a clinician as attempting to patronize or mimic his or her beliefs. Rather, the therapist should explain that these beliefs at times may engender feelings of distress, which in turn may interfere with later attempts to cope with a stressful problem. The clinician indicates that the purpose of this exercise is to facilitate the patient's adoption of a more positive orientation toward problems in living.

PROBLEM DEFINITION AND FORMULATION

The purposes of the next problem-solving task are to understand fully the nature of the problem and to identify a set of realistic goals and objectives. To accomplish this, patients are trained to (1) seek important facts and information concerning the problem; (2) describe these facts in clear and unambiguous terms; (3) differentiate objective facts from unverified inferences, assumptions, and interpretations; (4) identify the factors and circumstances that make the situation a problem; and (5) set a series of realistic problem-solving goals. Emphasis is placed on accuracy and comprehensiveness in defining and formulating a particular problem.

According to our model, clients are taught to be systematic and orderly when approaching problems—that is, to gather information, use concrete language, and separate facts from inferences and assumptions. Essentially, individuals learn to ask a wide variety of the five specific "W" questions: *who* ("Who is involved in this problem?" "Who is responsible for this problem?"); *what* ("What I am feeling about this problem?" "What is happening that is making me feel sad?" "What am I thinking about in reaction to this problem?" "What will happen if I don't solve this problem?"); *where* ("Where is this problem occurring?"); *when* ("When did this problem begin?" "When am I supposed to solve this problem?"); and *why* ("Why did this problem occur?" "Why am I feeling so sad?"). We have found certain occupations to be useful analogies when training patients to use this approach. For example, patients are encouraged to think of themselves in the roles of investigative reporters, detectives, or scientists.

In asking these "W" questions, patients are encouraged to use concrete and unambiguous language in order to minimize the likelihood of confusion and distortions of information. Clients are also taught to identify and correct the types of inferences, assumptions, and misconceptions that they may be making while answering these queries (e.g., selective attention and overgeneralization). Again, various cognitive restructuring strategies, such as the reverse-advocacy role-play strategy described earlier, can be helpful in this process.

In defining and formulating problems, patients are taught to delineate further specific goals and objectives that they would like to reach. Again, these goals are specified in concrete and unambiguous terms to minimize confusion. Clients are especially encouraged to state goals or objectives that are realistic and attainable. It is often the case that a client identifies a series of subgoals that work as steps to reach the overall problem-solving goal. For example, a client may state that an overall goal is to have a satisfying, long-term relationship with a member of the opposite sex. Important subgoals may include (1) ameliorating any personal skill deficits (e.g., communication problems) that may be contributing to difficulties with relationships; (2) meeting more people in general; (3) dating more frequently; and (4) minimizing the amount of distress associated with disappointments and feelings of rejection when they occur.

In specifying goals, two general types can be identified: problem-focused and emotion-focused goals. Problem-focused goals involve objectives that relate to actual changes in the problem itself. These are particularly relevant for situations that are possible to change, such as getting a new job. On the other hand, emotion-focused goals relate to objectives that are aimed at reducing or minimizing the impact of the distress associated with the experience of a problem. These relate to situations that are appraised as unchangeable, such as the death of a family member. In most cases, it is likely that both types of goals are important to identify in order to maximize effective problem-solving coping attempts. In the example above concerning relationships, the various subgoals encompass both types of goals.

The last step in problem definition and formulation training involves identifying those obstacles existing in a given situation that prevent a client from reaching specified goals. The factors that make a situation a problem may involve novelty, as when one moves to a new neighborhood; uncertainty, often experienced at the start of a new job; conflicting stimulus demands, as in arguments with a spouse/partner over issues of child rearing or money management; lack of resources, especially limited finances; or some other personal or environmental constraint or deficiency.

In identifying these obstacles, the therapist should be careful to help the patient accurately analyze the problem situation. Often, articulating these obstacles leads to a reevaluation of goals or a reappraisal of the situation. We have found that several presenting problems of depression, for example, which ultimately include goals of increasing one's self-esteem, actually can encompass a variety of subgoals (such as losing weight or improving physical appearance, job skills, and interpersonal relationships). Accurate identification of the obstacles and conflicts involved in a problem helps a patient deal better with complex problems and understand the "real problem" more clearly.

Within this context, clients are taught to consider alternative problem formulations. In some cases, the problem that was focused on initially may not be the "real" problem (i.e., the basic, primary, or most important problem). The basic problem in some cases may be an earlier problem in a current cause–effect problem chain, where problem A is causing problem B, which in turn is causing problem C. Another possibility is that the more important problem may be a broader or more complex problem, of which the specific problem focused on initially is only a part. Once this broader, more complex problem is identified, it can then be dealt with as a whole, or it may be solved more effectively by breaking it down into more manageable subproblems and working on each of them one at a time.

GENERATION OF ALTERNATIVE SOLUTIONS

The overall objective of the next problem-solving operation is to make available as many alternative solutions to the problem as possible, to increase the likelihood that the most effective ones will eventually be identified. In generating these alternatives, individuals are taught to use three general brainstorming principles: quantity, deferment of judgment, and variety.

According to the quantity principle, the more ideas one produces, the higher the likelihood that effective or good-quality options will be among those generated. Clients are encouraged to produce as many ideas as possible for each of the subgoals (both problem-focused and emotion-focused goals). The second principle, deferment of judgment, suggests that the quantity rule can best be carried out if one withholds judgment about the quality or effectiveness of any idea until a comprehensive list is produced. The only criterion that may be applied is relevance to the problem at hand; otherwise, evaluation of any option is reserved for the decision-making component. The last brainstorming rule, the variety principle, encourages individuals to think of a wide range of possible solutions across as many strategies or classes of approaches as possible, instead of focusing on only one or two narrow ideas. In generating solution options, individuals are encouraged to continue to use concrete and unambiguous terms.

Clinical Example. Mary was a 51-year-old woman who had recently been diagnosed with breast cancer. Since the diagnosis, she had experienced clinical symptoms of depression that were unrelated to the medical procedures. In working with her, we discovered that her fears of being ill or dying were accompanied by additional concerns. Mary was a widow, living alone, with her adult children nearby. Wanting to remain independent and strong, however, she minimized her need for visitors and support from her friends and family. Respecting her needs, her loved ones made a sincere effort to give Mary "her space" during the recovery process. However, this often left her feeling lonely. During PST, this problem was defined as "wanting to have loved ones in her company more often."

During several brainstorming sessions, Mary generated the following alternative solutions to this problem:

- Request that others visit by writing them letters
- Buy a pet
- Have a party
- Visit others when feeling well
- Invite members of my family to a session so we can problem-solve as a team
- Go to the local community center and see if volunteers can come to my home
- Talk to my friends and family and ask them to visit more often
- Meet new people and forget my family
- Start a reading group at the local bookstore
- Invite friends at church to house
- Buy a computer and send e-mails to family members
- Join local support groups
- Call family and friends more often on the phone

It was only after Mary began generating these ideas that she began to experience hope that she could solve this problem and feel better.

DECISION MAKING

After developing a list of possible alternative solutions, the problem solver's next objective is to choose among these options in order to develop an overall solution plan. To accomplish this process, patients are first encouraged to identify potential consequences of these alternatives. This involves identifying both short-term and long-term consequences, as well as both personal and social consequences.

Personal consequences that can be used as criteria involve effects on one's emotional well-being, amount of time and effort involved, and effects on one's physical well-being and personal growth. Social outcomes entail the consequences associated with the well-being of other individuals and their interpersonal relationships with a patient.

In addition, clients are taught to estimate the likelihood both that a given alternative will be effective in reaching their goals and that they will actually be able to implement the solution optimally. Estimating the latter involves evaluating their unique ability and desire to carry out a solution, regardless of its effect on the problem.

Overall, patients learn first to conduct a rough screening of the list of alternatives previously generated and to eliminate those that are obviously inferior because of associated unacceptable risks or because they are not feasible to implement. Next, they are taught to evaluate each alternative according to the major criteria above, as a means of deciding which alternatives to implement in the real-life setting. The overall cost–benefit ratio for each coping option can be calculated according to a simple rating scale (e.g., −3 = "very unsatisfactory" to +3 = "very satisfactory"). An idea that appears to have a large number of positive consequences and minimal costs may be rated as +2 or +3. Conversely, an alternative that is expected to yield few positive outcomes and a large number of negative consequences may be rated as −2 or −3.

Using these ratings, individuals may then develop an overall solution plan by first comparing the ratings of the various alternative solutions. If only a small number of ideas appear to be rated as potentially satisfactory, then a problem solver must ask several evaluative questions: "Do I have enough information?" "Did I define the problem correctly?" "Are my goals too high?" "Did I generate enough options?" At this point, the patient may need to go back and engage again in the previous problem-solving tasks.

If several effective or satisfactory alternatives are identified, then the client is encouraged to include a combination of potentially effective coping options for each subgoal, in order to "attack" the problem from a variety of perspectives. Furthermore, a contingency plan complete with alternative coping options is often useful in the event that the first group of options fails.

SOLUTION IMPLEMENTATION AND VERIFICATION

The first part of the last problem-solving task involves the actual performance of the chosen solution plan. In essence, the patient may be able to develop an effective solution plan hypothetically; however, if it is never actually carried out, then the problem will never get resolved, nor will the individual receive important "natural" feedback (i.e., problem-solving success or failure).

Clinical Example. At times, some patients inhibit their willingness to implement a solution plan because of fear of failure or poor self-efficacy beliefs. In such cases, we suggest that patients complete a "comparison worksheet," which requires them to list the consequences that will occur if the problem is *not* solved versus the consequences if the problem *is* resolved successfully. The following clinical example, adapted from Nezu et al. (1989), demonstrates this approach.

THERAPIST: Okay, Freda. Last session I had requested that you complete the worksheet that I gave you. Did you have a chance to do it this week?

FREDA: I guess I was supposed to list some of the consequences if my problem of getting a new job wasn't solved, right?

THERAPIST: Yes, as well as listing some of the positive consequences that you thought of when we first began looking at the various options.

FREDA: I did that also.

THERAPIST: Great! Let's start with the consequences if you don't get a new job, okay?

FREDA: Sure. Let's see what I wrote. First, I guess that I would feel horrible about myself. I know that I should get out of my present job. I guess if I don't, I'll be the biggest chicken ever!

THERAPIST: So one of the possible consequences is that you would evaluate yourself negatively. Is that correct?

FREDA: Yeah . . . I really wouldn't feel good about myself at all!

THERAPIST: Okay. Freda, are there any other consequences?

FREDA: Actually, I thought of a whole bunch of them! Another one is that I would continue to have a lousy salary! Without an increase in incoming funds, I'll never be able to get a place of my own and will continue to have problems with my crazy roommate, Hanna. Like I told you before, even though she seems nice on the outside, she always stabs people in the back, saying nasty things about them. I caught her several times doing that about me!

THERAPIST: Okay. Staying put in your current job, then, prevents you from having more money that can be used to get a place of your own.

FREDA: Yeah, that's a real big mess!

THERAPIST: Any others?

FREDA: I've got a few more. In general, though, they all have to do with my crazy roommate.

THERAPIST: Okay, then. Let's go over the possible consequences if you actually carry out your solution plan that we already discussed.

FREDA: Well, it's like the exact opposite! If I get a better-paying job, which I know exists out there, I'll feel better about myself. I'd feel more self-confident. Like you said, my life will never be "problem-free," but I do believe that a better job is a step closer in the right direction!

THERAPIST: Be a little more specific, Freda.

FREDA: Sure. Like I was saying, it's the opposite of the other list. If I get a new job, I can make more money. I would then be able to get a small apartment on my own. I would feel happier and finally feel like I can take risks, even though they are sometimes scary!

THERAPIST: I can certainly understand how you feel. Freda, let me ask you this question now. When you look over both lists of consequences, what's your reaction?

FREDA: I started to realize that I have always looked at it differently, only on the side of how scary risks are. I actually start to get mad at myself for not trying in the past. But I feel like if I keep thinking about the possible good consequences, I will be able to achieve some of my goals. If I don't solve this problem—nobody will do it for me! If I keep on going on like this, I will only get down on myself and get depressed, like usual!

THERAPIST: Okay, Freda. Based on that, what do you think you are going to do?

FREDA: Carry out my solution plan and give myself a chance for a change!

THERAPIST: Good for you!

The second aspect entails the careful monitoring and evaluation of the actual solution outcomes. After the solution plan is carried out, individuals are encouraged to monitor the real-life consequences that occur as a function of the implemented solution. Clients are taught to develop self-monitoring methods relevant to a given problem, which include (1) ratings of the solution outcome themselves (e.g., "Did the plan achieve the specified goals?" "What were the positive consequences?" "What were the negative consequences?"); (2) evaluative ratings of the clients' emotional reactions to these outcomes (e.g., "How do I feel about these outcomes?" "Do they make me happy?" "Am I less anxious?"); and (3) ratings of the degree to which outcomes match the consequences previously anticipated during the decision-making process (e.g., "Did what I predict was going to happen actually happen?")

If the match is satisfactory, then the problem solver is encouraged to administer some form of self-reinforcement, such as self-statements of congratulation or a tangible gift or reward. On the other hand, if the match is unsatisfactory, then he or she is encouraged either to implement the previously identified contingency plan or to recycle through the entire problem-solving process. Particular care should be exercised to differentiate between difficulties with the *performance* or implementation of a coping option and difficulties with the problem-solving *process* itself.

To underscore the importance of a therapist's ability to conduct PST competently and veridically, we have previously offered various "dos and don'ts" for conducting this treatment approach (D'Zurilla & Nezu, 1999; Nezu et al., 1998). These recommendations are presented in Table 7.1.

Empirical Status of PST

During the past two decades, rapidly increasing numbers of outcome studies have provided support for the efficacy of PST for a variety of different client populations and clinical problems, as either the sole treatment, part of a larger treatment package, a maintenance strategy, or a prevention program. For example, studies have focused on the following problems: psychiatric disorders requiring hospitalization, clinical depression, suicidality, anxiety disorders, emotional and behavioral problems in persons with mental retardation, marital/couple problems, parent–adolescent conflicts, parenting problems, substance abuse, weight control problems, severe medical problems, caregiving problems, stress management, competence enhancement, and community problems. Because of space limitations, we are unable to describe all of these outcome studies here. For a complete, critical review of this literature, the reader is referred to D'Zurilla and Nezu (1999). However, because the evidence for the efficacy of PST for clinical depression is particularly strong, we would like to highlight these investigations below.

PST FOR DEPRESSION

Hussian and Lawrence (1981) compared PST with a social reinforcement (SR) program for the treatment of depression in a group of geriatric patients living in a nursing home. Thirty-six patients who scored in the se-

TABLE 7.1. Dos and Don'ts When Conducting PST

1. *Don't* present PST in a mechanistic manner. PST should not be conducted in a rote fashion, devoid of a therapeutic atmosphere. Training in problem-solving skills should be as interactive as possible, consistently focusing on the importance of a positive patient–therapist relationship.

2. *Do* make PST relevant to a particular patient. All training examples should be specific and relevant to the client at hand. The therapist needs to adapt PST to the specific needs of a given patient (group, couple).

3. *Do* include homework assignments. Because practice is an important component of PST, clients should be encouraged to practice as much as possible between sessions.

4. *Do* focus on the patient, as well as the treatment. Although correctly implementing PST is important to ensure its effectiveness, patients themselves should always be the primary focus of attention.

5. *Don't* focus only on superficial problems. PST therapists need to use their own effective problem-solving skills to assess whether the problems being discussed are in fact the most crucial for a given client; otherwise, the effectiveness of treatment will be limited (Nezu & Nezu, 1989).

6. *Do* focus on solution implementation. The patient should be encouraged to implement as many solutions as possible during training in order to experience either success (i.e., problem resolution) or the need to recycle (i.e., troubleshooting and problem solving again if initial solution attempt is unsuccessful).

7. *Don't* ignore emotions in training. PST is geared to achieve not only "problem-focused goals," but "emotion-focused goals" as well.

8. *Do* use handouts as adjuncts to training. Written handouts help clients to remember and practice the skills between sessions. Often it may be useful to encourage patients to purchase a looseleaf notebook to store such handouts for current and future reference. In addition, such handouts need to be relevant to a given target population (e.g., see Nezu et al., 1998, for examples of PST handouts for cancer patients).

Note. These dos and don'ts are adapted from Nezu et al. (1998).

verely depressed range on the Beck Depression Inventory (BDI; Beck, Ward, Mendelson, Mock, & Erbaugh, 1961) were randomly divided into three groups: PST, SR, and a waiting-list control (WLC) group. Both treatment groups met for five 30-minute training sessions during a 1-week period of time. Training was carried out on an individual basis and involved discussion of each of the five stages of the D'Zurilla and Goldfried (1971) model, in addition to practicing solving real-life problems previously generated by the patients. The major objective of the SR program was to increase the rate of reinforcement the participants were receiving in their daily lives. Patients were prompted to engage in various activities such as arts and crafts, and were given SR for attendance, participation in a specific activity, perseverance, and interaction with other patients.

After the first week of treatment, each of the three groups was randomly divided in half to produce six subgroups. One PST subgroup received a second week of PST (PST-PST), whereas the second PST subgroup participated in the SR program (PST-SR). Similarly, one SR subgroup received a second week of SR (SR-SR), while the second SR subgroup received PST (SR-PST). Finally, one WLC subgroup remained on the waiting list for the second week (WLC-WLC), while the second WLC subgroup was changed to an informational control group (WLC-IC), meeting to discuss the various life changes that accompany aging.

At the end of the first week of treatment, both the PST and SR groups showed significantly less depression than did the WLC group. As expected, the PST group showed significantly better performance on a problem-solving test than did the SR group. Pre- to posttreatment assessment results showed a significant reduction in depression only for groups that received PST. The PST-PST group was significantly less depressed than both the WLC-IC and WLC-WLC groups, and the SR-PST group was significantly less depressed than the WLC-IC group. Differences between the SR-SR group and the control groups were not significant. The superiority of PST was maintained at a 2-week follow-up.

In an outcome study focusing on adult unipolar depression, Nezu (1986c) randomly assigned 26 clinically depressed individuals in an outpatient setting to one of three conditions: (1) PST; (2) problem-focused therapy (PFT); or (3) a WLC group. Both therapy conditions were conducted in a group setting over eight weekly sessions lasting from 1 1/2 to 2 hours. PST involved training in the problem-solving skills described by D'Zurilla and Nezu (1982). PFT involved discussions of the subjects' current life problems with a problem-solving goal, but no systematic training in problem-solving skills was provided. Dependent measures were obtained at pretreatment, posttreatment, and at a 6-month follow-up assessment. These measures included the BDI, the Depression scale of the Minnesota Multiphasic Personality Inventory (MMPI-D; Hathaway & McKinley, 1967), the PSI (Heppner & Petersen, 1982), and the Internal–External Locus of Control Scale (Rotter, 1966).

Both traditional statistical analyses and an analysis of the clinical significance of the results indicated substantial reductions in depression in the PST group that were maintained over the 6-month follow-up period, as measured by both the BDI and the MMPI-D. Moreover, the improvement in depression in the PST condition was significantly greater than in the PFT and WLC conditions. The superiority of PST over PFT was maintained at the 6-month follow-up evaluation. Further results revealed that PST participants increased significantly more than the other two groups in self-appraisal of problem-solving effectiveness, and also changed significantly in locus-of-control orientation from external to internal. These improvements were also maintained at the 6-month follow-up. Overall, these results provide support for the basic assumption that PST produces its effects by increasing problem-solving ability and strengthening personal control expectations.

The purpose of a subsequent study by Nezu and Perri (1989) was twofold: (1) to provide for a partial replication of the Nezu (1986c) investigation, and (2) to assess the relative contribution of the problem orientation component in treating depressed individuals. A dismantling research strategy was used to address these goals by randomly assigning 39 individuals who had been reliably diagnosed, according to the Research Diagnostic Criteria (RDC; Spitzer, Endicott, & Robins, 1978), as experiencing major depressive disorder to one of three conditions: (1) PST; (2) abbreviated PST (APST); and (3) a WLC group. In addition to the BDI, the Hamilton Rating Scale for Depression (HRSD; Hamilton, 1960), a measure completed by an independent clinician rater, was used to assess depression. Both treatment conditions included 10 therapy sessions lasting 2 hours each, conducted in groups by pairs of therapists counterbalanced by condition. Participants in the PST condition received training in all five components of the model. APST participants were provided with a similar package, with the exception of training in the problem orientation component. Subjects in the WLC condition were requested to wait until the program was able to accommodate them at a later date. In this manner, the degree to which training in problem orientation contributed to a positive treatment outcome could be determined by such a component analysis.

Pre- to posttreatment analyses indicated that individuals in the PST condition were significantly less depressed at posttreatment, according to both the BDI and HRSD, than were the APST and WLC participants. Furthermore, APST subjects reported significantly lower posttreatment depression scores than WLC participants. Decreases in depressive symptoms were also significantly correlated with increases in problem-solving ability. Furthermore, these results were clinically significant according to a metric whereby a "recovered" individual was defined as a treated subject (i.e., PST and APST participants) who had a posttreatment score two standard deviations beyond the mean of the dysfunctional population (i.e., untreated subjects or WLC participants). When this approach was utilized, over 85% of PST subjects, 50% of APST participants, and only 9% of WLC subjects experienced clinically meaningful decreases in depressive symptoms as measured by the BDI. As measured by the HRSD, these percentages were found to be 79%, 50%, and 9%, respectively.

A 6-month follow-up assessment revealed no significant differences between posttreatment and follow-up scores for either treatment condition. In other words, the therapeutic benefits obtained by participants in both treatment conditions were maintained 6 months after completion of treatment. In general, these overall results provide further support for the efficacy of PST for major depression, as well as underscoring the importance of including training in the problem orientation component.

Continuing this line of research, Arean et al. (1993) applied the Nezu et al. (1989) intervention model of depression specifically to an older population. Seventy-five individuals meeting inclusion criteria—that is, being older than 55 years; meeting RDC for a diagnosis of major depression; and scoring 20 or greater on the BDI, 10 or greater on the Geriatric Depression Scale (GDS; Yesavitch et al., 1983), and at least 18 on the HRSD—were randomly assigned to either PST, reminiscence therapy (RT), or a WLC group.

Both PST and RT were conducted within a group format with one of three therapists who were trained in both treatment approaches. Each group met for 12 weekly sessions lasting approximately 11/2 hours. Participants in the PST condition were trained in the five components of the problem-solving model contained in the Nezu et al. (1989) treatment manual. RT involved reviewing one's life history in order to gain perspective on and satisfaction with major positive and negative life events, and was based on a psychodynamic formulation that had previously received some empirical support for its efficacy for geriatric depression.

Overall results indicated that participants in both therapy conditions were significantly less depressed on all three measures of depression at posttreatment than were individuals in the WLC group. Moreover, the effects found at posttreatment for the PST and RT conditions were maintained 3 months after the completion of treatment. However, individuals in the PST condition reported significantly lower depression at posttreatment than RT participants on two of the three depression measures (i.e., the HRSD and GDS). Moreover, at posttreatment, a significantly greater proportion of individuals in the PST condition (88%), compared with participants in the RT (40%) and WLC (10%) groups, no longer met the RDC for major depression.

Mynors-Wallis, Gath, Lloyd-Thomas, and Tomlinson (1995) compared PST with a antidepressant medication regimen for the treatment of depression in a primary care population. Ninety-one adults with major depression were randomly assigned to PST, amitriptyline, or a drug placebo. Inclusion criteria involved meeting RDC for major depression and scoring 13 or more on the HRSD. In all three treatment conditions, participants were offered six or seven sessions lasting from 30 to 60 minutes over 3 months. Therapists included a psychiatrist and two general practitioners who were trained in PST and drug administration. In both "medication" conditions, patients and therapists were unaware of the accurate nature of the capsules.

In addition to the HRSD, two other outcome measures were employed—the BDI and a self-report measure of social functioning and adjustment. Results indicated that at 6 and 12 weeks posttreatment, the PST group was significantly less depressed on both measures of depression and more socially adjusted than was the placebo group. No significant differences were found between the PST and amitriptyline conditions, which suggests that PST is as effective as a psychopharmacological intervention for the treatment of depression.

CONCLUSIONS AND FUTURE DIRECTIONS

Although methodological problems in many of the outcome studies on PST limit the conclusions that can be drawn, the preponderance of the data support the efficacy of PST as a clinical intervention method for a variety of different psychological, behavioral, and health problems. The evidence indicates that PST not only produces immediate treatment benefits, but also contributes to the maintenance of treatment gains as well as the prevention of future difficulties. At the present time, the strongest treatment efficacy data relate to PST for clinical depression. In addition, the evidence is also very strong for PST as a maintenance strategy following behavioral weight control programs (see D'Zurilla & Nezu, 1999).

As we look ahead, there appears to be a growing trend toward applying PST to new populations and in innovative ways. One major area of research involves applications of PST with medical patients. Investigators at the University of Pittsburgh (Charlotte Brown) and in England (Laurence Mynors-Wallis, Dennis Gath, and their associates) are studying the efficacy of PST in the treatment of medical patients with emotional disorders in primary care settings. In addition, a number of outcome studies are in progress that focus on PST for patients with cancer or their caregivers. Studies on patients with cancer are being conducted at Brown University (Vincent Mor and Susan Allen), MCP Hahnemann University (Arthur Nezu and Christine Nezu), and Pennsylvania State University College of Medicine (Peter Houts). Under the direction of O. J. Sahler and James Varni, studies are being conducted at several different sites across the country on the use of PST to enhance the coping and caregiving abilities of mothers of children with cancer. At the University of Alabama–Birmingham, Timothy Elliott and Richard Shewchuk are evaluating the efficacy of PST for caregivers of patients with spinal cord injuries. At Johns Hopkins University, Matt Loscalzo and James Zabora are focusing on caregivers of three chronically ill populations: patients with cancer, patients with cardiac problems, and people with severe respiratory problems.

Another innovative application of PST is currently being investigated by Christine Nezu and Arthur Nezu at MCP Hahnemann University. These researchers are assessing the efficacy of PST as a means of improving the arousal management skills of sexual offenders and reducing their deviant sexual behavior.

Finally, more research is needed on the study of PST as a prevention strategy for populations at risk for the occurrence of psychological, behavioral, and/or health problems, such as the elderly, adolescents, individuals with health-compromising behavior patterns (e.g., substance abuse, poor diet, lack of exercise), and individuals experiencing high levels of environmental stress (e.g., job stress).

NOTE

1. In this chapter, the abbreviation "PST" refers to either "problem-solving therapy" or "problem-solving training."

2. Copyright 1996 by Marcel Dekker Inc. Adapted from Nezu, Nezu, Rothenberg, and D'Zurilla (1996) by courtesy of Marcel Dekker, Inc.

REFERENCES

Arean, P. A., Perri, M. G., Nezu, A. M., Schein, R. L., Christopher, F., & Joseph, T. X. (1993). Comparative effectiveness of social problem-solving therapy and reminiscence therapy as treatments for depression in older adults. *Journal of Consulting and Clinical Psychology, 61,* 1003–1010.

Beach, L. R., & Mitchell, T. R. (1978). A contingency model for the selection of decision strategies. *Academy of Management Review, 3,* 439–449.

Beck, A. T., Rush, A. J., Shaw, B. F., & Emery, G. (1979). *Cognitive therapy of depression.* New York: Guilford Press.

Beck, A. T., Ward, C. H., Mendelson, M., Mock, L., & Erbaugh, J. (1961). An inventory for measuring depression. *Archives of General Psychiatry, 4,* 561–571.

Bloom, B. L. (1985). *Stressful life event theory and research: Implications for primary prevention* (DHHS Publication No. AMD 85–1385). Rockville, MD: National Institute of Mental Health.

Burks, N., & Martin, B. (1985). Everyday problems and life change events: Ongoing vs. acute sources of stress. *Journal of Human Stress, 11,* 27–35.

Burns, L. R., & D'Zurilla, T. J. (1999). Individual differences in perceived information processing in stress and coping situations: Development and validation of the Perceived Modes of Processing Inventory. *Cognitive Therapy and Research, 23,* 345–371.

Cormier, W. H., Otani, A., & Cormier, S. (1986). The effects of problem-solving training on two problem-solving tasks. *Cognitive Therapy and Research, 10,* 95–108.

Davis, G. A. (1966). Current status of research and theory in human problem solving. *Psychological Bulletin, 66,* 36–54.

D'Zurilla, T. J. (1990). Problem-solving training for effective stress management and prevention. *Journal of Cognitive Psychotherapy: An International Quarterly, 4,* 327–355.

D'Zurilla, T. J., & Goldfried, M. R. (1971). Problem solving and behavior modification. *Journal of Abnormal Psychology, 78,* 107–126.

D'Zurilla, T. J., & Maydeu-Olivares, A. (1995). Conceptual and methodological issues in social problem-solving assessment. *Behavior Therapy, 26,* 409–432.

D'Zurilla, T. J., & Nezu, A. (1980). A study of the generation-of-alternatives process in social problem solving. *Cognitive Therapy and Research, 4,* 67–72.

D'Zurilla, T. J., & Nezu, A. (1982). Social problem solving in adults. In P. C. Kendall (Ed.), *Advances in cognitive-behavioral research and therapy* (Vol. 1, pp. 201–274). New York: Academic Press.

D'Zurilla, T. J., & Nezu, A. M. (1990). Development and preliminary evaluation of the Social Problem-Solving Inventory (SPSI). *Psychological Assessment: A Journal of Consulting and Clinical Psychology, 2,* 156–163.

D'Zurilla, T. J., & Nezu, A. M. (1999). *Problem-solving therapy: A social competence approach to clinical intervention* (2nd ed.). New York: Springer.

D'Zurilla, T. J., Nezu, A. M., & Maydeu-Olivares, A. (in press). *Manual for the Social Problem-Solving Inventory—Revised.* North Tonawanda, NY: Multi-Health Systems.

Edwards, W. (1961). Behavioral decision theory. *Annual Review of Psychology, 12,* 473–498.

Ellis, A., & Dryden, W. (1997). *The practice of rational emotive behavior therapy* (rev. ed.). New York: Springer.

Folkman, S., & Lazarus, R. S. (1988). Coping as a mediator of emotion. *Journal of Personality and Social Psychology, 54,* 466–475.

Frauenknecht, M., & Black, D. R. (1995). Social Problem-Solving Inventory for Adolescents (SPSI-A): Development and psychometric evaluation. *Journal of Personality Assessment, 64,* 522–539.

Freedman, B. I., Rosenthal, L., Donahoe, C. P., Schlundt, D. G., & McFall, R. M. (1978). A social-behavioral analysis of skill deficits in delinquent and nondelinquent adolescent boys. *Journal of Consulting and Clinical Psychology, 46,* 1448–1462.

Getter, H., & Nowinski, J. K. (1981). A free response test of interpersonal effectiveness. *Journal of Personality Assessment, 45,* 301–308.

Goddard, P., & McFall, R. M. (1992). Decision-making skills and heterosexual competence in college women: An information-processing analysis. *Journal of Social and Clinical Psychology, 11,* 401–425.

Hamilton, M. (1960). A rating scale for measuring depression. *Journal of Neurology, Neurosurgery and Psychiatry, 23,* 56–62.

Hathaway, S. R., & McKinley, J. C. (1967). *The Minnesota Multiphasic Personality Inventory.* New York: Psychological Corporation.

Heppner, P. P. (1988). *The Problem-Solving Inventory.* Palo Alto, CA: Consulting Psychologists Press.

Heppner, P. P., & Petersen, C. H. (1982). The development and implications of a personal problem solving inventory. *Journal of Counseling Psychology, 29,* 66–75.

Hussian, R. A., & Lawrence, P. S. (1981). Social reinforcement of activity and problem-solving training in the treatment of depressed institutionalized elderly patients. *Cognitive Therapy and Research, 5,* 57–69.

Kanner, A. D., Coyne, J. C., Schaefer, C., & Lazarus, R. S. (1981). Comparison of two modes of stress measurement: Daily hassles and uplifts versus major life events. *Journal of Behavioral Medicine, 4,* 1–39.

Kant, G. L., D'Zurilla, T. J., & Maydeu-Olivares, A. (1997). Social problem solving as a mediator of stress-related depression and anxiety in middle-aged and elderly community residents. *Cognitive Therapy and Research, 21,* 73–96.

Kendall, P. C., & Hollon, S. D. (Eds.). (1979). *Cognitive-behavioral interventions: Theory, research, and procedures.* New York: Academic Press.

Lazarus, R. S. (1999). *Stress and emotion: A new synthesis.* New York: Springer.

Lazarus, R. S., & Folkman, S. (1984). *Stress, appraisal, and coping.* New York: Springer.

McFall, R. M. (1982). A review and reformulation of the concept of social skills. *Behavioral Assessment, 4,* 1–33.

Marx, E. M., Williams, J. M. G., & Claridge, G. C. (1992). Depression and social problem solving. *Journal of Abnormal Psychology, 101,* 78–86.

Maydeu-Olivares, A., & D'Zurilla, T. J. (1996). A factor-analytic study of the Social Problem-Solving Inventory: An integration of theory and data. *Cognitive Therapy and Research, 20,* 115–133.

Maydeu-Olivares, A., & D'Zurilla, T. J. (1997). The factor structure of the Problem-Solving Inventory. *European Journal of Psychological Assessment, 13,* 206–215.

Mooney, R. L., & Gordon, L. V. (1950). *Manual: The Mooney Problem Checklist.* New York: Psychological Corporation.

Mynors-Wallis, L. M., Gath, D. H., Lloyd-Thomas, A. R., & Tomlinson, D. (1995). Randomised controlled trial comparing problem solving treatment with amitriptyline and placebo for major depression in primary care. *British Medical Journal, 310,* 441–445.

Nezu, A., & D'Zurilla, T. J. (1979). An experimental evaluation of the decision-making process in social problem solving. *Cognitive Therapy and Research, 3,* 269–277.

Nezu, A., & D'Zurilla, T. J. (1981a). Effects of problem definition and formulation on decision making in the social problem-solving process. *Behavior Therapy, 12,* 100–106.

Nezu, A., & D'Zurilla, T. J. (1981b). Effects of problem definition and formulation on the generation of alternatives in the social problem-solving process. *Cognitive Therapy and Research, 6,* 265–271.

Nezu, A. M. (1986a). Effects of stress from current problems: Comparisons to major life events. *Journal of Clinical Psychology, 42,* 847–852.

Nezu, A. M. (1986b). Negative life stress and anxiety: Problem solving as a moderator variable. *Psychological Reports, 58,* 279–283.

Nezu, A. M. (1986c). Efficacy of a social problem solving therapy approach for unipolar depression. *Journal of Consulting and Clinical Psychology, 54,* 196–202.

Nezu, A. M. (1987). A problem-solving formulation of depression: A literature review and proposal of a pluralistic model. *Clinical Psychology Review, 7,* 121–144.

Nezu, A. M., & D'Zurilla, T. J. (1989). Social problem solving and negative affective conditions. In P. C. Kendall & D. Watson (Eds.), *Anxiety and depression: Distinctive and overlapping features* (pp. 285–315). New York: Academic Press.

Nezu, A. M., & Nezu, C. M. (Eds.). (1989). *Clinical decision making in behavior therapy: A problem solving perspective.* Champaign, IL: Research Press.

Nezu, A. M., Nezu, C. M., Faddis, S., DelliCarpini, L. A., & Houts, P. S. (1995, November). *Social problem solving as a moderator of cancer-related stress.* Paper presented at the annual convention of the Association for Advancement of Behavior Therapy, Washington, DC.

Nezu, A. M., Nezu, C. M., Friedman, S. H., Faddis, S., & Houts, P. S. (1998). *Helping cancer patients cope: A problem-solving approach.* Washington, DC: American Psychological Association.

Nezu, A. M., Nezu, C. M., & Perri, M. G. (1989). *Problem-solving therapy for depression: Therapy, research, and clinical guidelines.* New York: Wiley.

Nezu, A. M., Nezu, C. M., Rothenberg, J. L., & D'Zurilla, T. J. (1996). Problem-solving therapy. In J. S. Kantor (Ed.), *Clinical depression during addiction recovery: Process, diagnosis, and treatment* (pp. 187–219). New York: Dekker.

Nezu, A. M., Nezu, C. M., Saraydarian, L., Kalmar, K., & Ronan, G. F. (1986). Social problem solving as a moderator variable between negative life stress and depressive symptoms. *Cognitive Therapy and Research, 10,* 489–498.

Nezu, A. M., & Perri, M. G. (1989). Social problem solving therapy for unipolar depression: An initial dismantling investigation. *Journal of Consulting and Clinical Psychology, 57,* 408–413.

Nezu, A. M., & Ronan, G. F. (1985). Life stress, current problems, problem solving, and depressive symptomatology: An integrative model. *Journal of Consulting and Clinical Psychology, 53,* 693–697.

Nezu, A. M., & Ronan, G. F. (1988). Stressful life events, problem solving, and depressive symptoms among university students: A prospective analysis. *Journal of Counseling Psychology, 35,* 134–138.

Osborn, A. (1963). *Applied imagination: Principles and procedures of creative problem solving* (3rd ed.). New York: Scribner.

Platt, J. J., Husband, S. D., Hermalin, J., Cater, J., & Metzger, D. (1993). A cognitive problem-solving employment readiness intervention for methadone clients. *Journal of Cognitive Psychotherapy: An International Quarterly, 7,* 21–33.

Platt, J. J., & Spivack, G. (1975). *Manual for the Means–Ends Problem-Solving Procedure (MEPS): A measure of interpersonal cognitive problem-solving skills.* Philadelphia: Hahnemann Community Mental Health/Mental Retardation Center.

Platt, J. J., Taube, D. O., Metzger, D. S., & Duome, M. J. (1988). Training in interpersonal problem solving (TIPS). *Journal of Cognitive Psychotherapy: An International Quarterly, 2,* 5–34.

Rotter, J. B. (1966). Generalized expectancies for internal versus external control of reinforcements. *Psychological Monographs, 80*(1, Whole No. 609).

Schotte, D. E., & Clum, G. A. (1987). Problem-solving skills in suicidal psychiatric patients. *Journal of Consulting and Clinical Psychology, 55,* 49–54.

Skinner, B. F. (1953). *Science and human behavior.* New York: Macmillan.

Spitzer, R. L., Endicott, J., & Robins, E. (1978). Research Diagnostic Criteria: Rationale and reliability. *Archives of General Psychiatry, 36,* 773–782.

Spivack, G., Platt, J. J., & Shure, M. B. (1976). *The problem-solving approach to adjustment.* San Francisco: Jossey-Bass.

Spivack, G., Shure, M. B., & Platt, J. J. (1985). *Means–Ends Problem Solving (MEPS): Stimuli and scoring procedures supplement.* Unpublished manuscript, Hahnemann University.

Weinberger, M., Hiner, S. L., & Tierney, W. M. (1987). In support of hassles as a measure of stress in predicting health outcomes. *Journal of Behavioral Medicine, 10,* 19–31.

Yesavitch, J., Brink, T., Rose, T., Lum, O., Hsuang, O., Adey, V., & Leier, V. (1983). Development and validation of a geriatric screening scale: A preliminary report. *Journal of Psychiatric Research, 17,* 37–49.

8

Cognitive-Behavioral Therapy with Youth

LAUREN BRASWELL
PHILIP C. KENDALL

The field of cognitive-behavioral therapy (CBT) with children and adolescents has experienced both expansion and refinement over the past decade. Since the publication of the original version of this chapter, there have been edited volumes focusing on CBT with youth (e.g., Finch, Nelson, & Ott, 1993; Kendall, 2000; Reinecke, Dattilio, & Freeman, 1996; Wilkes, Belsher, Rush, Frank, & Associates, 1994), various review articles (e.g., Ager & Cole, 1991; Kendall, 1993; Kendall & Panichelli-Mindel, 1995; Spence, 1994), meta-analyses (e.g., Baer & Nietzel, 1991; Durlak, Fuhrman, & Lampman, 1991), and an ever-burgeoning literature on the efficacy of various forms of CBT with young people. There continues to be a tremendous need for carefully executed treatment outcome studies with children (Kendall, 1998; Kendall, Flannery-Schroeder, & Ford, 1999; Weisz, Huey, & Weersing, 1998). Relative to a decade ago, however, the CBT outcome literature with children has greater breadth—and, in the case of some childhood disorders, depth—than had been the case. More specific approaches for adolescents have also been developed (Holmbeck, Calder, Shapera, Westhoven, Kenealy, & Updegrove, 2000). As will be discussed, some approaches that appeared as promising 10 years ago can now be recommended with confidence, whereas other treatments have not measured up to their early promise.

It is useful to view CBT with youth in its historical context. Such a historical perspective is presented in the definition of CBT originally offered by Kendall and Hollon (1979): CBT is "a purposeful attempt to preserve the demonstrated effectiveness of behavior modification within a less doctrinaire context and to incorporate the cognitive activities of the client in the effort to produce therapeutic change" (p. 1). Cognitive-behavioral (CB) strategies with children and adolescents use enactive, performance-based procedures as well as cognitive interventions to produce changes in thinking, feeling, and behavior (Kendall, 2000). Various forms of CBT with youth share the common goal of helping young people develop a world view that is characterized by a constructive problem-solving attitude. As described by Kendall and Panichelli-Mindel (1995), the problem-solving orientation can also be referred to as a "coping template." Through the provision of carefully planned experiences, CBT helps young people and their families build an adaptive, problem-solving perspective.

The CB therapist working with children and adolescents is called upon to fulfill the roles of diagnostician, consultant, and educator (Kendall, 2000). As a diagnostician, the therapist integrates data about a particular young client from a variety of sources, and combines this information with knowledge of psychopathology and normal child developmental processes to create a problem formulation. As a consultant, the therapist shares the problem formulation and the knowledge of the costs and expected benefits of different treatment options with the family members, to help them prioritize treatment goals and make choices about treatment strategies. Depending upon the treatment options selected, the therapist then provides education about the child's or adolescent's disorder and training in the needed skill areas for the young client and/or parents. In general, the CB therapist can describe him- or herself as functioning like a *coach* for the young person and/or the family (Kendall, 2000). The coaching analogy helps the child or adolescent understand that the therapist may be intensively involved with him or her for a given period of time, but, except in more unusual cases, is unlikely to be part of the family's support system for years to come.

Although there are similarities in the activities of CB therapists working with youth and with adults, in the sections that follow, the theoretical streams of influence more unique to youth-oriented CBT and differences in working with youth versus adults are considered. Next, the major content areas of CBT with children and adolescents are described, followed by a discussion of applications of CBT with specific juvenile disorders. The chapter concludes with a consideration of unresolved issues and questions for further research.

THEORETICAL INFLUENCES
ON THE DEVELOPMENT OF CBT WITH YOUTH

The theoretical lines of influence that gave rise to CB methods used with adults, such as the development of behaviorists' interest in the phenomenon of self-control and the emergence of cognitive learning theories of psychotherapy, also contributed to the rise of CBT with children and adolescents (Kendall & Hollon, 1979). In addition, CBT with youth benefited from the contributions of developmental psychology, including study of the development of self-control, social cognition, learning and memory, metacognitive skills, and attributional processes.

The study of both the development of self-control and the factors interfering with self-control played an interesting role in the emergence of certain CBT methods with children. The work of Luria (1961) and Vygotsky (1962), for instance, provided an initial theoretical formulation for understanding the emergence of verbal self-regulation or mediation of behavior. Mischel (1974) articulated the role of self-instructions and self-praise in reducing children's level of frustration in delay-of-gratification tasks, while Patterson and Mischel (1976) examined the role of verbal strategies in helping children resist distraction. Together, these bodies of work strongly influenced the development of the verbal self-instructional procedures originally employed by Meichenbaum and Goodman (1971).

The study of the development of social-cognitive processes played a role in the emergence of cognitive theories of juvenile disorders. The term "social cognition" (Shantz, 1983) refers to internal events or processes that are thought to mediate actions related to other people and their affairs. Although Piaget (1926) began to study social perspective taking in young children over 70 years ago, developmentalists did not display intense research interest in this area until the 1970s (Chandler, 1973; Hudson, 1978; Selman & Byrne, 1974; Selman, 1980; Shantz, 1975). Building on this research, Dodge (1986) proposed a social-cognitive information-processing model that explores and clarifies the particular social-cognitive factors associated with the emergence of problems with aggression in children. For example, Dodge and colleagues have observed that children who display aggressive behavior perceive and encode cues from their social environment in a manner different from that of nonaggressive peers. Those who tend to be aggressive display a pattern of attending to fewer cues before interpreting the behavior of others, and they tend to perceive others as being hostile in circumstances in which nonaggressive children perceive benign or neutral intentions (Dodge & Frame, 1982; Dodge & Newman, 1981; Dodge, Pettit, McClaskey, & Brown, 1986). Aggressive children also display a tendency to underperceive their own level of aggression (Lochman, 1987). Such efforts highlight the importance of cognitive as well as behavioral processes that may characterize a particular childhood difficulty. Research on social-cognitive processes has also begun to examine how a child's family may enhance certain social-cognitive factors, such as interpretation of an ambiguous social situation (Barrett, Rapee, Dadds, & Ryan, 1996).

A closely related line of research has explored the expectations and attributional processes of children and adolescents (Braswell, Koehler, & Kendall, 1985; Gladstone, Kaslow, Seeley, & Lewinsohn, 1997; Kortlander, Kendall, & Panichelli-Mindel, 1997; Mattis & Ollendick, 1997). The results of this literature suggest that young people's attributions for specific events and their preferences for particular kinds of explanations (i.e., their attributional style) have important therapeutic implications. Interestingly, a young client's attributional style seems to affect the therapy process and outcome, yet attributions can also be targets of intervention. As one might predict, however, some evidence also suggests that young children's attributional styles are not as "set" as those of older adolescents and adults (Turner & Cole, 1994). Research on parents' attributions about the causes and controllability of various child behaviors also has relevance for designing interventions that incorporate parents in maximally effective ways (Johnston & Patenaude, 1994; Smith & O'Leary, 1995).

The study of children's learning and memory processes has also influenced the use of certain CB strategies with such children (Cohen & Schleser, 1984; Reeve & Brown, 1985). As discussed by Kimball, Nelson, and Politano (1993), children's learning of information presented by modeling is clearly influenced by the development of attentional and retentional capacities. For example, young children may attend to only one aspect of a problem without integrating information that is presented sequentially. They may be likely to attend to aspects of a presentation that are sensational but perhaps peripheral to the central content to be delivered.

This brief listing of areas of developmental research merely illustrates the impact of developmental psychology upon CBT, and only highlights a few of the bodies of knowledge that have been integrated. It is hoped that future CBT efforts will remain guided by developmental research and theory.

DIFFERENCES IN WORKING
WITH YOUTH VERSUS ADULTS

Although there are obvious differences in conducting treatment with youth versus adults, factors relevant to how one conducts CBT include (1) the need for careful attention to a young client's level of cognitive and affective development, (2) use of age-appropriate modes of delivery of the therapy content, (3) the recognition of the differences in how young clients come to treatment, and (4) recognition of the extent to which a young client is embedded in his or her social context.

Attention to the cognitive and affective development of the client is important for any therapist; when one works with children and adolescents, it is crucial. An understanding of a youth's memory capacity is important for successful intervention, as well as an understanding of factors such as attentional capacity, verbal fluency and comprehension, and the capacity for conceptual reasoning. Some of the cognitive strategies that would be appropriate for use with adult clients may not be fully understood or managed by young clients, especially younger children. For example, the successful application of Ellis's rational emotive behavior therapy (Ellis, 1970; Dryden & Ellis, Chapter 9, this volume) or Beck's cognitive therapy for depression (Beck, Rush, Shaw, & Emery, 1979; DeRubeis, Tang, & Beck, Chapter 10, this volume) assumes that the client has the cognitive capacity to distinguish between rational and irrational thinking once this distinction has been discovered and identified by the therapist and client. A young child may be likely to perceive an Ellis-like confrontation of irrational thinking as scolding, as well as to find it difficult to comprehend the intended philosophical change.

Given the young client's developmental status, a CB therapist must also be apprised of age-appropriate modes of delivery of information. Or, in plainer language, when working with children, a therapist must be able to teach in a playful manner and play in a way that teaches (Kendall, Chu, Gifford, Hayes, & Nauta, 1998). Some children are not ready for a treatment that relies on verbal discourse as the only form of communication. The therapist must be comfortable with acting out important concepts through the use of puppets, manipulation of toys, or involvement in role play. The child therapist should also be able to help children develop visual representations of the ideas being addressed through artwork; drawing together on a blackboard; or the use of books, workbooks, or other visual aids. Simple, repetitive play activities, such as kneading clay, may also be useful when a child is able to talk but needs something to do with his or her hands to continue to feel comfortable. The play methods are not the primary concern, but the therapist needs to be prepared to engage the child in a developmentally appropriate manner, whatever that therapist's theoretical allegiance.

Work with children and adolescents also differs in terms of the typical method of referral for treatment. Perhaps a small number of adult clients are ordered into treatment by authorities, such as the court system, but the majority of adults choose to receive psychotherapy. Children and adolescents, however, do not phone to initiate their own appointments for treatment, even when they are in great psychological pain. Rather, their treatment is a result of the concern of adults around them—in most cases, their parents or teachers. Research suggests that both a parent's emotional state (Conrad & Hammen, 1989; Webster-Stratton & Hammond, 1988) and the degree of parental contribution to a child's difficulties (Reid, Kavanagh, & Baldwin, 1987) may influence the parent's tendency to perceive the child as having a difficulty requiring treatment. The gatekeeping role of adults can influence which types of young people are most likely to be brought in for mental health services. Adults are more likely to refer themselves for conditions that are causing them personal pain, such as depression or anxiety. At least in the United States, adults are more likely to seek treatment for youth who are displaying symptoms of disruptive behavior, such as vandalism, stealing, and aggression (Weisz & Weiss, 1991). In other words, adults tend to bring in young persons who are causing pain to adults, rather than youth who are necessarily experiencing pain themselves. Fortunately, parents and teachers are becoming more sensitive to recognizing the treatment needs of children and adolescents who are depressed and/or anxious, but these types of youth still represent an underserved group.

As illustrated in the preceding discussion, a young client is much more embedded in the social context of his or her family and school than is typically the case for an adult client (Craighead, Meyers, & Craighead, 1985). This state of affairs has implications both for the identification of the ongoing causes of the youth's difficulties and for the development of the treatment plan. The recognition of the role of the parents and other powerful people in the young person's life, and the inclusion of these individuals in some aspect of the intervention process, is often crucial for the successful treatment of the young client. As discussed by Braswell (1991), previous CBT efforts have varied widely in the extent to which parents were explicitly incorporated in the treatment process, but the current trend is toward the inclusion of parents in the treatment of virtually all forms of youth mental and behavioral health concerns.

COMMON TREATMENT COMPONENTS

Although CBT varies according to the age of the young client and the presenting problem, several strategies are generally considered common to this approach to treatment (Kendall, 1993). In this section, we discuss problem solving, cognitive restructuring, self-regulation, affective education, relaxation training, modeling, role plays, and behavioral contingencies. Following these discussions, we consider the applications of the strategies to specific juvenile disorders.

Problem-Solving Orientation and Training

Problem solving characterizes the general orientation of the therapist, regardless of the specific strategies being trained, and is common across different types of juvenile disorders. The CB clinician approaches the young client's or family's difficulties as problems to be solved, rather than as inevitable outcomes of a specific disease process or family circumstance. CBT recommends that the therapist use the problem-solving orientation not only when addressing the client's presenting complaint, but also when confronting a variety of dilemmas that may occur during the course of treatment. For example, the therapist not only can assist a family in problem solving regarding parent–child conflicts, but can also actively use problem solving to handle issues such as poor attendance at therapy sessions, client behavior during the session, or difficulty locating suggested supportive resources. The therapist models problem solving when handling issues related to the therapist's behavior (e.g., misplacement of keys for the office or difficulty locating needed testing or play materials). Such modeling is not enacted in an effort to have the therapist appear incompetent, but rather to provide a real-life demonstration of the pragmatic value of problem-solving strategies for the client and family.

Problem-solving training as a specific treatment component has a rich history of applications with both youth and adults. The 1970s brought a dramatic increase in attempts to formulate problem solving as a set of skills relevant for clinical endeavors (e.g., D'Zurilla & Goldfried, 1971; Mahoney, 1977). Spivack, Shure, Platt, and their associates hypothesized that effective interpersonal cognitive problem solving demands a number of subskills, such as sensitivity to human problems, the ability to generate alternative solutions, the capacity to conceptualize the appropriate means to achieve a given solution, and a sensitivity to consequences and cause–effect relationships in human behavior (Shure & Spivack, 1978; Spivack, Platt, & Shure, 1976).

Many formulations of specific problem-solving steps are consistent with the subskills articulated by Spivack, Shure, and their colleagues. A typical problem-solving training format might include teaching the young client and/or family to become more skilled at recognizing or identifying problems ("Slow down. What's the problem?"), at generating alternatives ("What are my choices?"), at evaluating emotional and behavioral consequences ("What would happen with this choice? How might I feel?"), at selecting and implementing a choice or solution ("Now how do I carry out the best choice?"), and finally at evaluating the success of the selected alternative ("How did that choice work? Should I make another choice next time?"). In some problem-solving approaches, clients are encouraged to use specific language, whereas in others the problem-solving steps are presented as an outline to guide problem discussion. Table 8.1 presents an example of a problem-solving outline suggested by Arthur L. Robin (personal communication, January 5, 2000) for use with parents and adolescents.

As will be detailed in the section on applications, problem-solving training approaches have attained positive outcomes when used as a component in the treatment of a variety of emotional and behavioral difficulties experienced by children and adolescents. Although the problem-solving process may be similar across different types of difficulties, the focus of problem-solving efforts may vary. In situations involving parent–adolescent conflict, problem-solving training may be used to create a reasonable set of expectations for the adolescents' home and/or school behavior and to clarify how unmet expectations can be corrected. Similarly, parents and their teenage children may need to use a problem-solving process to discover

---

TABLE 8.1. Problem-Solving Steps for Adolescents and Parents

I. Define the problem.
   A. You each tell the others what they are doing that bothers you and why.
      1. Be brief.
      2. Be positive, not accusing.
   B. You each repeat the others' statements of the problem to check out your understanding of what they said.
II. Generate alternative solutions.
   A. You take turns listing possible solutions.
   B. You follow three rules for listing solutions:
      1. List as many ideas as possible.
      2. Don't evaluate the ideas.
      3. Be creative; suggest crazy ideas.
   C. You won't have to do it just because you say it.
III. Evaluate/decide upon the best idea.
   A. You take turns evaluating each idea.
      1. Would this idea solve the problem for you?
      2. Would this idea solve the problem for others?
      3. Rate the idea "plus" or "minus" on a worksheet.
   B. You select the best idea.
      1. Look for ideas rated "plus" by all.
         a. Select one such idea.
         b. Combine several such ideas.
      2. If no ideas are rated "plus" by all, see where you came closest to agreement and negotiate a compromise.
         If two parents are participating, look for ideas rated "plus" by one parent and the teenager.
IV. Plan to implement the selected solution.
   A. You decide who will do what, when, where, and how.
   B. Plan reminders for task completion.
   C. Plan consequences for compliance or noncompliance.

Note. From A. L. Robin (personal communication, January 5, 2000). Reprinted with permission.

new, more age-appropriate ways to have fun together as a family, while still respecting the teenagers' need for time with peers. Problem-solving with a child or adolescent displaying aggression may focus on determining more appropriate ways to communicate anger, acquire desired objects from others, and/or attain legitimate power within the peer group. With a depressed young client, problem-solving training may be used to explore how to put more pleasurable events into the client's life, how to attain more positive peer contacts, or how to develop greater skill in an area where the client would like to experience feelings of mastery. For anxious youth, problem-solving training might be directed toward creating an action plan for a situation that has previously been viewed as threatening or overwhelming.

In addition to differences in the kinds of problems to be addressed with youth manifesting different disorders, different disorders are associated with certain difficulties with the problem-solving process. For example, youth prone to aggression and other acting-out difficulties may need special training and support in the problem formulation phase, due to their tendency to misperceive the intentions of others and overperceive hostility in their social environment. They may also need help slowing themselves down during the alternative generation phase, so they can generate more nonaggressive alternatives for addressing the problem situation. Children and adolescents who are depressed may also need special encouragement when asked to generate a variety of alternatives, for they may be struggling with depressive rigidity in their thinking (Stark, 1990). Depressed youth also need help learning to refrain from prematurely dismissing a possible solution before it has been thoroughly evaluated (Stark, Rouse, & Livingston, 1991). As illustrated in these examples, problem-solving training is conceptualized as a flexible vehicle that can be easily adapted to the needs of individual clients and their families. It is not so much an end as a means to guide clients and their families to identify even more specific skill needs that could/should be addressed.

Cognitive Restructuring

Research suggests that children displaying emotional and behavioral concerns engage in various forms of negative thinking about the self (Crick & Dodge, 1994; Hammen, 1988; Kendall, Stark, & Adam, 1990; Rabian, Peterson, Richters, & Jensen, 1993). The field is moving beyond simply identifying that, for example, depressed youth make certain negative attributions about themselves, to formulations that explore the interconnections between negative cognitive representations and the youth's social world (Rudolph, Hammen, & Burge, 1997). Cognitive restructuring methods (e.g., Beck et al., 1979; Ellis & Harper, 1975) were developed as a means of addressing these negative cognitive representations, whether they be expectations, beliefs, or self-statements. As illustrated in many of the chapters of this volume, cognitive restructuring activities remain at the core of much of CBT conducted with adults. There are various types of cognitive restructuring, but all variations involve first helping the client become aware of self-statements, expectancies, or beliefs that reflect unhelpful ways of thinking about the self, the world, and/or the future. The therapist then guides the client to consider the connection between these negative thoughts and the client's emotional experience. Finally, the therapist and client collaborate in various ways to identify, create, and test more adaptive ways of thinking.

In work with children or adolescents, the basic elements of cognitive restructuring are similar to those used with adult clients, but the clinician must give careful consideration to the young client's developmental level. Harter (1982) has noted that children younger than 5 or 6 years of age are usually not interested in or capable of dispassionate reflection upon their thoughts and/or thinking processes. Over the elementary school years, this capacity for self-reflection develops, with children first being able to examine thoughts about issues that are highly salient and current in their lives. It is probably not until adolescence, and/or the achievement of a cognitive-developmental level comparable to Piaget's stage of formal operations, that clients can fully examine thoughts as examples of broader schemata that have developed over time and as a result of specific experiences. Of course, a young person is in the process of schema formation, so it makes sense that it would be difficult to identify consistent world views and expectancies in one too young!

When conducting cognitive restructuring with a child, a therapist often introduces the notion of examining one's thinking by having the child fill in "thought bubbles" over the heads of cartoon characters facing various scenarios (see Kendall, 1990; Kendall, Chansky, et al., 1992). When the child seems to understand the concept of how thoughts accompany actions and feeling states, the therapist may then ask the child to keep a simple self-statement log or diary of a particular kind of thought, such as a self-putdown or other type of negative self-statement relevant to the child's presenting concerns. Several programs for children recommend presenting the idea of being a "thought detective," to help a child understand the task of discovering when these negative thoughts are occurring (Stark, 1990; Stark et al., 1996). The therapist then guides the child to consider the connection between these negative thoughts and unpleasant emotions, perhaps having the child conduct mood ratings in connection with their thought monitoring. Through guided questioning and designing and conducting behavioral experiments, the clinician then introduces the possibility that one could choose to think differently about the matter at hand, and that thinking differently could lead to feeling differently.

Attribution retraining is an example of early efforts at cognitive restructuring with children (Dweck, 1975). This form of cognitive restructuring was based upon the cognitive theories of motivation espoused by Bandura (1969) and Weiner (1979). These theories emphasized how the child's causal explanations for why he or she was performing well or poorly had implications for his or her behavioral persistence, expectancies for future performance, and affective reactions to success and failure. Most efforts at attribution retraining attempt to create a training environment in which the child learns to take more individual credit for his or her academic or other achievements, thus encouraging the child's experience of positive control and/or self-efficacy. Dweck (1975), for example, worked with failure-prone elementary-school-age children who tended to be debilitated by their academic difficulties. In Dweck's attribution retraining condition, these children received repeated practice in solving math problems. When they experienced some failure, they were told that "failure means you should try harder." In contrast to a success-only training group, the children receiving the attribution retraining displayed increased persistence in attempting to solve problems and a shift in their belief system about failure, with an increased tendency to attribute failure to lack of effort rather than lack of ability. Further research suggested that this form of attribution retraining is most likely to be successful when used with students who are not applying the knowledge or skills they already possess, or when used in conjunction with teaching new problem-solving strategies (Clifford, 1984; Schunk, 1983).

In addition to uniquely child-focused examples of cognitive restructuring, such as attribution retraining, efforts more like those associated with Beck's cognitive therapy for depression have also been employed with children and adolescents (Dudley, 1997; Stark, 1990; Wilkes et al., 1994). As with adults, the therapist elicits negative self-statements in various ways. Once these self-statements have been identified, the young client and the therapist then collaborate in examining the evidence that supports or refutes this negative interpretation. The question "What's the evidence to support this view?" may be one of the most basic tools of cognitive restructuring, followed by the question "Is there another way of looking at or explaining this observation?" With this second question, the therapist helps the child or adolescent explore alternative explanations that could account for his or her troubling observations (e.g., a friend did not say hello when passed in the hallway). A third common question used in cognitive restructuring involves asking "What if . . . ?" or, put another way, "Even if the observation is true and there's not an alternative explanation, is this really so terrible?" (e.g., "Your friend didn't say hello. She may or may not be mad at you, but even if she *is* mad, is that so catastrophic?"). As discussed by Stark (Stark, 1990; Stark, Boswell, & Hoke, 2000), clinicians working with children and adolescents must be cautious in the use of "What if . . . ?"

questions, for if there is not a solid therapist–client relationship or the statement is made in a sarcastic manner, the client may feel that the therapist is mocking him or her. Beyond using these standard questions for discussion, the therapist may also help the client formulate a behavioral experiment to gather evidence for or against a particular viewpoint. Wilkes et al. (1994) present a number of examples of such experiments, including one in which a learning-disabled teenager was helped to test his belief that if he asked questions in school, his peers would think he was "dumb." With the help of the therapist, he created a plan to note the number of questions being asked in the classroom by individuals he viewed as "smart" versus those he considered "not so smart." In this way, he was able to surprise himself with data indicating that more questions were asked by people he viewed as "smart."

The targets of cognitive restructuring tend to vary with the presenting difficulties of the child or adolescent. As noted by Kendall, Kortlander, Chansky, and Brady (1992), given the anticipatory nature of anxiety, the therapist is likely to engage in careful exploration of maladaptive expectations related to upcoming events. With depressed clients, there is more of a tendency to ruminate and form misattributions about events in the past. Feindler and colleagues (Feindler, 1991; Feindler & Ecton, 1986) noted that youth with serious anger control difficulties may need cognitive restructuring that addresses their hostile interpretations of interactions, their beliefs in the legitimacy of aggression and retaliation, and their expectations of being immune from consequences.

The use of age-appropriate materials can be very helpful is accomplishing the very abstract task of examining and changing distorted thinking. Dudley (1997) has developed a curriculum for group cognitive therapy with depressed children or adolescents that includes many charts, graphs, stories, and illustrations depicting youth of varying cultural and ethnic backgrounds. Such visual aids, as well as the use of appropriate workbook-type materials (Kendall, 1992; Nelson & Finch, 1996; Stark et al., 1996), can be extremely valuable in helping the CB clinician communicate about complex cognitive constructs with school-age and adolescent clients.

When working with a young client, one must be equally attuned to the cognitive processing of the parents, for their expectancies and beliefs about their child's situation will have direct impact on their parenting behavior and their choices of treatment for their child and/or family. In particular, the CB clinician must strive to be sensitive to the parents' beliefs about the cause of their child's difficulties; otherwise, it may be difficult for the parents to fully endorse or enthusiastically participate in a treatment plan that is not consistent with the parents' understanding of the problem. For example, Anastopoulos (1996) has observed that the inconsistency of performance and situational variability of symptoms in a child with attention-deficit hyperactivity disorder (ADHD) may lead to the development of beliefs in the parents or teachers that the child's difficulties are just the result of being lazy or not exerting sufficient effort. Changing this belief requires proper education about the disorder in question, and without such information the parents are unlikely to endorse some of the most effective behavioral and pharmacological interventions for ADHD.

As illustrated in the preceding example, unhelpful cognitions can be addressed through simple discussion and education. In other cases, more intensive or formalized efforts at cognitive restructuring may be necessary. Such efforts could take the form of relabeling or reframing the young client's behavior (or the parents' response to their child's behavior) to reduce blame-oriented beliefs that may be interfering with the pursuit of positive action. In particular, the therapist may be working to guide parents or other adults away from endorsing global, stable, internal attributions for the young person's behavior, and to move them toward explanations that are relatively more local, unstable, and external. For example, rather than endorsing an explanation of a child's aggressive behavior that implies the child is innately destructive, the CB therapist may offer an alternative conceptualization that also fits the available data, such as "I notice he is most likely to shove other children when the classroom is very crowded and the children are expected to share a small number of supplies." The latter view offers hints at possible intervention in the very way the problem is described, while the former view could be interpreted as presenting fewer options (short of a personality transplant). CB clinicians also accomplish simple yet useful reframes with parents and their children when they shift their discussion from the deficits or difficulties a child is presenting to a consideration of what positive skills need to be trained and encouraged in the child in order to eliminate the areas of concern. Based upon their work with conflicted parents and teens, Robin (1998) and Robin and Foster (1989) provide useful examples of common unreasonable beliefs and their more reasonable reframes, as well as specific suggestions for approaching this topic with both parents and teens. In presenting such reframes, the CB therapist helps parents understand that these choices of problem formulation are not a matter of truth versus falsehood, but rather a matter of which conceptualization is most likely to encourage constructive efforts to cope with the problem at hand.

Self-Control/Self-Regulation Approaches

The class of treatment techniques referred to as "self-control" or "self-regulation" is a transitional link between traditional behavioral approaches and perspectives that include greater attention to cognitive factors. Interest in self-regulation methods blossomed following the studies by Kanfer

(1970, 1971) that outlined a model of self-regulation including the components of self-monitoring, self-recording, self-evaluation, and self-reinforcement. "Self-monitoring" refers to the act of observing the occurrence of a defined cognitive or behavioral event, such as noting on-task behavior, tracking negative self-statements, or noting a change in mood. "Self-recording" refers to the process of making some type of record of the observed event, whether this be a notation on a chart, a check mark on a form, or a more elaborate entry in a mood diary. "Self-evaluation" involves comparing one's recorded behavior against some previously established standard, and then "self-reinforcement" is enacted if a predetermined goal has been achieved.

Self-regulation methods have been applied as the sole treatment for addressing discrete behavioral concerns, as well as being employed as one component of more comprehensive disorder-specific programs. Carter (1993) has presented a successful application of a simple self-monitoring approach designed to help a student decrease his frequency of blurting out in class by increasing the number of times he raised his hand and waited to be called on by the teacher, and self-monitoring coupled with self-evaluation and reinforcement has been used to increase on-task behavior in both elementary and secondary students with learning difficulties (Hallahan, Lloyd, Kneedler, & Marshall, 1982; Hughes & Hendrickson, 1987; Prater, Joy, Chilman, Temple, & Miller, 1991). Teaching youth to self-monitor or become more aware of internal arousal and emotional reactions is a common element of treatment for young clients struggling with aggressive behavior (Lochman, White, & Wayland, 1991; Nelson & Finch, 1996), as well as for those experiencing serious anxiety disorders or depression. In the case of anxious youth, they are taught to monitor early signs of fear or distress and use these emotional signals as cues to enact their coping skills (see Kendall, 1992, 1994, 1998, 2000). CBT for depressed youth virtually always involves asking the children or teenagers to monitor their moods and/or certain types of thoughts. In addition, the clients may be asked to monitor their involvement in pleasure or mastery-oriented events. Some treatment programs for depressed children and adolescents also address the overly rigid or unrealistic standards for self-evaluation that such youth may manifest (Stark, 1990).

Affective Education

Helping youth learn how to accurately recognize and label their own emotional experiences, as well as the emotions of others, is an important component of CBT with children and teens displaying a variety of difficulties. In some cases, young clients may be keenly aware of their emotional state but need help in developing a vocabulary for discussing these experiences, or, as

Southam-Gerow and Kendall (2000) have reported, need help in recognizing that emotions are modifiable. They may also need information to understand and normalize the physiological symptoms that accompany the experience of strong emotions. Other clients may need help in understanding the range and intensity of emotional expression. In particular, these children and adolescents often need training in learning to recognize the early physiological cues of emotional distress, so they can respond to the problem creating this distress while their emotions are still at relatively low intensity, rather than waiting until they experience some type of emotional meltdown. Still other youth need additional help in understanding the connection between thoughts and feelings. They benefit from learning how self-talk has the potential to increase or decrease the intensity of an emotional response. Again, the workbook materials developed to accompany the treatment of specific childhood disorders, such as those written by Kendall (1992) for the treatment of anxiety disorders and simple guided exercises can help young clients examine their emotions in a nonthreatening manner and make the connection between thoughts and feelings more concrete.

As part of affective education, the CB therapist may also explain that strong emotions tend to have a disorganizing effect on thinking in both children and adults. This makes it difficult to exhibit new learning or behavior patterns when one is extremely upset, unless these new behavioral responses have been well practiced. Ideally, this practice will occur first in a very nonthreatening context that provides much support for trying out new behavior (i.e., therapy), and then will occur in ever more challenging environments. Sports or coaching analogies can be useful for communicating this concept. The therapist can explain that learning to use a new self-management skill is much like trying out a new soccer or basketball move. First the young client must work on the skill in practice and receive a lot of coaching; then the move can be tried out in scrimmages; and finally the client is ready to begin to use the new move in a game situation.

Relaxation Training

Teaching children and adolescents more effective ways to relax is another major component of CBT for a variety of juvenile concerns. Historically, relaxation training has been a key element in the behavioral treatment of internalizing difficulties in youth (Barrios & O'Dell, 1989; Morris & Kratochwill, 1983). Rather than viewing relaxation as an alternative conditioned response, however, CB therapists present relaxation as a coping skill to be developed and consciously enacted whenever needed. Relaxation training has also become an important element in the treatment of children and adolescents with anger management difficulties (Feindler & Ecton,

1986; Lochman et al., 1991). Stark (1990) has cautioned that youth may not understand the rationale for relaxation training as well as adult clients. Younger children in particular may feel intimidated by the procedures, so it is important for the clinician to provide adequate information to both parents and children about the purpose and appropriate uses of relaxation methods.

Relaxation training with youth has been implemented in many forms. Both Stark (1990) and Kendall, Chansky, et al. (1992) have recommended the use of Ollendick and Cerny's (1981) modification of deep muscle relaxation training with youth. In this classic approach to relaxation training, young clients learn to tense and relax various muscle groups, and become more adept at perceiving the physiological indicators of muscle tension. The goal is for clients then to use this awareness to respond to early cues of muscle tension by enacting their relaxation procedures. Koeppen (1974) created a series of guided images to help school-age children be able to tense and relax various muscle groups, and Cautela and Groden (1978) developed modifications of relaxation procedures for use with young children or children with special needs.

In addition to these examples of more involved relaxation training, there are a number of simple procedures that clinicians can use with preschool and school-age children. For example, we (Kendall & Braswell, 1993) have described the "robot–ragdoll game," in which the therapist and child first move around the room like robots, making their arms and legs very stiff and tense. Upon the therapist's signal, the child is then instructed to flop gently in a nearby chair and allow his or her arms and legs to be relaxed and loose. The therapist then points out the differences in these two bodily states. Children can also be taught brief inductions to slow, deep breathing, such as having the child hold an index finger in front of his or her mouth as though it were a candle. The child is told to take a deep breath, hold the breath, and then let it out so slowly that an imaginary candle flame on the end of a finger will flicker but not be extinguished. Other brief methods include backward counting or the selection and use of calm self-talk. It is usually advised to present a variety of different options for achieving relaxation, and then to have the child select and practice the methods he or she prefers. After relaxation skills have been taught and practiced in the session, the therapist can create an audiotape of the child's preferred methods for use at home. Although relaxation training is typically employed as one component in a multifaceted treatment plan, Kahn, Kehle, Jenson, and Clark (1990) reported that relaxation training alone was as effective as CBT involving self-monitoring, cognitive restructuring, and problem solving in decreasing depressive symptomatology and increasing self-esteem.

Modeling

In therapy, as in the rest of life, people do not have to rely upon trial-and-error learning to discover most of what they need to know. Fortunately, humans are primed to be able to learn by observing others, and this form of learning is referred to as "observational learning" or "modeling." Modeling as an intervention in its own right has been demonstrated as effective in achieving the elimination of behavioral deficits, the reduction of excessive fears, and the facilitation of social behavior (Bandura, 1969, 1971; Rosenthal & Bandura, 1978). Virtually all effective CB interventions with youth involve some form of modeling as a means of training desired coping skills. As a component in CB interventions, modeling has been presented in a number of different forms, including filmed modeling, symbolic modeling, graduated modeling, participant modeling, and covert or cognitive modeling.

The phenomenon of modeling has received significant research attention. As summarized by Goldstein (1995), a learner's response to modeling is influenced by at least three classes of factors: features of the model, features of the learner, and the consequences associated with the modeled behavior. For example, having models verbalize their thoughts and actions while engaging in the behavior results in superior learning relative to models who do not verbalize (Meichenbaum, 1971). As the models verbalize, they provide learners with a demonstration of how to think themselves through a particular problem or situation, and talking aloud provides the learners with auditory as well as visual cues. Providing verbal labels for actions may be particularly important in work with younger children, for, as summarized by Kimball et al. (1993), younger children have greater difficulty differentiating central from peripheral information and may miss subtle but important cues provided by context. Children, like adults, are also more likely to imitate the behavior of someone they perceive as similar to themselves in some way, and all humans are more likely to model behavior displayed by individuals who are liked and admired. For some types of learning, "coping models" may be superior to "mastery models." A mastery model demonstrates successful task performance without indications of anxiety or difficulty. A coping model may demonstrate task performance that includes some mistakes, and the model may display some anxiety or discomfort, yet he or she is able to fulfill the task requirements with persistent effort. Coping modeling shows a client not only how to execute the necessary behaviors, but also how to cope with thoughts, emotions, and behaviors that might interfere with task performance. The more the model is able to include the learner in the modeling, the more likely the learner is to imitate the behavior (Kazdin, 1974; Meichenbaum, 1971; Sarason, 1975). Thus participant live-action modeling by a person highly similar to the learner is most likely to achieve the desired effect (Barrios & O'Dell, 1989), but when this option is not available, cognitive modeling coupled with some form of symbolic modeling may be a useful substitute. Youth can be helped to create their own covert cognitive models. As part of the treatment of anxious children, Kendall, Chu, Pimentel, and Choudhury (2000) recommend having a child imagine how a favorite TV cartoon or movie character might handle a feared situation. The use of such models may also serve as a comforting, counterconditioning agent, as proposed decades ago by Lazarus and Abramovitz (1962).

In CBT, the clinician also works with parents and teachers to help them become more conscious models of the skills they would like to see developed in the young clients. Adults working with acting-out children and adolescents, in particular, may need special encouragement and reinforcement from the therapist to be conscious of how important it is that they model good frustration tolerance skills when attempting to cope with the exceedingly challenging behavior of these youth. The therapist can also offer guidance in helping the parents select desired symbolic models, in the form of books, stories, videos, TV programs, and audiotapes that present compelling examples of the desired behaviors/skills. The reader is referred to Strayhorn (1988) for a particularly creative discussion of the use of desirable models in stories and play.

Role Playing

Like modeling, role playing is more of a training delivery method than a specific content area, but nonetheless it is a common element of CB interventions. Through role-playing exercises, the CB therapist can provide the client with performance-based learning experiences. In addition to serving as a vehicle for training, role playing provides a means of ongoing assessment of the extent to which a client is able to produce the newly learned behavior, although research suggests that role-play situations may elicit more social behaviors than are observed in similar but more naturalistic interactions (Beck, Forehand, Neeper, & Baskin, 1982). In-session role plays can, however, help the therapist detect any gaps in knowledge or incomplete behavioral information that has been provided to the client. Role plays typically involve the therapist and client; however, there is an increasing tendency to design interventions so that youth can participate in role-playing situations with age-appropriate peers (Albano & Barlow, 1996; Frankel, Cantwell, & Myatt, 1996). The use of role playing with videotaped feedback is another means of potentially increasing the impact of this training method (Chandler, 1973; Sarason & Ganzer, 1973). Depending upon how they are structured, role-playing situations can certainly be used to help clients attain a more realistic level of emotional arousal. For example,

Hinshaw and colleagues (Hinshaw, Buhrmester, & Heller, 1989; Hinshaw, Henker, & Whalen, 1984a) adapted a technique originally developed by Goodwin and Mahoney (1975) called the "circle game" to help boys with ADHD develop skills of anger control in response to verbal taunts by their peers.

Behavioral Contingencies

The range and type of behavioral contingencies used within CBT are limited only by the imagination of the therapist and (one would hope) by the findings of the relevant treatment outcome literature. Behavioral contingencies are most likely to be effective in serving the goals of the therapy when their choice is informed by an awareness of developmental considerations and an understanding of features of the young client's disorder and the parents' status that might increase or decrease the effectiveness of behavioral methods.

Although this information is hardly new, it still appears that many CB interventions underutilize behavioral contingencies and are somewhat insensitive to developmental factors in the choice of contingencies. The implications of developmental findings for key behavioral tools such as reward and punishment have been clearly articulated by Furman (1980), who advised researchers and clinicians using positive reinforcement methods to be aware of developmental changes in the value of social approval, accuracy feedback, mastery incentives, and tangible versus symbolic reinforcers. For example, Furman (1980) summarized findings indicating that for preschoolers and young elementary-school-age children, rewards have meaning for the social approval they connote. As children get older, they still care about social approval, but mastery incentives become increasingly important. In other words, by later elementary school age rewards become more meaningful when they signify that the child not only has earned adult approval but has also achieved some type of goal. This shift toward the increased importance of mastery motivation is also mirrored in the shift from tangible to more symbolic rewards. Again, younger children tend to be more responsive to tangible rewards, but with increasing cognitive age, rewards with more symbolic meaning increase in value.

Sensitivity to features of a young client's disorder can also lead to the selection of more appropriate rewards. Youth with ADHD, for example, exhibit a seeming need for stimulation and a quick satiation to material or events that are viewed as repetitive (Zentall, 1995). As a group, these youth tend to respond best in reward conditions in which there is very frequent feedback about behavior, many opportunities for reward, and prudent negative consequences for the display of inappropriate behaviors (Pfiffner & Barkley, 1998). In addition, reward systems are better able to maintain

their motivational impact if there is an ever-changing array of backup rewards and/or an element of chance in terms of the particular reward provided. When working with depressed youth, one may have very different
challenges in implementing a functional reward system, including helping
the clients identify what would (or at least used to be) pleasurable for them.
As discussed by Stark (1990), the therapist may need to address any overly
rigid or restrictive beliefs on the part of a client or family about the use of
rewards.

The effective implementation of contingencies in the home setting requires having a parent who is able to attend to such matters in a reasonably
consistent manner. Parents may need education about the full range of
available contingencies. In particular, parents may not be fully aware of the
reinforcing power of their attention. Some families may benefit from very
explicit instruction in learning to give attention to desirable behavior and
remove attention from inappropriate behavior. Fortunately, such training is
a common element in a number of behavioral child management programs
with demonstrated success (Barkley, 1997; Forehand & McMahon, 1981;
Webster-Stratton, 1984). Strayhorn (1988) also presents an excellent discussion of how parents can be primed to use the power of their attention to
encourage the display of more desirable behavior by their child. Beyond the
use of their attention, parents may need guidance in the use of explicit rewards for the occurrence of desired behavior or rewards for time intervals
without the display of undesirable behavior (e.g., fighting with siblings or
inappropriate language). Punishment methods, such as response cost, may
be valuable when tackling situations that involve the impulsive display of
undesirable behavior. Bloomquist's (1996) skills training guide for parents
and therapists is a helpful resource filled with charts and graphs that can
guide the implementation of behavioral methods to support change on the
part of children and/or parents.

When a child is approximately 7 or 8 years of age, he or she may be
developmentally able to participate in contingencies that involve greater
self-evaluation and self-reward. Such activities might involve having the
child rate his or her own behavior in the context of a therapy session, as we
have illustrated elsewhere (Kendall & Braswell, 1993). Hinshaw and
Erhardt (1991) have described a similar self-evaluation procedure for use in
small-group settings, referred to as the "match game." Each child in the
group is working on an individualized behavioral goal, and at random intervals throughout group, one of the leaders halts the ongoing activity and
asks the children to rate how they are doing on their individual goals, using
a 5-point scale. As the initial training goal is accuracy of self-ratings, children can earn bonus points if their self-ratings are within 1 point of the
therapist's ratings of their behavior, even if the behavior has not been appropriate. When the leader shares his or her ratings, there is specific feed-

back provided to the children, so it is clear how the leader derived his or her ratings. Over time, as the children become more accurate, then the standards are raised, and the children must both match the leader's rating and be exhibiting reasonably appropriate behavior in order to earn bonus points.

In a playground application of self-evaluation procedures, Hinshaw, Henker, and Whalen (1984b) trained children with ADHD to accurately evaluate their own social behavior, and then compared the effects of this training with traditional external reinforcement in the presence and absence of conjoint medication treatment. At posttest, the group receiving both self-evaluation training and medication exhibited the most appropriate behavior, and the group receiving self-evaluation training only was observed to be better behaved than the group receiving traditional external reinforcement. Training appropriate self-evaluation and self-reinforcement skills is important not only in work with more acting-out children, but also in work with children experiencing anxiety and depression (Kendall, Chansky, et al., 1992; Stark, 1990). In either case, attempting to help the children become more involved in the science of their own behavior change seems highly consistent with the CBT goal of developing a coping orientation.

APPLICATIONS WITH SPECIFIC JUVENILE DISORDERS

Common elements suggest that CBT is somewhat uniform in its application, but this is not the case. Despite these common components, treatments are designed for specific disorders, and the strategies are used differentially to be consistent with the nature of each disorder. In this section, we describe some disorder-specific programs and related research findings.

Aggressive Behavior

Aggressive behavior in children and adolescents, along with other forms of acting-out and disruptive behavior, is the leading cause of referral for mental health services in the United States (Achenbach & Howell, 1993). Aggressive behavior is frequently observed in the context of other symptoms associated with the diagnoses of oppositional defiant disorder and conduct disorder; however, given its aversive nature, aggressive behavior can lead a young person to be rejected and avoided by others, even in the absence of other symptomatology. As previously discussed, Dodge and colleagues have identified how youth who tend to exhibit reactive aggression make certain types of social information-processing errors that affect functions such as how they interpret the social behaviors of others and themselves, and how much information they take in before formulating actions. They also appear to be deficient in their ability to generate nonaggressive alternatives to social problem situations. Although the detection of these social-cognitive deficiencies and distortions is concerning, a review of the CBT literature suggests that aggressive children are responsive to CB interventions. There is a healthy tradition of success with both school- and clinic-based interventions for youth exhibiting aggressive behavior.

We consider school-based treatments first. Decades ago, Robin and colleagues (Robin & Schneider, 1974; Robin, Schneider, & Dolnick, 1976) created an intervention called the "turtle technique" for use with emotionally disturbed elementary school children who were exhibiting difficulties with aggression. Children were first trained to do the "turtle response" of pulling in their limbs and lowering their heads in provoking situations. Next, the children were trained to use relaxation skills while "doing the turtle." Social problem-solving skills of generating alternative solutions and examining their consequences were then introduced. Finally, the targeted children and their classmates were given social rewards for cueing and supporting each other when someone was "doing the turtle." Thus this intervention involved relaxation training, problem-solving training, and behavioral support for skills use. It was found to be effective in the target environment, which in this case was the classroom.

The work of Lochman and colleagues (Lochman et al., 2000; Lochman, Burch, Curry, & Lampron, 1984; Lochman & Curry, 1986; Lochman, Lampron, Gemmer, Harris, & Wyckoff, 1989) provides another example of a successful programmatic school-based intervention. This group program includes training and practice in the use of problem-solving steps, training in the recognition of physiological cues of arousal, and practice in the use of self-calming talk during provocation situations. The addition of behavioral goal setting was found to result in a further improvement in treatment impact. In this circumstance, the goal setting involved having a child state a goal in group while the classroom teacher monitored progress on the goal on a daily basis, with contingent reinforcement for successful goal attainment. In a 3-year follow-up of boys treated in this anger coping program, Lochman (1992) reported that, relative to untreated controls, treated children had lower rates of drug and alcohol involvement and higher levels of social problem-solving skills and self-esteem. The groups were equivalent, however, in rates of reported delinquent behavior, leading Lochman (1992) to suggest the need for interventions of greater intensity that also permit greater parental involvement.

CB interventions have also been successful with more severely impaired samples, as illustrated by the work of Kazdin and colleagues (Kazdin, Bass, Siegel, & Thomas, 1989; Kazdin, Esveldt-Dawson, French, & Unis, 1987a, 1987b; Kazdin, Siegel, & Bass, 1992) with 7- to 13-year-old children hospitalized for severe conduct-disordered behavior. The CBT emphasized problem-solving training, and treatment effects were improved by the addition of more *in vivo* opportunities for skills practice and by behavioral child management training for the parents. Kazdin et al. (1992) reported that the combination of problem-solving training and parent management training was the most successful at moving children from clinical to normative levels of functioning as assessed by rating scale measures. Kazdin and Crowley (1997) observed that children with greater academic dysfunction and with more symptoms at study outset across a range of different diagnostic categories appeared to benefit less from CBT. In addition, parent, family, and contextual factors such as economic disadvantage, parental history of antisocial behavior, and poor child-rearing practices were associated with poorer outcomes.

When positive findings from these selected examples of programmatic efforts are combined with other reports of successful applications of social-cognitive skills training with youth exhibiting delinquent or conduct-disordered behavior (Kendall, Reber, McLeer, Epps, & Ronan, 1990; Kolko, Loar, & Sturnick, 1990; Sarason & Ganzer, 1973), one sees a consistent pattern of positive effects. Nevertheless, not all treated cases result in total success. Given the social impact of aggressive behavior, it is hoped that future treatment studies will be able to achieve persistent as well as positive results in improving the social adaptation of aggressive youth.

Anxiety Disorders

Experiencing some fears or anxieties is part of normal growth for most children (Miller, Barrett, & Hampe, 1974). Treatment may be needed, however, if and when the severity or duration of these fears begins to impinge upon a child's accomplishment of key developmental tasks, such as making friends, attending school, and tolerating age-appropriate separations from parents. Without treatment, it appears that anxiety disorders in childhood and adolescence may have a chronic course and are associated with anxiety disorders in adulthood (Keller et al., 1992). Fortunately, within the domain of CB interventions for youth, no area has evidenced more exciting development than that of the treatment of anxiety disorders. In the first edition of this chapter, the discussion of anxiety disorders involved a brief description of a CBT program for school phobia (Kendall, Howard, & Epps, 1988), which, we had to note, had at that point no empirical evaluation. Over a decade later, there is a much more rich and interesting literature to inform both researchers and clinicians.

Building upon the results of a promising case study (Kane & Kendall, 1989), Kendall (1994) conducted a randomized clinical trial comparing 16 sessions of CBT with a waiting-list control for the treatment of children meeting *Diagnostic and Statistical Manual of Mental Disorders,* third edition, revised (DSM-III-R) criteria for the diagnoses of overanxious disorder, separation anxiety disorder, or avoidant disorder. The manualized treatment (Kendall, 1992) includes individual therapy sessions focused on helping children recognize anxious feelings and somatic reactions to anxiety, clarify unrealistic or negative beliefs or expectations about anxiety-provoking situations, develop a plan to cope with the situation, and evaluate their performance and administer self-reinforcement as appropriate. Manuals for group treatment (Flannery-Schroeder & Kendall, 1997) and family treatment (Howard et al., 1999) are also available.

Table 8.2 presents the four-step plan (the first letters of the four steps form the acronym "FEAR") that is used in this program to guide processing of anxiety experiences. The coping skills needed to perform these steps are trained via modeling, role playing, *in vivo* exposure, and the use of behavioral contingencies. In addition, the children receive training in relaxation methods. The first eight sessions of the treatment involve education in the cognitive constructs just described, whereas the last eight sessions involve imaginal, analogue, and *in vivo* use of the trained skills. The results of Kendall (1994) indicated that at both posttest and 1-year follow-up, many treated participants had improved so much that they no longer qualified for a clinical diagnosis. Perhaps even more exciting, an extended follow-up (average of 3 1/2 years) found that positive outcomes were still being maintained (Kendall & Southham-Gerow, 1996). Using DSM-IV diagnostic categories and a larger sample, Kendall et al. (1997) replicated and extended the results of Kendall (1994), finding that comorbidity for other DSM-IV diagnoses did not affect treatment outcome. In an interesting analysis of the role of the two segments of the training, it was observed that significant change on the outcome measures followed the second, enactment-

---

TABLE 8.2. FEAR Plan for Use with Anxious Youth

1. Feeling nervous?
   Are you feeling nervous? How can you tell?

2. Expecting bad things to happen?
   Tune into your self-talk. What is it that is worrying you in this situation?

3. Attitudes and actions can help.
   What are some others ways to think about this situation? What are some actions I can take to make this situation better?

4. Results and rewards.
   How did I do? Was I able to help myself take action and feel better?
   Way to go!

Note. From Kendall (1992). Copyright 1992 by Philip C. Kendall. Reprinted with permission.

oriented phase of treatment. In an exploration of possible mechanisms associated with change, Treadwell and Kendall (1996) reported that reductions in children's anxious self-talk did seem to mediate treatment-related change. As discussed by Kendall and Treadwell (1996), this research program has also been responsible for developing a broader array of assessment tools for examining the self-talk, self-perceptions, coping abilities, and level of treatment satisfaction of children experiencing anxiety disorders.

Creating their own 12-week group treatment adaptation of the Kendall (1992) program, Mendlowitz et al. (1999) also obtained reductions in symptoms of anxiety and depression and changes in coping strategy use in children meeting criteria for one or more DSM-IV anxiety disorders. The impact of parental involvement in treatment was examined by having children assigned to one of three conditions: child group only, parent group only, and child and parent groups. Children in the child and parent treatment condition reported greater use of active coping strategies at posttest and were rated by their parents as displaying greater improvement in their emotional well-being.

Drawing upon a successful program for adults with social phobia (Heimberg et al., 1990), Albano and Barlow (1996) have developed CBT groups for socially anxious teenagers. The key program components include cognitive restructuring to identify and change the cognitive distortions that perpetuate the anxiety, social skills training to address areas of deficit, and problem-solving training. Albano and Barlow (1996) note that problem-solving training is needed because these teens have long favored coping styles characterized by behavioral avoidance and escape from aversive situations, so they have little practice in proactive planning. Albano, Marten, Holt, Heimberg, and Barlow (1995) have reported positive results in an empirical evaluation of this approach.

A CB approach to the treatment of children presenting with phobias and other anxiety disorders has also been elaborated by Silverman, Ginsburg, and Kurtines (1995). This approach is similar to that presented by Kendall, Chansky, et al. (1992) and includes separate and conjoint child and parent sessions. Treatment includes three phases: education, application, and relapse prevention. Evaluating this treatment through a multiple-baseline design across subjects, Eisen and Silverman (1993, 1998) found significant improvement on child and parent self-report measures, as well as on clinician ratings and physiological measures. Treatment gains were maintained at a 6-month follow-up.

A promising example of cognitive-behavioral treatment of obsessive–compulsive disorder (OCD) in children has been developed by March and colleagues (March, 1995; March & Mulle, 1998; March, Mulle, & Herbel, 1994). The treatment protocol has the irresistible title *How I Ran OCD off My Land* and uses traditional behavioral approaches of exposure, response prevention, and extinction, coupled with an anxiety management component that includes relaxation training, controlled breathing, and cognitive restructuring (March & Mulle, 1998). March et al. (1994) conducted an open trial with patients already stabilized on pharmacological treatments and achieved further improvements at both immediate posttest and 6-month follow-up. Booster behavioral treatments allowed medication discontinuation in six of nine asymptomatic patients without relapse after 6 months of follow-up.

In addition to this increase in the number of treatment outcome studies exploring the impact of CBT for anxiety disorders, investigators have also begun to explore other factors related to remaining in treatment. In an analysis of treatment completers and terminators, Kendall and Sugarman (1997) found that whereas socioeconomic status and parental educational level were not associated with ending treatment prematurely, being from a single-parent home and being a member of an ethnic minority group were associated with terminating rather than completing treatment. In contrast to studies with acting-out youth, in which those leaving treatment tend to be more severely impaired, terminators indicated fewer anxiety symptoms in self-report measures. Considering the value for both maintaining young clients in treatment and improving their outcome, Kendall, MacDonald, and Treadwell (1995) have argued for pursuing an increased role for parents in the treatment of their children's anxiety disorders. In addition to providing valuable information about their children's functioning, parents could serve as coping models, function as coaches for *in vivo* exposure sessions, and, if needed, learn new parenting techniques and alter their own unhelpful expectations or beliefs that might be interfering with their children's progress. Indeed, the findings of both Barrett, Dadds, and Rapee (1996) and Mendlowitz et al. (1999) indicate the potential value of adding a parent training component to anxiety treatment programs.

As discussed by Kazdin and Weisz (1998), the outcome literature on CBT for anxiety disorders in children is noteworthy, for it includes treatment studies that (1) focus on cases serious enough to meet formal diagnostic criteria; (2) include assessments of clinical significance; (3) conduct assessments over longer follow-up periods than is commonly the case, with the demonstration of persisting effects; and (4) demonstrate that positive results can be achieved by different research teams (see also Ollendick & King, 2000).

Depression

In the first edition of this chapter, we speculated about the possible value of CBT for the treatment of depression in children and adolescents, but there was very little empirical work to support this view. Informative, highly descriptive books and chapters have since been published that articulate how various CB procedures can be applied with children and adolescents. Wilkes et al. (1994) present a detailed account of how one can apply Beck's cognitive therapy for depression with adolescent clients. Dudley (1997) offers a detailed curriculum for conducting group therapy with depressed children. Her program includes creative charts, drawings, and stories for helping children understand key cognitive constructs. As an alternative to programmatic treatment approaches, Shirk and Harter (1996) have used the "case formulation" approach of Persons (1991) to illustrate how a CB therapist develops a working hypothesis about the processes underlying a child's presenting problems and then utilizes specific interventions to address these processes. Rotheram-Borus, Piacentini, Miller, Graae, and Castro-Blanco (1994) have presented a structured approach to CBT for adolescents who have attempted suicide and their families. These works make excellent reading for the clinician interested in learning to apply CB techniques with depressed children and adolescents. The past decade has yielded an increased number of controlled outcome studies with depressed adolescents; however, the number of studies with younger children remains small, and the studies are fairly diverse in terms of the CBT approaches being examined.

One body of work has examined the impact of school-based group interventions with children selected on the basis of self-report measures and, in some cases, teacher referral. Working with fifth- and sixth-graders, Butler, Miezitis, Friedman, and Cole (1980) compared the effectiveness of a treatment emphasizing social skills training through role playing with an approach emphasizing cognitive restructuring. Both treatment conditions were compared with an attention-placebo control and a waiting-list control, yielding four groups. Children across all four groups reported significant pre- to posttest improvement on the Children's Depression Inventory (Kovacs, 1981). Those receiving the role-playing treatment evidenced the greatest improvement on self-report and teacher report measures, followed by the cognitive restructuring group.

Reynolds and Coats (1986) compared the effectiveness of CBT emphasizing self-monitoring, self-evaluation, and self-reinforcement with a relaxation training condition in which the adolescent clients were trained in progressive muscle relaxation methods and urged to use these methods when coping with stressful events. Relative to a waiting-list control condition, both active treatments yielded significant change on self-report measures, and these changes were maintained at a 5-week follow-up.

Stark, Kaslow, and Reynolds (1987) contrasted a self-control intervention based on the work of Fuchs and Rehm (1977) with a behavioral social skills condition based on Lewinsohn's (1974) model of depression. In the self-control condition, the 9- to 12-year-old subjects were taught how to set more realistic standards for self-evaluation of performance, to set subgoals for larger tasks, to increase their use of self-reinforcement, to decrease their frequency of self-punishment, and to examine their own attributions. Training in self-monitoring, with special attention to the monitoring of pleasant events, was also included. The behavioral approach also included self-monitoring training, as well as scheduling of pleasant events, problem solving about social situations, and discussion of the relationship between feelings and social behavior. After 12 group sessions, both treated groups displayed significant improvement relative to a waiting-list control. The self-control group displayed the greatest positive change. The self-control intervention reported in this study was also found to yield significant positive change in an uncontrolled trial conducted with an ethnically diverse population of fourth- and fifth-graders, as described in Rehm and Sharp (1996). Combining elements of the self-control condition and the behavioral social skills condition along with training in cognitive restructuring, Stark (1990) evaluated the effects of this multicomponent CBT intervention with that of a nonspecific psychotherapy control condition for the treatment of fourth- through seventh-graders exhibiting elevated levels of depressive symptomatology. Children in both groups reported significant reductions in symptoms of depression and fewer depressive cognitions at posttest. These results were maintained at a 7-month follow-up. Between-group comparisons indicated that the CBT group reported significantly fewer symptoms of depression in a structured interview and had fewer depressive cognitions.

Working with severely depressed adolescents, Lewinsohn and colleagues (Lewinsohn, Clarke, Hops, & Andrews, 1990; Lewinsohn, Clarke, & Rohde, 1994; Lewinsohn, Clarke, Rohde, Hops, & Seeley, 1996) have conducted two randomized clinical trials of their CBT program, referred to as the Adolescent Coping With Depression program. This group program trains skills emphasized in cognitive formulations of depression (such as learning to recognize depressogenic patterns of thinking and substituting more constructive cognitions), along with skills associated with more behavioral formulations (such as increasing client behaviors that elicit positive reinforcement and avoid negative reinforcement from the environment). Accomplishing the change in reinforcement pattern often requires the training of social and other coping skills. Training is accomplished through structured group sessions that emphasize role playing, homework assignment, and rewards and contracts. A companion group education program for the parents of the depressed teens has also been developed (Lewinsohn, Rohde, Hops, & Clarke, 1991). Both clinical trials yielded evidence for change as a result of treatment. Interestingly, adding parent group participation did not appear to yield outcomes significantly better than those achieved when only the adolescents formally participated in the program (Lewinsohn et al., 1990). Also, an attempt to clarify the most effective pattern of booster sessions following group completion did not yield results in favor of one pattern over another (Lewinsohn et al., 1994). Clarke, Rohde, Lewinsohn, Hops, and Seeley (1998) also demonstrated the effectiveness of group CBT over a waiting-list control, with improvement rates not significantly different for adolescent participation only or adolescent plus parent participation.

Also working with depressed adolescents, Brent and colleagues (Brent et al., 1997; Brent et al., 1998; Brent, Kolko, Birmaher, Baugher, & Bridge, 1999), compared the effectiveness of CBT with systemic–behavioral family therapy and nondirective supportive therapy. CBT resulted in more rapid and complete relief of depressive symptoms than the other two treatments following the end of the acute treatment phase (Brent et al., 1997). CBT demonstrated a particular treatment advantage with patients comorbid for anxiety (Brent et al., 1998), but CBT's relative efficacy decreased in cases where maternal depression was present. Despite the superior results observed during the initial 12-week clinical trial, patients in the CBT condition were just as likely as those in the other two conditions to receive or be recommended for additional treatment during the 24-month follow-up period (Brent et al., 1999), with need for follow-up treatment best predicted by the continuing severity of depressive symptoms at the end of the acute phase and the presence of disruptive behavior and family difficulties. Brent et al. (1999) speculate that with adolescent patients, CBT may be superior for initial reduction of depressive symptomatology, but approaches providing some form of family involvement may be of greater value in addressing residual behavioral disruption and/or ongoing family conflicts.

In a fascinating approach to school-based prevention, Clarke et al. (1995) identified ninth-graders considered to be at risk for but not yet experiencing an episode of depression, based upon self-report measures and follow-up structured diagnostic interview. These students then participated in 15 after-school group sessions lasting 45 minutes each, in which students were taught cognitive techniques for identifying and challenging unhelpful thinking that might increase feelings of depression. Using survival analysis, the investigators then examined how many cases of major depressive disorder or dysthymia emerged in the treated group versus a usual-care control group of teens. At a 12-month follow-up, rates of depression were 14.5% for the treated group compared to 25.7% for the controls. Thus some evidence supportive of a preventive effect was obtained.

Prevention or reduction of risk for relapse or recurrence of depression following successful treatment is also an important concern in work with children and adolescents who have experienced major depressive disorder. Kroll, Harrington, Jayson, Fraser, and Gowers (1996) conducted a pilot study examining the value of maintenance CBT for adolescents whose major depressive disorder was in remission. Relative to controls, adolescents in the maintenance CBT condition exhibited a lower cumulative risk of relapse over a 6-month period (0.2 vs. 0.5). In contrast, Clarke et al. (1998) found that booster sessions did not reduce rate of recurrence during a 24-month follow-up period, for overall rates of recurrence were low for all conditions. Booster sessions did, however, appear to accelerate recovery among those adolescents who were still displaying symptoms of depression at the end of the acute treatment phase.

As these studies indicate, CBT for depressed children and adolescents is a promising treatment. There is, however, a striking need for the treatment packages within this domain to be carefully evaluated by research teams that are independent from the creators of these approaches.

Attention-Deficit/Hyperactivity Disorder

As discussed by Braswell (1998), the evolution in thinking about the usefulness of CBT in the treatment of ADHD provides an interesting example in the cycle of science (see also Hinshaw, 2000). Often a new approach is enthusiastically greeted, widely applied, and then found to be less useful than was originally believed. Youth who meet criteria for a diagnosis of ADHD present with levels of inattention, impulsivity, and in some cases hyperactivity that are inappropriately high for their age and cognitive level. When interacting with such youth, it is common for adults to think how much easier life would be if the youth could just pause a bit to stop and think about what they are doing *before* getting themselves into problematic situations. Given this common-sense observation, as well as the findings of previous research on the cognitive deficiencies associated with ADHD-type behavior (August, 1987; Douglas, 1983; see also Kendall & McDonald, 1993), there would seem to be a natural match between the explicit goals of certain types of CBT (such as problem-solving approaches that train explicit forms of self-instructions) and the needs of children with ADHD. Following the positive outcomes achieved by Meichenbaum and Goodman (1971) in their application of verbal self-instructional training with impulsive kindergarten and first-grade children, CBT methods for working with children exhibiting ADHD-type behaviors received phenomenal research attention (see reviews by Braswell & Bloomquist, 1991; Kendall & Braswell, 1993). As summarized in these articles, positive outcomes were achieved with teacher-identified impulsive children. In their meta-analytic review of the CB outcome literature with impulsive children, Baer and Nietzel (1991) concluded that CBT was associated with improvements of approximately one-third to three-quarters of a standard deviation in treated children relative to untreated controls, but the targeted groups had scores that fell close to comparison group means, both before and after treatment. Thus the severity of the behavioral issues of these children must be questioned, and the efficacy with impulsiveness may not generalize to formally diagnosed ADHD.

Consistent with this concern, researchers conducting interventions with children who met full criteria for ADHD (or its diagnostic equivalent at the time of each study) were not achieving positive results on either social or academic outcome measures (see reviews by Abikoff, 1985, 1991; Kendall & Braswell, 1993). In addition, when CBT was combined with psychostimulant medication treatment, there was little evidence of effects beyond those achieved with medication alone (Abikoff et al., 1988; Brown, Borden, Wynne, Schleser, & Clingerman, 1986; Brown, Wynne, & Medenis, 1985). Braswell et al. (1997) evaluated the effects of a 2-year school-based child group training program that targeted children selected by parents and teachers on the basis of their disruptive behavior. Two-thirds of this sample met DSM-III-R criteria for ADHD. Treated children received 28 training groups over a 2-year period, and their parents and teachers participated in groups in which they received information about ADHD and behavior management. The results of this multicomponent intervention were compared to those of a control condition in which parents and teachers received information but the children received no direct service. Both conditions displayed improvement at the first posttest, and subsequent follow-up data indicated no significant difference in the functioning of the two groups. Thus, despite these authors' initial enthusiasm for the use of these methods, the findings of others as well as our own more recent findings force the conclusion that problem-solving training efforts should not be considered a treatment for the primary symptoms of ADHD. As noted by Goldstein and Goldstein (1998), children with ADHD appear to need interventions at the point of performance, rather than interventions that train skills in one setting and provide few or no prompts and reinforcements for skill use in the target environment.

This observation is consistent with the finding that when problem-solving CBT was implemented to address conflict between adolescents with ADHD and their parents, this form of intervention performed as well as the other psychosocial interventions examined (Barkley, Guevremont, Anastopoulos, & Fletcher, 1992). In this application, the adolescents with ADHD were trained in and practiced the use of problem-solving skills with the very people with whom they were expected to employ these skills (i.e., their parents). When CBT is dealing with conditions that are as "hardwired" or neurologically based as appears to be the case with ADHD (Goldstein & Goldstein, 1998), it may be the case that CBT applications have not been implemented with an intensity that matches the true treatment needs of the clients.

Although cognitive problem-solving approaches may not be the most appropriate interventions for the primary symptoms of ADHD, these approaches may be suitable for treatment of adjunctive issues (such as parent–child conflict), and for treatment of coexisting concerns (including aggressive behavior, anxiety, and depression). The Multimodal Treatment Study of Children with Attention-Deficit/Hyperactivity Disorder (MTA Cooperative Group, 1999a) provides an interesting model in this regard. The results of the 14-month randomized trial indicate that carefully titrated medication treatment appears to have the greatest positive impact on the core symptoms of ADHD, while combined medication and intensive behavioral intervention demonstrated additional positive effect on coexisting issues, including symptoms of oppositional defiant disorder, internalizing symptoms, and parent–child relationship concerns. Behavioral treatment without medication was only significantly better than standard community care for those children who manifested ADHD and symptoms of anxiety (MTA Cooperative Group, 1999b).

Other Domains of Application

Although we have been attempting to highlight major areas of application of CBT methods with children, it must also be noted that these methods have been applied with other areas of concern. An extensive body of research within the educational literature has explored the use of self-instructional methods, in particular, with academic concerns (Deshler, Alley, Warner, & Schumaker, 1981; Leon & Pepe, 1983; Harris & Graham, 1996), and self-monitoring/self-regulation interventions have been effective in helping learning-disabled students improve behaviors essential for academic success, such as attention to task (Prater et al., 1991; Shapiro & Cole, 1994). Various types of behavioral medicine concerns, including chronic pain in general (Masek, Russo, & Varni, 1984) and more specific issues such as recurrent abdominal pain (Sanders et al., 1989), have been successfully addressed via CBT methods. Elements of CB skills training have also been included in prevention efforts (Tremblay, Pagani-Kurtz, Masse, Vitaro, & Phil, 1995; Weissberg, Caplan, & Harwood, 1991) and as one component of Henggeler's multisystemic treatment for serious juvenile offenders (Henggeler, Melton, & Smith, 1992). Thus CBT has been advanced, broadly and successfully applied, and considered efficacious or promising with a variety of childhood concerns.

CONCLUSIONS AND FUTURE DIRECTIONS

The treatment outcome literature examining interventions with children and adolescents provides evidence that CBT has displayed continued positive growth during the 1990s (Kazdin & Kendall, 1998; Kazdin & Weisz, 1998; Ollendick & King, 2000). Specific forms of CBT can be recommended with reasonable confidence as treatments for aggressive 7- to 13-year-olds and for anxious and/or depressed children and adolescents. Other reviews of the field have deemed several of these approaches as probably efficacious (Brestan & Eyberg, 1998; Kaslow & Thompson, 1998; Ollendick & King, 1998). Yet, as always, research questions and pragmatic concerns about implementation remain.

Role of Parental Involvement

In recent years, the field has moved beyond the simple call for parental involvement in the treatment of childhood difficulties, with many of the studies cited herein involving parents in creative and substantive ways. In addition to the previously cited examples, it has been established that adding certain forms of CB skill training for parents can enhance the effectiveness of other types of treatment for childhood disorders. For example, adding problem-solving training about issues that affect the parents has been found to improve the outcomes of behavioral child management training (Griest et al., 1982; Pfiffner, Jouriles, Brown, Etscheidt, & Kelly, 1990). Nevertheless, there is still much to understand about when, how, and for whom parents are best involved. With preschoolers and school-age children, building in a strong role for parents would seem to be clearly preferred; for adolescents, however, further study is needed to understand whether or not greater impact is achieved by efforts to involve (or change) peers relative to efforts to enhance parental involvement. When parents are involved, is it best to do so via parent groups, or do family sessions in which content can be better adapted to the needs of particular parents and children have greater impact? To maximize effectiveness, should parental involvement precede, follow, or occur conjointly with child treatment? Do the answers to these questions vary with the particular type of juvenile difficulty being treated? Clearly, many questions about the form of parental involvement remain.

The effective transformation of parental expectancies and beliefs also seems to be an important area for future inquiry. It is well established that parental beliefs and expectancies about various aspects of child behavior influence parents' emotions and behavioral responses toward their children (Bugental & Cortez, 1988; Dix, Ruble, Gresec, & Nixon, 1986; Johnston & Patenaude, 1994; Roehling & Robin, 1986). The field now seems poised to examine how changing parental perceptions, expectations, or attitudes can result in observable changes in behavior. Interestingly, a model for such exploration may be provided by the work of the behaviorist Wahler and colleagues (Wahler, 1990; Wahler, Carter, Fleischman, & Lambert, 1993; Wahler & Dumas, 1989). In their attempts to understand why some mothers were able to make and sustain positive treatment-induced changes in their child management practices, whereas others either could not make the same changes or failed to sustain change following the end of treatment, Wahler and Dumas (1989) hypothesized that multiple stressors in the lives of some mothers make it difficult for them to track their children's behavior accurately. This difficulty and preoccupation with other concerns lead these mothers to respond inconsistently and indiscriminately to their children's behavior. Through a process Wahler et al. (1993) have referred to as "synthesis teaching," such a mother is guided to see the similarities *and* differences in the way in which she interacts with her child and with others with whom she may have coercive relationships, in an effort to help her perceive child behavior more objectively. The results of Wahler et al. (1993) also suggest the value of addressing parental perceptions as a means of fostering the effectiveness of traditional child behavior management Strassberg's (1997) work on the cognitive bases of maternal discipline dysfunction further highlights the need to explore and address parental interpretations of child behavior—particularly how maternal overinterpretation of defiant intent on the part of the child may contribute to the genesis of coercive parent–child interactions.

Programmatic versus Prescriptive Intervention

It is common for review articles to call for greater attention to the match between client characteristics and features of the treatment, in an effort to avoid the frequently noted client uniformity myth (Kiesler, 1966). Now that several treatment programs have demonstrated efficacy with their target populations, the field has the opportunity for examining the extent to which programmatic versus prescriptive applications of these treatments yield better results. Although programmatic implementation allows some individualizing of content, it is generally the case that each client receives training in the same set of CB skill components. In contrast, prescriptive or idiographic treatment involves tailoring the treatment to the individual skill needs of the client. Eisen and Silverman (1993, 1998) explored this issue in the treatment of anxiety disorders in children, and obtained results suggesting that prescriptive treatment yielded superior levels of change. For example, anxious children whose primary symptoms involved worry responded most positively to cognitive therapy, while those for whom somatic complaints were their primary symptoms responded most positively to relaxation training, with both treatment groups also engaging in exposure-based activities. From a descriptive rather than an empirical standpoint, Shirk and Harter (1996) present a case formulation approach to the development of prescriptive CBT for children with self-esteem issues. Future research that clarifies the best matches between treatment components and symptom groups will have tremendous practical value for clinicians as they struggle

to provide interventions that are both time-efficient *and* empirically supported.

Transportability

As discussed by Kazdin and Kendall (1998), demonstrating that CBT is efficacious in research contexts is the first step, but it cannot be assumed that
these methods will yield similar outcomes in community-based clinics,
where features of the setting, therapists, and clients may be quite different.
Recognition of this issue highlights the need for treatment outcome researchers to strive to conduct experimental trials with clients of severity
levels and cultural backgrounds similar to those seen in community-based
settings. Such research must also consider a wide variety of highly practical
issues, such as how participation and outcome are affected when clients (or
their parents) are responsible for paying for each session, or how successfully manualized treatments are implemented by clinicians with only a minimum of training in a particular approach. Transportability is also affected
by the extent to which practicing clinicians perceive a treatment as valid
and acceptable. Understanding of how child and family therapists view
CBT methods will be an important step in promoting the widespread use of
those methods that have demonstrated efficacy.

Integration of Findings across Domains

Although demonstrating the efficacy of a particular approach demands
great specificity of methods, it is hoped that future treatment efforts will
also strive to do a better job of integrating existing and emerging knowledge from the domains of child development, education, and psychopathology, as well as the treatment outcome literature. Contingencies
within academics tend to favor researchers that develop their own approach to a condition, often with an accompanying jargon that heightens
the perceived uniqueness of the approach. Advancement in our understanding depends, however, upon the integration and validation of knowledge
rather than just the discovery of unique facts. Validation efforts require that
researchers test each other's proposed treatments. Even more importantly,
researchers and clinicians alike must screen proposed treatments to be sure
that both the form and content of these interventions are consistent with
what is already known about how children of certain ages are most likely
to learn, retain, and be motivated to use new skills. Are developmentally
appropriate skills being trained? Is the mode of training age-appropriate?
Are there accompanying behavioral contingencies to support the learning
process, and are these contingencies consistent with the age of the child and
what is already established about the particular disorder being treated?

Through such questioning and integration of knowledge across domains, the field of CBT with children will be able to move forward, rather than risk being caught in redundant cycles of "discovery" of findings that have already been accepted and/or rejected based upon work in other domains of inquiry.

REFERENCES

Abikoff, H. (1985). Efficacy of cognitive training interventions in hyperactive children: A critical review. *Clinical Psychology Review, 5,* 479–512.

Abikoff, H. (1991). Cognitive training in ADHD children: Less to it than meets the eye. *Journal of Learning Disabilities, 24,* 205–209.

Abikoff, H., Ganales, D., Reiter, G., Blum, C., Foley, C., & Klein, R. G. (1988). Cognitive training in academically deficient ADHD boys receiving stimulant medication. *Journal of Abnormal Child Psychology, 16,* 411–432.

Achenbach, T. M., & Howell, C. T. (1993). Are American children's problems getting worse?: A 13-year comparison. *Journal of the American Academy of Child and Adolescent Psychiatry, 32,* 1145–1154.

Ager, C. L., & Cole, C. L. (1991). A review of cognitive-behavioral interventions for children and adolescents with behavioral disorders. *Behavioral Disorders, 16,* 276–287.

Albano, A. M., & Barlow, D. (1996). Breaking the vicious cycle: Cogntive-behavioral group treatment for socially active youth. In E. D. Hibb & P. S. Jensen (Eds.), *Psychosocial treatments for child and adolescent disorders: Empirically based strategies for child clinical practice* (pp. 43–62). Washington, DC: American Psychological Association.

Albano, A. M., DiBartolo, P. M., Heimburg, R. G., & Barlow, D. (1995). Children and adolescents: Assessment and treatment. In R. G. Heimburg, M. R. Leibowitz, D. A. Hope, & F. Schneier (Eds.), *Social phobia: Diagnosis, assessment and treatment* (pp. 387–425). New York: Guilford Press.

Anastopoulos, A. D. (1996). Facilitating parental understanding and management of attention deficit/hyperactivity disorder. In M. A. Reinecke, F. M. Dattilio, & A. Freeman (Eds.), *Cognitive therapy with children and adolescents: A casebook for clinical practice* (pp. 327–343). New York: Guilford Press.

August, G. J. (1987). Production deficiencies in free recall: A comparison of hyperactive learning-disabled and normal children. *Journal of Abnormal Child Psychology, 15,* 429–440.

Baer, R. A., & Nietzel, M. T. (1991). Cognitive and behavioral treatment of impulsivity in children: A meta-analytic review of the outcome literature. *Journal of Clinical Child Psychology, 20,* 400–412.

Bandura, A. (1969). *Principles of behavior modification.* New York: Holt, Rinehart & Winston.

Bandura, A. (1971). Psychotherapy based upon modeling procedures. In A. Bergin & S. Garfield (Eds.), *Handbook of psychotherapy and behavior change* (pp. 621–658). New York: Wiley.

Barkley, R. A. (1997). *Defiant children (2nd ed.): A clinician's manual for assessment and parent training.* New York: Guilford Press.

Barkley, R. A., Guevremont, D. C., Anastopoulos, A. D., & Fletcher, K. E. (1992). A comparison of three family conflicts in adolescents with attention deficit hyperactivity disorder. *Journal of Consulting and Clinical Psychology, 60,* 450–462.

Barrett, P. M., Dadds, M. M., & Rapee, R. M. (1996). Family treatment of childhood anxiety: A controlled trial. *Journal of Consulting and Clinical Psychology, 64,* 333–342.

Barrett, P. M., Rapee, R. M., Dadds, M. M., & Ryan, S. M. (1996). Family enhancement of cognitive style in anxious and aggressive children. *Journal of Abnormal Child Psychology, 24,* 187–203.

Barrios, B. A., & O'Dell, S. L. (1989). Fears and anxieties. In E. J. Mash & R. A. Barkley (Eds.), *Treatment of childhood disorders* (pp. 167–221). New York: Guilford Press.

Beck, A. T., Rush, A. J., Shaw, B. F., & Emery, G. (1979). *Cognitive therapy of depression.* New York: Guilford Press.

Beck, S., Forehand, R., Neeper, R., & Baskin, C. H. (1982). A comparison of two analogue strategies for assessing children's social skills. *Journal of Consulting and Clinical Psychology, 50,* 596–597.

Bloomquist, M. L. (1996). *Skills training for children with behavior disorders.* New York: Guilford Press.

Braswell, L. (1991). Involving parents in cognitive-behavioral therapy with children and adolescents. In P. C. Kendall (Ed.), *Child and adolescent therapy: Cognitive-behavioral procedures* (pp. 316–351). New York: Guilford Press.

Braswell, L. (1998). Self-regulating training for children with ADHD: Response to Harris and Schmidt. *The ADHD Report, 6,* 1–3.

Braswell, L., August, G., Bloomquist, M. L., Realmuto, G. M., Skare, S., & Crosby, R. (1997). School-based secondary prevention for children with disruptive behavior: Initial outcomes. *Journal of Abnormal Child Psychology, 25,* 197–208.

Braswell, L., & Bloomquist, M. L. (1991). *Cognitive-behavioral therapy with ADHD children: Child, family, and school interventions.* New York: Guilford Press.

Braswell, L., Koehler, C., & Kendall, P. C. (1985). Attributions and outcomes in child psychotherapy. *Journal of Social and Clinical Psychology, 3,* 458–465.

Brent, D. A., Holder, D., Kolko, D. A., Birmaher, B., Baugher, D. A., Roth, C., Iyengar, S., & Johnson, B. A. (1997). A clinical psychotherapy trial for adolescent depression comparing cognitive, family, and supportive treatments. *Archives of General Psychiatry, 54,* 877–885.

Brent, D. A., Kolko, D. J., Birmaher, B., Baugher, M., & Bridge, J. (1999). A clinical trial for adolescent depression: Predictors of additional treatment in the acute and follow-up phases of the trial. *Journal of the American Academy of Child and Adolescent Psychiatry, 38,* 263–271.

Brent, D. A., Kolko, D. J., Birmaher, B., Baugher, M., Bridge, J., Roth, C., & Holder, D. (1998). Predictors of treatment efficacy in a clinical trial of three psychosocial treatments for adolescent depression. *Journal of the American Academy of Child and Adolescent Psychiatry, 37,* 906–914.

Brestan, E. V., & Eyberg, S. M. (1998). Effective psychosocial treatments of conduct disordered children and adolescents: 29 years, 82 studies, and 5,272 kids. *Journal of Clinical Child Psychology, 27,* 180–189.

Brown, R. T., Borden, K. A., Wynne, M. E., Schleser, R., & Clingerman, S. R. (1986). Methylphenidate and cognitive therapy with ADD children: A methodological reconsideration. *Journal of Abnormal Child Psychology, 13,* 69–87.

Brown, R. T., Wynne, M. E., & Medenis, R. (1985). Methylphenidate and cognitive therapy: A comparison of treatment approaches with hyperactive boys. *Journal of Abnormal Child Psychology, 13,* 69–87.

Bugental, D. B., & Cortez, V. L. (1988). Physiological reactivity to responsive and unresponsive children as moderated by perceived control. *Child Development, 59,* 686–693.

Butler, L., Miezitis, S., Friedman, R., & Cole, E. (1980). The effects of two school-based intervention programs on depressive symptoms in preadolescents. *American Educational Research Journal, 17,* 111–119.

Carter, J. F. (1993, Spring). Self-management: Education's ultimate goal. *Teaching Exceptional Children,* 28–31.

Cautela, J. R., & Groden, J. (1978). *Relaxation: A comprehensive manual for adults, children, and children with special needs.* Champaign, IL: Research Press.

Chandler, M. (1973). Egocentrism and anti-social behavior: The assessment and training of social perspective-taking skills. *Developmental Psychology, 9,* 326–332.

Clarke, G. N., Hawkins, W., Murphy, M., Sheeber, L. B., Lewinsohn, M., & Seeley, J. R. (1995). Targeted prevention of unipolar depressive disorder in an at-risk sample of high school adolescents: A randomized trial of a group cognitive interview. *Journal of the American Academy of Child and Adolescent Psychiatry, 34,* 312–321.

Clarke, G. N., Rohde, P., Lewinsohn, P. M., Hops, H., & Seeley, J. R. (1998). Cognitive-behavioral treatment of adolescent depression: Efficacy of acute group treatment and booster sessions. *Journal of the American Academy of Child and Adolescent Psychiatry, 38,* 272–279.

Clifford, M. M. (1984). Thoughts on a theory of constructive failure. *Educational Psychology, 19,* 108–120.

Cohen, R., & Schleser, R. (1984). Cognitive development and clinical interventions. In A. W. Meyers & W. E. Craighead (Eds.), *Cognitive behavior therapy with children* (pp. 45–68). New York: Plenum Press.

Conrad, M., & Hammen, C. (1989). Role of maternal depression in perceptions of child maladjustment. *Journal of Consulting and Clinical Psychology, 57,* 663–667.

Craighead, W. E., Meyers, A. W., & Craighead, L. W. (1985). A conceptual model for cognitive-behavior therapy with children. *Journal of Abnormal Child Psychology, 13,* 331–342.

Crick, N., & Dodge, K. (1994). A review and reformulation of social information-processing mechanisms in children's social adjustment. *Psychological Bulletin, 115,* 74–101.

Deshler, D. D., Alley, G. R., Warner, M. M., & Schumaker, J. B. (1981). Instructional practices for promoting skill acquisition and generalization in severely learning disabled adolescents. *Learning Disability Quarterly*, 6, 231–234.

Dix, T. H., Ruble, D. M., Gresec, J. E., & Nixon, S. (1986). Mothers' implicit theories of discipline: Child effects, parent effects, and the attribution process. *Child Development*, 57, 879–894.

Dodge, K. A. (1986). A social information processing model of social competence in children. In M. Perlmutter (Ed.), *Minnesota Symposia on Child Psychology: Vol. 18. Cognitive perspectives on children's social and behavioral development* (pp. 77–125). Hillsdale, NJ: Erlbaum.

Dodge, K. A., & Frame, C. L. (1982). Social cognitive biases and deficits in aggressive boys. *Child Development*, 53, 620–635.

Dodge, K. A., & Newman, J. P. (1981). Biased decision-making processes in aggressive boys. *Journal of Abnormal Psychology*, 90, 375–379.

Dodge, K. A., Pettit, G. S., McClaskey, C. C., & Brown, M. M. (1986). Social competence in children. *Monographs of the Society for Research in Child Development*, 51(2, Serial No. 213).

Douglas, V. I. (1983). Attention and cognitive problems. In M. Rutter (Ed.), *Developmental neuropsychiatry* (pp. 280–329). New York: Guilford Press.

Dudley, C. D. (1997). *Treating depressed children: A therapeutic manual of cognitive behavioral interventions*. Oakland, CA: New Harbinger.

Durlak, J. A., Fuhrman, T., & Lampman, C. (1991). Effectiveness of cognitive-behavior therapy for maladapting children: A meta-analysis. *Psychological Bulletin*, 110, 204–214.

Dweck, D. S. (1975). The role of expectations and attributions in the alteration of learned helplessness. *Journal of Personality and Social Psychology*, 25, 109–116.

D'Zurilla, T. J., & Goldfried, M. R. (1971). Problem-solving and behavior modification. *Journal of Abnormal Psychology*, 78, 107–126.

Eisen, A. R., & Silverman, W. K. (1993). Should I relax or change my thought?: A preliminary examination of cognitive therapy, relaxation training, and their combination with overanxious children. *Journal of Cognitive Psychotherapy: An International Quarterly*, 7, 265–279.

Eisen, A. R., & Silverman, W. K. (1998). Prescriptive treatment for generalized anxiety disorder in children. *Behavior Therapy*, 29, 105–121.

Ellis, A. (1970). *The essence of rational psychotherapy: A comprehensive approach to treatment*. New York: Institute for Rational Living.

Ellis, A., & Harper, R. (1975). *A new guide to rational living*. North Hollywood, CA: Wilshire Books.

Feindler, E. L. (1991). Cognitive strategies in anger control interventions for children and adolescents. In P. C. Kendall (Ed.), *Child and adolescent therapy: Cognitive-behavioral procedures* (pp. 66–97). New York: Guilford Press.

Feindler, E. L., & Ecton, R. B. (1986). *Adolescent anger control: Cognitive-behavioral techniques*. New York: Pergamon Press.

Finch, A. J., Nelson, W. M., & Ott, E. S. (Eds.). (1993). *Cognitive-behavioral procedures with children and adolescents: A practical guide*. Needham Heights, MA: Allyn & Bacon.

Flannery-Schroeder, E., & Kendall, P. C. (1997). *Cognitive-behavioral therapy for anxious children: Therapist manual for group treatment*. Ardmore, PA: Workbook.

Forehand, R., & McMahon, R. J. (1981). *Helping the noncompliant child: A clinician's guide to parent training*. New York: Guilford Press.

Frankel, F., Cantwell, D. P., & Myatt, R. (1996). Helping ostracized children: Social skills training and parent support for socially rejected children. In E. D. Hibb & P. Jensen (Eds.), *Psychosocial treatments for child and adolescent disorders: Empirically based strategies for clinical practice* (pp. 595–617). Washington, DC: American Psychological Association.

Fuchs, C. Z., & Rehm, L. P. (1977). A self-control behavior therapy program for depression. *Journal of Consulting and Clinical Psychology, 45,* 206–215.

Furman, W. (1980). Promoting social development: Developmental implications for treatment. In B. B. Lahey & A. E. Kazdin (Eds.), *Advances in clinical child psychology* (Vol. 3, pp. 1–40). New York: Plenum Press.

Gladstone, T. R. G., Kaslow, N. J., Seeley, J. R., & Lewinsohn, P. M. (1997). Sex differences, attributional style, and depressive symptoms among adolescents. *Journal of Abnormal Child Psychology, 25,* 297–305.

Goldstein, S. (1995). *Understanding and managing children's classroom behavior.* New York: Wiley.

Goldstein, S., & Goldstein, M. (1998). *Managing attention deficit hyperactivity disorder in children: A guide for practitioners.* New York: Wiley.

Goodwin, S., & Mahoney, M. J. (1975). Modifications of aggression through modeling: An experimental probe. *Journal of Behavior Therapy and Experimental Psychiatry, 6,* 200–202.

Griest, D. L., Forehand, R., Rogers, T., Breiner, J., Furey, W., & Williams, C. A. (1982). Effects of parent enhancement therapy on the treatment outcome and generalization of a parent training program. *Behaviour Research and Therapy, 20,* 429–436.

Hallahan, D. P., Lloyd, J. W., Kneedler, R. D., & Marshall, K. J. (1982). A comparison of the effects of self- versus teacher-assessment of on-task behavior. *Behavior Therapy, 12,* 715–723.

Hammen, C. (1988). Self cognitions, stressful events, and the prediction of depression in children of depressed mothers. *Journal of Abnormal Child Psychology, 16,* 347–360.

Harris, K., & Graham, S. (1996). *Making the writing process work: Strategies for composition and self-regulation.* Cambridge, MA: Brookline Books.

Harter, S. (1982). A developmental perspective on some parameters of self-regulation in children. In P. Karoly & F. H. Kanfer (Eds.), *Self-management and behavior change: From theory to practice* (pp. 165–204). New York: Pergamon Press.

Heimberg, R. G., Dodge, C. S., Hope, D. A., Kennedy, C. R., Zollo, L. J., & Becker, R. J. (1990). Cognitive behavioral group treatment for social phobia: Comparison with a credible placebo control. *Cognitive Therapy and Research, 14,* 1–23.

Henggler, S. W., Melton, G. B., & Smith, L. A. (1992). Family preservation using multisystemic therapy: An effective alternative to incarcerating serious juvenile offenders. *Journal of Consulting and Clinical Psychology, 60,* 953–961.

Hinshaw, S. P. (2000). Attention-deficit/hyperactivity disorder: The search for viable treatments. In P. C. Kendall (Ed.), *Child and adolescent therapy: Cognitive-behavioral procedures* (pp. 88–128). New York: Guilford Press.

Hinshaw, S. P., Buhrmester, D., & Heller, T. (1989). Anger control in response to verbal provocation: Effects of stimulant medication for boys with ADHD. *Journal of Abnormal Child Psychology, 17*, 393–407.

Hinshaw, S. P., & Erhardt, D. (1991). Attention-deficit hyperactivity disorder. In P. C. Kendall (Ed.), *Child and adolescent therapy: Cognitive-behavioral procedures* (pp. 98–128). New York: Guilford Press.

Hinshaw, S. P., Henker, B., & Whalen, C. K. (1984a). Self-control in hyperactive boys in anger-inducing situations: Effects of cognitive-behavioral training and of methylphenidate. *Journal of Abnormal Child Psychology, 12*, 55–77.

Hinshaw, S. P., Henker, B., & Whalen, C. K. (1984b). Cognitive-behavioral and pharmacologic interventions for hyperactive boys: Comparative and combined effects. *Journal of Consulting and Clinical Psychology, 52*, 739–749.

Holmbeck, G., Calder, C., Shapera, W., Westhoven, V., Kenealy, L., & Updegrove, A. (2000). Working with adolescents: Guides from developmental psychology. In P. C. Kendall (Ed.), *Child and adolescent therapy: Cognitive-behavioral procedures* (2nd ed., pp. 334–385). New York: Guilford Press.

Howard, B., Chu, B., Krain, A., Marrs-Garcia, A., & Kendall, P. C. (1999). *Cognitive-behavioral family therapy for anxious children* (2nd ed.). Ardmore, PA: Workbook.

Hudson, L. M. (1978). On the coherence of role-taking abilities: An alternative to correlational analysis. *Child Development, 49*, 223–227.

Hughes, C. A., & Hendrickson, J. M. (1987). Self-monitoring with at-risk students in the regular class setting. *Education and Treatment of Children, 10*, 236–250.

Johnston, C., & Patenaude, R. (1994). Parent attributions for inattentive–overactive and oppositional–defiant child behaviors. *Cognitive Therapy and Research, 18*, 261–275.

Kahn, J. S., Kehle, T. J., Jenson, W. R., & Clark, E. (1990). Comparison of cognitive-behavioral, relaxation, and self-modeling interventions for depression among middle-school students. *School Psychology Review, 19*, 196–208.

Kane, M. T., & Kendall, P. C. (1989). Anxiety disorders in children: A multiple baseline evaluation of a cognitive-behavioral treatment. *Behavior Therapy, 20*, 499–508.

Kanfer, F. H. (1970). Self-monitoring: Methodological limitations and clinical applications. *Journal of Consulting and Clinical Psychology, 35*, 148–152.

Kanfer, F. H. (1971). The maintenance of behavior by self-generated reinforcement. In A. Jacobs & L. G. Sachs (Eds.), *The psychology of private events* (pp. 39–59). New York: Academic Press.

Kaslow, N. J., & Thompson, M. P. (1998). Applying the criteria for empirically supported treatments to studies of psychosocial interventions for child and adolescent depression. *Journal of Clinical Child Psychology, 27*, 146–155.

Kazdin, A. E. (1974). Covert modeling, model similarity, and reduction of avoidance behavior. *Behavior Therapy, 5*, 325–340.

Kazdin, A. E., Bass, D., Siegel, T., & Thomas, C. (1989). Cognitive-behavioral therapy and relationship therapy in the treatment of children referred for antisocial behavior. *Journal of Consulting and Clinical Psychology, 57,* 522–535.

Kazdin, A. E., & Crowley, M. J. (1997). Moderators of treatment outcome in cognitively based treatment of antisocial children. *Cognitive Therapy and Research, 21,* 185–207.

Kazdin, A. E., Esveldt-Dawson, K., French, N. H., & Unis, A. S. (1987a). Effects of parent management training and problem-solving skills training combined in the treatment of antisocial child behavior. *Journal of the American Academy of Child and Adolescent Psychiatry, 26,* 416–424.

Kazdin, A. E., Esveldt-Dawson, K., French, N. H., & Unis, A. S. (1987b). Problem-solving skills training and relationship therapy in the treatment of antisocial child behavior. *Journal of Consulting and Clinical Psychology, 55,* 76–85.

Kazdin, A. E., & Kendall, P. C. (1998). Current progress and future plans for developing effective treatments: Comments and perspectives. *Journal of Clinical Child Psychology, 27,* 217–226.

Kazdin, A. E., Siegel, T. C., & Bass, D. (1992). Cognitive problem-solving skills training and parent management training in the treatment of antisocial behavior in children. *Journal of Consulting and Clinical Psychology, 60,* 733–747.

Kazdin, A. E., & Weisz, J. R. (1998). Identifying and developing empirically supported child and adolescent treatments. *Journal of Consulting and Clinical Psychology, 66,* 19–36.

Keller, M. B., Lavori, P., Wunder, J., Beardslee, W. R., Schwartz, C. E., & Roth, J. (1992). Chronic anxiety disorders in children and adolescents. *Journal of the American Academy of Child and Adolescent Psychiatry, 31,* 595–599.

Kendall, P. C. (1992). *Coping cat workbook.* Ardmore, PA: Workbook.

Kendall, P. C. (1993). Cognitive-behavioral therapies with youth: Guiding theory, current status, and emerging developments. *Journal of Consulting and Clinical Psychology, 61,* 235–247.

Kendall, P. C. (1994). Treating anxiety disorders in youth: Results of a randomized clinical trial. *Journal of Consulting and Clinical Psychology, 62,* 100–110.

Kendall, P. C. (1998). Empirically supported psychological therapies. *Journal of Consulting and Clinical Psychology, 66,* 1–3.

Kendall, P. C. (Ed.). (2000). *Child and adolescent therapy: Cognitive-behavioral procedures* (2nd ed.). New York: Guilford Press.

Kendall, P. C., & Braswell, L. (1993). *Cognitive-behavioral therapy for impulsive children* (2nd ed.). New York: Guilford Press.

Kendall, P. C., Chansky, T. E., Kane, M., Kim, R., Kortlander, E., Ronan, K., Sessa, F., & Siqueland, L. (1992). *Anxiety disorders in youth: Cognitive-behavioral interventions.* Needham Heights, MA: Allyn & Bacon.

Kendall, P. C., Chu, B., Gifford, A., Hayes, C., & Nauta, M. (1998). Breathing life into a manual. *Cognitive and Behavioral Practice, 5,* 177–198.

Kendall, P. C., Chu, B., Pimentel, S., & Choudhury, M. (2000). Treating anxiety disorders in youth. In P. C. Kendall (Ed.), *Child and adolescent therapy: Cognitive-behavioral procedures* (2nd ed., pp. 235–287). New York: Guilford Press.

Kendall, P. C., Flannery-Schroeder, E., & Ford, J. (1999). Therapy outcome research methods. In P. C. Kendall, J. Butcher, & G. Holmbeck (Eds.), *Hand-*

book of research methods in clinical psychology (pp. 330–363). New York: Wiley.

Kendall, P. C., Flannery-Schroeder, E., Panichelli-Mindel, S. M., Southam-Gerow, M., Henin, A., & Warman, M. J. (1997). Therapy for youth with anxiety disorders: A second randomized clinical trial. *Journal of Consulting and Clinical Psychology, 65,* 366–380.

Kendall, P. C., & Hollon, S. D., (Eds.). (1979). *Cognitive-behavioral interventions: Theory, research and procedures.* New York: Academic Press.

Kendall, P. C., Howard, B. L., & Epps, J. (1988). The anxious child: Cognitive-behavioral treatment strategies. *Behavior Modification, 12,* 281–310.

Kendall, P. C., Kortlander, E., Chansky, T. E., & Brady, E. U. (1992). Comorbidity of anxiety and depression in youth: Treatment implications. *Journal of Consulting and Clinical Psychology, 60,* 869–880.

Kendall, P. C., & MacDonald, J. P. (1993). Cognition in psychopathology of youth and implications for treatment. In K. S. Dobson & P. C. Kendall (Eds.), *Psychopathology and cognition* (pp. 387–432). San Diego, CA: Academic Press.

Kendall, P. C., MacDonald, J. P., & Treadwell, K. R. H. (1995). The treatment of anxiety disorders in youth: Future directions. In A. R. Eisen, C. A. Kearney, & C. E. Schaefer (Eds.), *Clinical handbook of anxiety disorder in children and adolescents* (pp. 573–597). Northvale, NJ: Aronson.

Kendall, P. C., & Panichelli-Mindel, S. M. (1995). Cognitive-behavioral treatments. *Journal of Abnormal Child Psychology, 23,* 107–124.

Kendall, P. C., Reber, M., McLeer, S., Epps, J., & Ronan, K. R. (1990). Cognitive-behavioral treatment of conduct-disordered children. *Cognitive Therapy and Research, 14,* 279–297.

Kendall, P. C., & Southam-Gerow, M. A. (1996). Long-term follow-up of a cognitive-behavioral therapy for anxiety disordered youth. *Journal of Consulting and Clinical Psychology, 64,* 724–730.

Kendall, P. C., Stark, K. D., & Adam, T. (1990). Cognitive deficit or cognitive distortion in childhood depression. *Journal of Abnormal Child Psychology, 18,* 255–270.

Kendall, P. C., & Sugerman, A. (1997). Attrition in the treatment of childhood anxiety disorder. *Journal of Consulting and Clinical Psychology, 65,* 883–888.

Kendall, P. C., & Treadwell, K. R. H. (1996). Cognitive-behavioral treatment for childhood anxiety disorders. In P. S. Jensen & E. D. Hibbs (Eds.), *Psychosocial treatment research with children and adolescents* (pp. 23–41). Washington, DC: American Psychological Association.

Kiesler, D. J. (1966). Some myths of psychotherapy research and the search for a paradigm. *Psychological Bulletin, 65,* 110–136.

Kimball, W., Nelson, W. M., & Politano, P. M. (1993). The role of developmental variables in cognitive-behavioral interventions with children. In A. J. Finch, W. M. Nelson, & E. S. Ott (Eds.), *Cognitive-behavioral procedures with children and adolescents: A practical guide* (pp. 25–66). Needham Heights, MA: Allyn & Bacon.

Koeppen, A. S. (1974). Relaxation training for children. *Elementary School Guidance and Counseling, 9,* 14–26.

Kolko, D. J., Loar, L. L., & Sturnick, D. (1990). Inpatient social-cognitive skills training groups with conduct disordered and attention deficit disordered children. *Journal of Child Psychology and Psychiatry, 31,* 737–748.

Kortlander, E., Kendall, P. C., & Panichelli-Mindel, S. (1997). Maternal expectations and attributions about coping in anxious children. *Journal of Anxiety Disorders, 11,* 297–315.

Kovacs, M. (1981). Rating scales to assess depression in school aged children. *Acta Paedopsychiatrica, 46,* 305–315.

Kroll, L., Harrington, R., Jayson, D., Fraser, J., & Gowers, S. (1996). Pilot study of continuation cognitive-behavioral therapy for major depression in adolescent psychiatric patients. *Journal of the American Academy of Child and Adolescent Psychiatry, 35,* 1156–1161.

Lazarus, A. A., & Abramovitz, A. (1962) The use of "emotive imagery" in the treatment of children's phobias. *Journal of Mental Science, 108,* 191–195.

Leon, J. A., & Pepe, H. J. (1983). Self-instructional training: Cognitive behavior modification for remediating arithmetic deficits. *Exceptional Children, 50,* 54–60.

Lewinsohn, P. M. (1974). A behavioral approach to depression. In R. M. Friedman & M. M. Katz (Eds.), *The psychology of depression: Contemporary theory and research.* New York: Wiley.

Lewinsohn, P. M., Clark, G. N., Hops, H., & Andrews, J. (1990). Cognitive-behavioral group treatment of depression in adolescents. *Behavior Therapy, 21,* 385–401.

Lewinsohn, P. M., Clark, G. N., & Rohde, P. (1994). Psychological approaches to the treatment of depression in adolescents. In W. M. Reynolds & H. F. Johnston (Eds.), *Handbook of depression in children and adolescents* (pp. 309–344). New York: Plenum Press.

Lewinsohn, P. M., Clark, G. N., Rohde, P., Hops, H., & Seeley, J. R. (1996). A course in coping: A cognitive-behavioral approach to the treatment of adolescent depression. In E. D. Hibbs & P. S. Jensen (Eds.), *Child and adolescent disorders: Empirically based strategies for clinical practice* (pp. 109–135). Washington DC: American Psychological Association.

Lewinsohn, P. M., Rohde, P., Hops, H., & Clark, G. (1991). *Leader's manual for parent groups: Adolescent Coping with Depression.* Eugene, OR: Castalia Press.

Lochman, J. E. (1987). Self and peer perceptions and attributional biases of aggressive and nonaggressive boys in dyadic interactions. *Journal of Consulting and Clinical Psychology, 55,* 404–410.

Lochman, J. E. (1992). Cognitive-behavioral intervention with aggressive boys: Three-year follow-up and preventive effects. *Journal of Consulting and Clinical Psychology, 60,* 426–434.

Lochman, J. E., Burch, P. R., Curry, J. F., & Lampron, L. B. (1984). Treatment and generalization effects of cognitive-behavioral and goal-setting interventions with aggressive boys. *Journal of Consulting and Clinical Psychology, 52,* 915–916.

Lochman, J. E., & Curry, J. F. (1986). Effects of social problem-solving training and self-instruction training with aggressive boys. *Journal of Consulting and Clinical Psychology, 15,* 159–164.

Lochman, J. E., Lampron, L. B., Gemmer, T. C., Harris, R., & Wyckoff, G. M. (1989). Teacher consultation and cognitive-behavioral interventions with aggressive boys. *Psychology in the Schools, 26,* 179–188.

Lochman, J. E., Whidby, J., & FitzGerald, D. (2000). Cognitive behavioral assessment and treatment with aggressive children. In P. C. Kendall (Ed.), *Child and adolescent therapy: Cognitive-behavioral procedures* (pp. 31–87). New York: Guilford Press.

Lochman, J. E., White, K. J., & Wayland, K. K. (1991). Cognitive-behavioral assessment and treatment with aggressive children. In P. C. Kendall (Ed.), *Child and adolescent therapy: Cognitive-behavioral procedures* (pp. 25–65). New York: Guilford Press.

Luria, A. R. (1961). *The role of speech in the regulation of normal and abnormal behaviors.* New York: Liveright.

Mahoney, M. J. (1977). Reflections in the cognitive–learning trend in psychotherapy. *American Psychologist, 32,* 5–18.

March, J. S. (1995). Behavioral psychotherapy for children and adolescents with obsessive compulsive disorder: A review of the literature and recommendation for treatment. *Journal of the American Academy of Child and Adolescent Psychiatry, 34,* 7–18.

March, J. S., & Mulle, K. (1998). *OCD in children and adolescents: A cognitive-behavioral treatment manual.* New York: Guilford Press.

March, J. S., Mulle, K., & Herbel, B. (1994). Behavioral psychotherapy for children and adolescents with obsessive–compulsive disorder: An open trial of a new protocol-driven treatment package. *Journal of the American Academy of Child and Adolescent Psychiatry, 33,* 333–341.

Masek, B., Russo, D. C., & Varni, J. W. (1984). Behavioral approaches to the management of chronic pain in children. *Pediatric Clinics of North America, 31,* 1113–1131.

Mattis, S. G., & Ollendick, T. H. (1997). Children's cognitive responses to the somatic symptoms of panic. *Journal of Abnormal Child Psychology, 25,* 47–51.

Meichenbaum, D. (1971). Examination of model characteristics in reducing avoidance behavior. *Journal of Personality and Social Psychology, 17,* 298–307.

Meichenbaum, D., & Goodman, J. (1971). Training impulsive children to talk to themselves: A means of developing self-control. *Journal of Abnormal Psychology, 77,* 115–126.

Mendlowitz, S. L., Manassis, K., Bradley, S., Scapillato, D., Miezitis, S., & Shaw, B. F. (1999). Cognitive-behavioral group treatments in childhood anxiety disorders: The role of parental involvement. *Journal of the American Academy of Child and Adolescent Psychiatry, 38,* 1223–1229.

Miller, L. C., Barrett, C. L., & Hampe, E. (1974). Phobias of childhood in a prescientific era. In S. David (Ed.), *Child personality and psychopathology* (pp. 89–134). New York: Wiley.

Mischel, W. (1974). Processes in delay of gratification. In L. Berkowitz (Ed.), *Advances in experimental social psychology* (Vol. 7, pp. 249–292). New York: Academic Press.

Morris, R. J., & Kratochwill, T. R. (1983). *Treating children's fears and phobias: A behavioral approach.* New York: Pergamon Press.

MTA Cooperative Group. (1999a). A 14-month randomized clinical trial of treatment strategies for attention-deficit/hyperactivity disorder. *Archives of General Psychiatry, 56*, 1073–1086.

MTA Cooperative Group. (1999b). Moderators and mediators of treatment response for children with attention-deficit/hyperactivity disorder. *Archives of General Psychiatry, 56*, 1088–1096.

Nelson, W. M., & Finch, A. J. (1996). *"Keeping your cool": The anger management workbook.* Ardmore, PA: Workbook.

Ollendick, T. H., & Cerny, J. A. (1981). *Clinical behavior therapy with children.* New York: Plenum Press.

Ollendick, T. H., & King, N. J. (1998). Empirically supported treatments for children with phobic and anxiety disorders: Current status. *Journal of Clinical Child Psychology, 27*, 156–167.

Ollendick, T. H., & King, N. J. (2000). Empirically supported treatments for children and adolescents: Guides from developmental psychology. In P. C. Kendall (Ed.), *Child and adolescent therapy: Cognitive-behavioral procedures* (2nd ed., pp. 386–425). New York: Guilford Press.

Persons, J. (1991). Psychotherapy outcome studies do not accurately represent current models of psychotherapy. *American Psychologist, 46*, 99–106.

Pfiffner, L., & Barkley, R. A. (1998). Treatment of ADHD in school settings. In R. A. Barkley (Ed.), *Attention-deficit hyperactivity disorder: A handbook for diagnosis and treatment* (2nd ed., pp. 458–490). New York: Guilford Press.

Pfiffner, L., Jouriles, E. N., Brown, N. B., Etscheidt, M. A., & Kelly, J. A. (1990). Effects of problem-solving therapy as outcomes of parent training on single-parent families. *Child and Family Behavior Therapy, 12*, 1–11.

Piaget, J. S. (1926). *The language and thought of the child.* New York: Harcourt, Brace.

Prater, M. A., Joy, R., Chilman, B., Temple, J., & Miller, S. R. (1991). Self-monitoring of on-task behavior with adolescents with learning disability. *Learning Disability Quarterly, 14*, 164–177.

Rabian, B., Peterson, R., Richters, J., & Jensen, P. (1993). Anxiety sensitivity among anxious children. *Journal of Clinical Child Psychology, 22*, 441–446.

Reeve, R. A., & Brown, A. L. (1985). Meta-cognition reconsidered: Implications for intervention research. *Journal of Abnormal Child Psychology, 13*, 343–356.

Rehm, L. P., & Sharp, R. N. (1996). Strategies for childhood depression. In M. A. Reinecke, F. M. Dattilio, & A. Freeman (Eds.), *Cognitive therapy with children and adolescents: A casebook for clinical practice* (pp. 103–123). New York: Guilford Press.

Reid, J. B., Kavanagh, K., & Baldwin, D. V. (1987). Abusive parents' perceptions of child problem behaviors: An example of parental bias. *Journal of Abnormal Child Psychology, 15*, 457–466.

Reinecke, M. A., Dattilio, F. M., & Freeman, A. (1996). *Cognitive therapy with children and adolescents: A casebook for clinical practice.* New York: Guilford Press.

Reynolds, W. M., & Coats, K. I. (1986). A comparison of cognitive-behavioral therapy and relaxation training for the treatment of depression in adolescents. *Journal of Consulting and Clinical Psychology, 54*, 653–660.

Robin, A. L. (1998). Training families with ADHD adolescents. In R. A. Barkley, *Attention-deficit hyperactivity disorder: A handbook for diagnosis and treatment* (2nd ed., pp. 413–457). New York: Guilford Press.

Robin, A. L., & Foster, S. L. (1989). *Negotiating parent–adolescent conflict: A behavioral–family systems approach.* New York: Guilford Press.

Robin, A. L., & Schneider, M. (1974). *The turtle technique: An approach to self-control in the classroom.* Unpublished manuscript, State University of New York at Stony Brook.

Robin, A. L., Schneider, M., & Dolnick, M. (1976). The turtle technique: An extended case study of self-control in the classroom. *Psychology in the Schools, 13,* 449–453.

Roehling, P. V., & Robin, A. L. (1986). Development and validation of the Family Belief Inventory: A measure of unrealistic beliefs among parents and adolescents. *Journal of Consulting and Clinical Psychology, 54,* 693–697.

Rosenthal, T., & Bandura, A. (1978). Psychological model: Theory and practice. In S. L. Garfield & A. E. Bergin (Eds.), *Handbook of psychotherapy and behavior change* (2nd ed., pp. 621–658). New York: Wiley.

Rotheram-Borus, M. J., Piacentini, J., Miller, S., Graae, F., & Castro-Blanco, D. (1994). Brief cognitive behavioral treatment for adolescent suicide attempters and their families. *Journal of the American Academy of Child and Adolescent Psychiatry, 33,* 508–517.

Rudolph, K. D., Hammen, C., & Burge, D. (1997). A cognitive–interpersonal approach to depressive symptoms in preadolescent children. *Journal of Abnormal Child Psychology, 25,* 33–45.

Sanders, M. R., Rebgetz, M., Morrison, M., Bor, W., Gordon, A., Dadds, M., & Shepherd, R. (1989). Cognitive-behavioral treatment of recurrent nonspecific abdominal pain in children: An analysis of generalization, maintenance, and side effects. *Journal of Consulting and Clinical Psychology, 57,* 294–300.

Sarason, I. G. (1975). Test anxiety and the self-disclosing model. *Journal of Consulting and Clinical Psychology, 43,* 148–153.

Sarason, I. G., & Ganzer, V. J. (1973). Modeling and group discussion in the rehabilitation of juvenile delinquents. *Journal of Counseling Psychology, 20,* 442–449.

Schunk, P. H. (1983). Ability versus effort attributional feedback: Differential effects on self-efficacy and achievement. *Journal of Educational Psychology, 75,* 848–856.

Selman, R. L. (1980). *The growth of interpersonal understanding: Developmental and clinical analyses.* New York: Academic Press.

Selman, R. L., & Byrne, D. A. (1974). A structural developmental analysis of levels of role-taking in middle childhood. *Child Development, 45,* 803–806.

Shapiro, E. S., & Cole, C. L. (1994). *Behavior change in the classroom: Self-management interventions.* New York: Guilford Press.

Shantz, C. V. (1983). Social cognition. In J. H. Flavell & E. Markman (Eds.), *Carmichael's manual of child psychology: Vol. 3. Cognitive development* (pp. 495–555). New York: Wiley.

Shirk, S., & Harter, S. (1996). Treatment of low self-esteem. In M. A. Reinecke, F. M. Dattilio, & A. Freeman (Eds.), *Cognitive therapy with children and adoles-*

cents: A casebook for clinical practice (pp. 175–198). New York: Guilford Press.

Shure, M. B., & Spivack, G. (1978). *Problem-solving techniques in childrearing.* San Francisco: Jossey-Bass.

Silverman, W. K., Ginsburg, G. S., & Kurtines, W. M. (1995). Clinical issues in treating children with anxiety and phobic disorders. *Cognitive and Behavioral Practice, 2*, 93–117.

Smith, A. M., & O'Leary, S. G. (1995). Attributions and arousal as predictors of maternal discipline. *Cognitive Therapy and Research, 19*, 459–471.

Southam-Gerow, M. A., & Kendall, P. C. (in press). Emotion understanding in youth referred for treatment of anxiety disorders. *Journal of Clinical Child Psychology.*

Spence, S. (1994). Practitioner review: Cognitive therapy with children and adolescents—from theory to practice. *Journal of Child Psychology and Psychiatry, 3*, 1191–1227.

Spivack, G., Platt, J. J., & Shure, M. B. (1976). *The problem-solving approach to adjustment.* San Francisco: Jossey-Bass.

Stark, K. D. (1990). *Childhood depression: School-based intervention.* New York: Guilford Press.

Stark, K. D., Sander, J. B., Yancy, M., Bronik, M., & Hoke, J. (2000). Treatment of depression in childhood and adolescence: Cognitive-behavioral procedures for the individual and family. In P. C. Kendall (Ed.), *Child and adolescent therapy: Cognitive-behavioral procedures* (2nd ed., pp. 173–234). New York: Guilford Press.

Stark, K. D., Kendall, P. C., McCarthy, M., Stafford, M., Barron, R., & Thomeer, M. (1996). *Taking action: A workbook for overcoming depression.* Ardmore, PA: Workbook.

Stark, K. D., Reynolds, W. M., & Kaslow, N. J. (1987). A comparison of the relative efficacy of self-control therapy and behavioral problem-solving therapy for depression in children. *Journal of Abnormal Child Psychology, 15*, 91–113.

Stark, K. D., Rouse, L., & Livingston, R. (1991). Treatment of depression during childhood and adolescence: Cognitive-behavioral procedures for the individual and family. In P. C. Kendall (Ed.), *Child and adolescent therapy: Cognitive-behavioral procedures* (pp. 165–208). New York: Guilford Press.

Strassberg, Z. (1997). Levels of analysis in cognitive bases of maternal disciplinary dysfunction. *Journal of Abnormal Psychology, 25*, 209–215.

Strayhorn, J. M. (1988). *The competent child: An approach to psychotherapy and preventive mental health.* New York: Guilford Press.

Treadwell, K. R. H., & Kendall, P. C. (1996). Self-talk in anxiety-disordered youth: States of mind, content specificity, and treatment outcome. *Journal of Consulting and Clinical Psychology, 64*, 941–950.

Tremblay, R. E., Pagani-Kurtz, L., Masse, L. C., Vitaro, F., & Phil, R. (1995). A bimodal preventive intervention for disruptive kindergarten boys: Its impact through mid-adolescence. *Journal of Consulting and Clinical Psychology, 63*, 560–568.

Turner, J. E., & Cole, D. A. (1994). Developmental differences in cognitive diatheses for child depression. *Journal of Abnormal Child Psychology, 22,* 15–32.

Vygotsky, L. (1962). *Thought and language.* New York: Wiley.

Wahler, R. G. (1990). Some perceptual functions of social networks in coercive mother–child interactions. *Journal of Social and Clinical Psychology, 9,* 43–53.

Wahler, R. G., Carter, P. G., Fleischman, J., & Lambert, W. (1993). The impact of synthesis teaching and parent training with mothers of conduct-disordered children. *Journal of Abnormal Child Psychology, 21,* 425–440.

Wahler, R. G., & Dumas, J. E. (1989). Attentional problems in dysfunctional mother–child interactions. *Psychological Bulletin, 105,* 116–130.

Webster-Stratton, C. (1984). Randomized trial of two parent-training programs for families with conduct disordered children. *Journal of Consulting and Clinical Psychology, 52,* 666–678.

Webster-Stratton, C., & Hammond, M. (1988). Maternal depression and its relationship to life stress, perceptions of child behavior problems, parenting behaviors, and child conduct problems. *Journal of Abnormal Child Psychology, 16,* 299–315.

Weiner, B. (1979). A theory of motivation of some classroom experience. *Journal of Educational Psychology, 71,* 3–25.

Weissberg, R. P., Caplan, M., & Harwood, R. (1991). Promoting competent young people in competence-enhancing environments: A systems-based perspective on primary prevention. *Journal of Consulting and Clinical Psychology, 59,* 830–841.

Weisz, J. R., Huey, S. J., & Weersing, V. R. (1998). Psychology outcome research with children and adolescents: The state of the art. In T. H. Ollendick & R. J. Prinz (Eds.), *Advances in clinical child psychology* (Vol. 20). New York: Plenum Press.

Weisz, J. R., & Weiss, B. (1991). "Studying the referability" of child clinical problems. *Journal of Consulting and Clinical Psychology, 59,* 266–273.

Wilkes, T. C. R., Belsher, G., Rush, A. J., Frank, E., & Associates. (1994). *Cognitive therapy for depressed adolescents.* New York: Guilford Press.

Zentall, S. S. (1995). Modifying classroom tasks and environments. In S. Goldstein, *Understanding and managing children's classroom behavior* (pp. 356–374). New York: Wiley.

9

Rational Emotive Behavior Therapy

WINDY DRYDEN
ALBERT ELLIS

Rational emotive behavior therapy (REBT) was founded by Albert Ellis in 1955 (Ellis, 1997a). As such, it has the longest history of any of the forms of cognitive-behavioral therapy (CBT) covered in the present handbook. Like many originators of new therapeutic systems of that time, Ellis had become increasingly disenchanted with the traditional psychoanalytic therapies as effective and efficient helping systems. Although this disillusionment was in part responsible for the creation of REBT, a number of other influences can be detected in this regard. Ellis had a long-standing interest in philosophy and was particularly influenced by the writings of Stoic philosophers such as Epictetus and Marcus Aurelius. In particular, the oft-quoted phrase of Epictetus, "People are disturbed not by things but by their view of things," crystallized Ellis's view that philosophical factors are more important than psychoanalytic and psychodynamic factors in accounting for psychological disturbance.

In addition to the influence of the Stoics, the impact of a number of other philosophers can be discovered in Ellis's ideas. For example, Ellis (1981a) has shown that he was influenced by Immanuel Kant's writings on both the power and the limitations of cognition and ideation, particularly those to be found in Kant's *Critique of Pure Reason*. From its inception, Ellis has argued that REBT is founded upon the tenets of logico-empirical methods of science, and in this respect has pointed to the writings of Popper (1959, 1963) and Reichenbach (1953) as having a distinct impact on his efforts to make these philosophical ideas core features of the therapeutic system of REBT. Interestingly, George Kelly (1955), the founder of personal construct therapy, was independently engaged in a very similar project at that same time.

REBT is closely identified with the tenets of ethical humanism (Russell, 1930, 1965). Furthermore, REBT has distinct existential roots; Ellis has said in this respect that he was particularly influenced by the ideas of Paul Tillich (1953) in the mid-1950s. Like other existentialists (e.g., Heidegger, 1949), REBT theorists agree that humans are "at the centre of their universe (but not of the universe) and have the power of choice (but not of unlimited choice) with regard to their emotional realm" (Dryden & Ellis, 1986, p. 130). Ellis (1984a) has claimed that REBT is doubly humanistic in its outlook, in that it

a) attempts to help people maximize their individuality, freedom, self-interest, and self-control at the same time that it, and
b) tries to help them live in an involved, committed, and selectively loving manner. It thereby strives to facilitate individual and social interest. (p. 23)

Although Ellis himself espouses atheistic values, a number of REBT theorists and practitioners do subscribe to religious faiths (Hauck, 1972; Powell, 1976). REBT is not against religion per se; rather, it opposes religiosity—a dogmatic and devout belief in faith by nature unfounded upon fact, which is deemed to lie at the heart of psychological disturbance (Ellis, 1983a). Indeed, REBT shares with the philosophy of Christianity the view that we would do better to condemn the sin but forgive (or, more accurately, accept) the sinner.

Finally, Ellis's ideas have been influenced by the work of the general semanticists (particularly Korzybski, 1933), who have argued that our psychological processes are to a great extent determined by our overgeneralizations and by the careless language we employ. Like Korzybski, Ellis holds that modification of the errors in our thinking and our language will have a marked effect on our emotions and actions.

Although Ellis has claimed that the creation of REBT owes more to the work of philosophers than to (pre-1959) psychologists, he was in fact influenced by the writings of a number of psychologists. Ellis was originally trained in psychoanalytic methods by a training analyst of the Karen Horney school; the influence of Horney's (1950) ideas on the "tyranny of the shoulds" is certainly apparent in the conceptual framework of REBT. However, while Horney saw that this mode of thought has a profound impact on the development and maintenance of neurotic problems, she did not, as Ellis later did, emphasize the dogmatic and absolutistic nature of these cognitions. Furthermore, while Horney saw that these "shoulds" had a tyrannical effect on psychological disturbance, she did not take a vigorous and active stance in helping people to challenge and change them, as is favored by REBT therapists.

Ellis (1973) states that REBT owes a unique debt to the ideas of Alfred Adler (1927), who held that a person's behavior springs from his or her ideas. Adler's concept of the important role played by feelings of inferiority in psychological disturbance predates Ellis's view that ego anxiety based on the concept of self-rating constitutes a fundamental human disturbance. As shown above, REBT emphasizes the role of social interest in determining psychological health—a concept central to the philosophy of Adler (1964). Other Adlerian influences on REBT are the importance humans attribute to goals, purposes, values, and meanings; the emphasis on active, directive teaching; the employment of a cognitive, persuasive form of therapy; and the teaching method of holding live demonstrations of therapy sessions before an audience. However, REBT differs from Adlerian therapy in that it gives more emphasis to the biological roots of human disturbance (Ellis, 1976a) and places less stress on the role of early childhood experience and birth order as factors in accounting for such disturbance. Furthermore, Adler did not discriminate among the various types of cognitions and did not mention the devout, absolutistic "musts" that are a central feature of the REBT perspective on psychological disturbance. Finally, while Adler was somewhat vague about distinct therapeutic methods and did not use behavioral techniques, REBT espouses many specific therapeutic techniques and methods, and is notably both cognitive and behavioral (Dryden, 1984a; Ellis, 1994b, 1998).

When Ellis first gave presentations on what was at that time called "rational psychotherapy" in the mid-1950s, he stressed the cognitive–philosophical aspects of the therapy to emphasize its differences with the psychoanalytic therapies. This stance led critics to accuse rational psychotherapy of neglecting its clients' emotions, which was not the case. Consequently, in 1961 Ellis decided to change the name of his approach to "rational–emotive therapy" (RET). This remained the name of the approach until 1993, when Ellis changed the name of the approach again to "rational emotive behavior therapy" (REBT), in reply to critics who argued that RET neglected clients' behaviors (Ellis, 1993a). However, REBT has always advocated the use of active behavioral methods, and in this regard, Ellis has acknowledged the influence of some of the earliest pioneers of behavioral therapy (Dunlap, 1932; Jones, 1924; Watson & Rayner, 1920) on his ideas and therapeutic practice. Also, from its inception, REBT has actively and systematically employed homework assignments to encourage clients to practice their newly acquired therapeutic insights in their own life situation. Ellis saw the importance of such assignments in his early work as a sex and marriage counselor (before creating REBT); in overcoming his own early anxieties about approaching women and speaking in public; and from the pioneering work of Herzberg (1945), who advocated the use of such assignments in his book *Active Psychotherapy.*

Students of the history of the development of psychotherapy will be interested to note that at the same time as Ellis was creating REBT, a number of other therapists, all working independently of each other, were developing therapeutic systems that all had some cognitive-behavioral emphasis (Eric Berne, George Kelly, Abraham Low, E. Lakin Phillips, and Julian Rotter). Of these, only REBT is today recognized as a major form of CBT and as such is represented in the present handbook.

BASIC THEORY

We begin by considering what image of the person is put forward by the REBT theoretical model. The theory's perspective on (1) the nature of psychological health and disturbance, (2) the acquisition of psychological disturbance, and (3) how such disturbance is perpetuated is then presented. REBT's theory of therapeutic change is next examined, and we conclude this section by discussing how the REBT theoretical model compares with those posited by other forms of CBT.

The Image of the Person

The theory behind REBT conceives of the person as a complex, biosocial organism with a strong tendency to establish and pursue a wide variety of goals and purposes. Although people differ enormously in *what* will bring them happiness, the fact that they do construct and pursue personally valued goals shows that they strive to bring a sense of meaning to their lives. Humans are thus seen as hedonistic, in that their major goals appear to be to stay alive and to pursue happiness. In this respect, they are further seen as having the related tasks of satisfying both their self-interests and their social interests. It is noted that humans normally do better at satisfying these twin interests by active than by passive pursuit.

The concept of "rationality" is central to an understanding of REBT's image of the person. Here "rational" means that which is true, is logical, and aids people in achieving their basic goals and purposes. Although people are motivated by hedonistic concerns, they often experience a clash between short-range and long-range goals. REBT theory holds that while people would do better to satisfy some of their short-range goals, they should adopt a philosophy of long-range hedonism if they are to achieve their basic goals and purposes. "Irrational," then, means that which is false, is illogical, and hinders or obstructs people from achieving their basic (long-range) goals and purposes. Rationality is thus not defined in any absolute sense in REBT theory, since that which aids or hinders this goal achievement is defined according to the individual in his or her own particular situation.

While REBT theory does stress the role played by cognitive factors in human functioning, cognition, emotion, and behavior are not viewed as separate psychological processes, but rather as processes that are highly interdependent and interactive. Thus, the statement "cognition leads to emotion" tends to accentuate a false picture of psychological separatism. In the famous "ABCs" of REBT, A has traditionally stood for an *activating* event; B for the way that this inferred event is evaluated (i.e., a person's *beliefs);* and C for the emotional, behavioral, and cognitive *consequences* that stem from B. As stated, however, this model does not emphasize the interactive nature of the psychological processes contained within it (Ellis, 1985a, 1994b). And yet, when humans adhere to a particular set of evaluative beliefs at B, this tends very much to influence the inferences they make and the environments they seek out at A. While beliefs do affect emotion and behavior, it is equally true that the way we feel and act has a profound effect on our beliefs. Our emotional and behavioral reactions help to create environments and skew our perceptions of these environments, which in turn have a constraining effect on our emotional and behavioral repertoires (as in the "self-fulfilling prophecy" effect). Thus it should be underscored that REBT theory sees the person as having overlapping intrapsychic processes and as being in constant interaction with his or her social and material environment.

When cognitive factors are considered from the vantage point of REBT's view of the person, Ellis (1976a, 1979a) has stressed that humans have two major biological tendencies. First, they have a strong tendency to think irrationally. According to REBT theory, they show great ease in converting their strong preferences into devout, absolutistic demands. Although Ellis (1984a) has acknowledged that there are social influences operating here, he has also noted that "even if everybody had had the most rational upbringing, virtually all humans would often irrationally transform their individual and social preferences into absolutistic demands on a) themselves, (b) other people, and (c) the universe around them" (p. 20).

Ellis (1976a, 1979a) has argued that the following constitutes evidence in favor of his hypothesis of the biological basis of human irrationality:

1. Virtually all humans, including bright and competent people, show evidence of major human irrationalities.
2. Virtually all the disturbance-creating irrationalities (absolutistic "shoulds" and "musts") that are found in our society are also found in just about all social and cultural groups that have been studied historically and anthropologically.
3. Many of the irrational behaviors that we engage in, such as procrastination and lack of self-discipline, go counter to the teachings of parents, peers, and the mass media.
4. Humans (even bright and competent people) often adopt other irrationalities after giving up former ones.
5. People who vigorously oppose various kinds of irrational behaviors often fall prey to these very irrationalities: Atheists and agnostics exhibit zealous and absolutistic philosophies, and highly religious individuals act immorally.
6. Insight into irrational thoughts and behaviors helps only partially to change them.
7. Humans often return to irrational habits and behavioral patterns, even though they have often worked hard to overcome them.
8. People often find it easier to learn self-defeating than self-enhancing behaviors. Thus people very easily overeat but have great trouble following a sensible diet.
9. Psychotherapists, who should presumably be good role models of rationality, often act irrationally in their personal and professional lives.
10. People frequently delude themselves into believing that certain bad experiences (e.g., divorce, stress, and other misfortunes) will not happen to them.

However, lest these hypotheses gives the impression that REBT has a gloomy image of humans, it is important to state that REBT theory stresses the existence of a second basic biological tendency. Here humans are seen as having both the ability to think about their thinking and the ability to exercise their power to choose to work toward changing their irrational thinking. Thus, people are by no means powerless slaves to their tendency toward irrational thinking; they can transcend (although not fully) its effects by deciding to work actively and continually toward changing this thinking, through employing cognitive, emotive, and behavioral challenging or disputational methods. In the final analysis, then, the REBT image of the person is quite an optimistic one.

The REBT view is that the person is by nature fallible and most probably not perfectible. Humans "naturally" make errors and, as described above, often seem to defeat and obstruct themselves in the pursuit of their long-range goals. Therapeutically, they are thus encouraged to accept themselves as fallible and to challenge their self-created demands for perfection and the self-depreciation that virtually always accompanies such demands (particularly when they are not met). REBT emphasizes that the person is also an incredibly complex organism and one that is constantly in flux. As such, REBT theory considers that humans have great potential to utilize the many opportunities they encounter to effect changes in the ways in which they think, feel, and act.

REBT is a constructivistic approach to psychotherapy, in that it holds that while people's preferences are influenced by their upbringing and their culture, they disturb themselves when their desires are not met by constructing irrational beliefs about such situations. However, REBT disagrees with constructivistic approaches that argue that all constructions are equally viable. By contrast, REBT theory holds that some constructions (i.e., rational beliefs) are more consistent with reality, more logical, and more functional than other constructions (i.e., irrational beliefs). Consequently, a major goal of REBT is to encourage clients to make rational constructions about aversive situations rather than irrational constructions.

In summary, Figure 9.1 shows where REBT theory stands on 10 personality dimensions put forward by Corsini (1977). A unidirectional symbol (ϕ or γ) indicates the pole that is stressed in the theoretical underpinnings of REBT (ϕ for the left-hand pole, γ for the right-hand pole). The sign v indicates that the theory encompasses both poles of the dimension equally.

The Nature of Psychological Disturbance and Health

REBT theory posits that at the heart of disturbance lies the tendency of humans to make devout, absolutistic evaluations of the perceived events in their lives. These evaluations are couched in the form of dogmatic "musts," "shoulds," "have to's," "got to's," and "oughts." Ellis (1983a) has argued that these absolutistic cognitions are at the core of a philosophy of a dogmatic religiosity that he claims to be the central feature of human emotional and behavioral disturbance. These beliefs are deemed to be irrational in REBT theory, in that they are rigid, are inconsistent with reality, are illogical, and usually impede people in the pursuit of their basic goals and purposes. Absolute "musts" do not invariably lead to psychological disturbance, because it is possible for a person to believe devoutly that he or she must succeed at all important projects, have confidence that he or she will be successful in these respects, and actually succeed in them and thereby not experience psychological disturbance. However, the person remains vulnerable because there is always the possibility that he or she may fail in the future. Thus, while on the grounds of probability REBT theory argues

Focus on explicit, observable behavior that can be counted and numbered.	OBJECTIVE	γ	SUBJECTIVE	Concern with the inner personal life of the individual—his or her ineffable self.
Person seen as composed of parts, organs, units, elements put together to make the whole.	ELEMENTARISTIC	γ	HOLISTIC	The person is seen as having a certain unity and the parts as aspects of the total entity. The individual is seen as indivisible.
Apersonal theories are impersonal, are statistically based, and consider generalities rather than individuals. They are based on group norms.	APERSONAL	γ	PERSONAL	Personal theories deal with the single individual. They are idiographic.
Focus on the measurement of units of behavior.	QUANTITATIVE	γ	QUALITATIVE	Behavior is seen as too complex to be measured exactly.
The individual is seen as a unit reactor, not a learner, filled with instincts and based on generalizations preestablished by heredity.	STATIC	γ	DYNAMIC	The individual is seen as a learner, with interactions between behavior and consciousness and between consciousness and unconsciousness.
The person is predominantly biologically based.	ENDOGENISTIC	φ	EXOGENISTIC	The person is predominantly influenced by social and environmental factors.
The individual is seen as not responsible for his or her behavior—as being the pawn of society, heredity, or both.	DETERMINISTIC	γ	INDETERMINISTIC	The person is seen as basically under his or her own direction. Control is within the person, and prediction is never completely possible.
The individual is seen in terms of what he or she has inherited or learned in the past.	PAST	PRESENT/FUTURE	FUTURE	The individual is seen as explained by his or her anticipations of future goals.
The person is seen as operating on an emotional basis and with the intellect at the service of the emotions.	AFFECTIVE	ν	COGNITIVE	The person is seen as essentially rational, with the emotions subserving the intellect.
The individual is seen as rational and affected by factors within his or her awareness span.	CONSCIOUS	ν	UNCONSCIOUS	The person is seen as having considerable investment below the level of awareness.

FIGURE 9.1. REBT described on 10 personality dimensions. γ means that the right-hand pole is stressed in REBT; φ means that the left-hand pole is stressed; and ν means that both poles are emphasized equally. Adapted from Corsini (1977). Copyright 1977 by F. E. Peacock, Publishers, Inc. Adapted with permission.

that an absolutistic philosophy will frequently lead to such disturbance, it does not claim that this is absolutely so. In this way, even with respect to its view of the nature of human disturbance, REBT adopts an antiabsolutistic position.

REBT theory goes on to posit that if humans adhere to a philosophy of "musturbation," they will strongly tend to make a number of irrational conclusions that are deemed to be derivatives of these "musts." These derivatives are viewed as irrational because they too are false, illogical, are extreme, and because they tend to sabotage a person's basic goals and purposes.

The first derivative is known as "awfulizing." This occurs when an event is rated as being more than 100% bad—a truly exaggerated and magical conclusion that stems from the belief "This must not be as bad as it is." The second derivative is known as "low frustration tolerance" (LFT), which means believing that one cannot experience virtually any happiness at all, under any conditions, if an event that must not happen actually occurs or threatens to occur. The third derivative, known as "depreciation," represents a tendency for humans to rate themselves and other people as subhuman or undeserving if they or the others do something that "must" not be done or fail to do something that "must" be done. Depreciation can also be applied to the world or life conditions that are rated as being "rotten" for failing to give the person what he or she must have.

Although Ellis (1984a) has argued that awfulizing, LFT, and depreciation are secondary irrational processes in that they stem from the philosophy of "musts," these processes can sometimes be primary. Indeed, Wessler (1984) has argued that they are more likely to be primary and that "musts" are often derived from them. However, the philosophy of "musts" on the one hand, and those of awfulizing, LFT, and depreciation on the other, are in all probability interdependent processes and often seem to be different sides of the same cognitive coin.

In summary, it is possible to discern two major categories of human psychological disturbance in REBT theory: ego disturbance and discomfort disturbance (Ellis, 1979b, 1980a). In ego disturbance, the person depreciates him- or herself as a result of making "musturbatory" demands on the self, others, and the world. In discomfort disturbance, the person again makes demands on the self, others, and the world, but these demands reflect the belief that comfort and comfortable life conditions must exist.

Ellis (1984a, 1985a) notes that humans also make numerous kinds of illogical assumptions when they are disturbed. In this respect, REBT agrees with cognitive therapists (Beck, Rush, Shaw, & Emery, 1979; Burns, 1980) that such cognitive distortions are a feature of psychological disturbance. However, REBT theory holds that such distortions almost always stem from the "musts." Some of the most frequent of them are listed in Table 9.1.

Although REBT clinicians at times discover all the illogicalities listed in Table 9.1 and a number of others that are less frequently found with clients, they particularly focus on the unconditional "shoulds," "oughts," and "musts" that seem to constitute the philosophical core of irrational beliefs leading to emotional disturbance. REBT clinicians hold that if they do not expose clients to and help them to relinquish these core beliefs, the clients will most probably continue to hold them and to create new irrational derivatives from them. At the same time, REBT therapists usually encourage their clients to have strong and persistent desires, wishes, and preferences, and to avoid feelings of detachment, withdrawal, and lack of involvement (Ellis, 1972a, 1973, 1984b, 1984c, 1994b, 1996a).

More importantly, REBT holds that unrealistic and illogical beliefs do

---

TABLE 9.1. Common Cognitive Distortions

1. *All-or-none thinking:* "If I fail at any important task, as I must not, I'm a *total* failure and *completely* unlovable!"

2. *Jumping to conclusions and negative non sequiturs:* "Since they have seen me dismally fail, as I *absolutely should* not have done, they will view me as an incompetent worm."

3. *Fortune telling:* "Because they are laughing at me for failing, they know that I *absolutely should* have succeeded, and they will despise me forever."

4. *Focusing on the negative:* "Because I *can't stand* things going wrong, as they *must* not, I can't see any good that is happening in my life."

5. *Disqualifying the positive:* "When they compliment me on the good things I have done, they are only being kind to me and forgetting the foolish things that I *absolutely should* not have done."

6. *Allness and neverness:* "Because conditions of living *ought* to be good and actually are so bad and so intolerable, they'll always be this way ,and I'll never have any happiness."

7. *Minimization:* "My accomplishments are the result of luck and are unimportant. But my mistakes, which I *absolutely should* never have made, are as bad as could be and are totally unforgivable."

8. *Emotional reasoning:* "Because I have performed so poorly, as I *absolutely should* not have done, I feel like a total nincompoop, and my strong feeling proves that I *am* no damned good."

9. *Labeling and overgeneralization:* "Because I must not fail at important work and have done so, I am a complete loser and failure!"

10. *Personalizing:* "Since I am acting far worse than I *absolutely should* act and they are laughing, I am sure they are only laughing at me, and that is *awful!*"

11. *Phonyism:* "When I don't do as well as I *ought* to do and they still praise and accept me, I am a real phony and will soon fall on my face and show them how despicable I am!"

12. *Perfectionism:* "I realize that I did fairly well, but I *absolutely should* have done perfectly well on a task like this, and am therefore really an incompetent!"

not in *themselves* create emotional disturbance. It is quite possible for people to believe unrealistically that because they frequently fail, they always do (i.e., perceived failure). It is also possible for them to believe illogically that because they have frequently failed, they always will (i.e., projected failure). But in both these instances, they can rationally conclude, "Too bad! Even though I often fail, there is no reason why I must succeed. I would prefer to, but I never *have to*, do well. So I'll manage to be as happy as I can be, even with my constantly failing." They would then rarely be emotionally disturbed.

To reiterate, REBT considers the essence of human emotional disturbance to consist of the absolutistic "musts" and "must nots" that people think about their failure, about their rejections, about their poor treatment by others, and about life's frustrations and losses. REBT therefore differs from other forms of CBT, such as those of Beck (1967, 1976), Bandura (1969, 1977), Goldfried and Davison (1976), Janis (1983), A. A. Lazarus (1981), R. Lazarus (1966), Mahoney (1977), Maultsby (1984), and Meichenbaum (1977), in that it particularly stresses therapists' looking for clients' dogmatic, unconditional "musts," differentiating the "musts" from clients' preferences, and teaching them how to relinquish the former and retain the latter (Bard, 1980; Dryden, 1984a; Ellis, 1962, 1977c, 1984c, 1985a; Ellis & Becker, 1982; Ellis & Harper, 1975; Grieger & Boyd, 1980; Grieger & Grieger, 1982; Phadke, 1982; Walen, DiGiuseppe, & Wessler, 1980; Wessler & Wessler, 1980).

If the philosophy of "musturbation" is at the core of much psychological disturbance, then what philosophy is characteristic of psychological health? REBT theory argues that a philosophy of relativism or "desiring" is a central feature of psychologically healthy humans. This philosophy acknowledges that humans have a large variety of desires, wishes, wants, preferences, and so on, but that if they refuse to transform these nonabsolute values into grandiose dogmas and demands, they will not become psychologically disturbed. They will, however, experience healthy negative emotions (e.g., sadness, regret, disappointment, healthy anger or annoyance) whenever their desires are not fulfilled. These emotions are considered to have constructive motivational properties, in that they help people to both remove obstacles to goal attainment and make constructive adjustments when their desires cannot be met.

Three major derivatives of the philosophy of desiring are postulated by REBT theory. They are deemed to be rational in that they are flexible, are consistent with reality, are sensible, and tend to help people reach their goals or formulate new goals if their old ones cannot be realized. The first derivative is known as "antiawfulizing." Here, if a person does not get what he or she wants, the person acknowledges that this is bad. However, because he or she does not believe "I have to get what I want," but holds his or her evaluation to a 0–100 continuum of badness, he or she does not therefore rate this situation as "awful." In general, when a person adheres to the desiring philosophy, the stronger his or her desire, the greater his or her rating of badness will be when the person does not get what he or she wants. The second derivative is known as "high frustration tolerance." Here the person (1) acknowledges that an undesirable event has happened (or may happen); (2) believes that the event should empirically occur if it does; (3) considers that the event can be and is worth tolerating; (4) attempts to change the undesired event or accepts the "grim" reality if it cannot be modified; and (5) actively pursues other goals even though the situation cannot be altered. The third derivative is known as "acceptance." Here the person accepts him- or herself and others as fallible human beings, who do not have to act other than they do. In addition, life conditions are accepted as they exist. People who have the philosophy of acceptance acknowledge fully that the world is highly complex and exists according to laws that are often outside their personal control. It is important to emphasize here that acceptance does not imply resignation. A rational philosophy of acceptance means that the person acknowledges that whatever exists empirically *should* exist, but does not absolutely *have to* exist forever. The person who is resigned to a situation usually does not attempt to modify it.

REBT theory argues that people can hold rational and irrational beliefs at the same time. Thus one may rationally believe "I want you to love me," and simultaneously (and irrationally) believe "Since I want you to love me, you must do so." REBT theory also makes unique distinctions between healthy and unhealthy negative emotions. Healthy negative emotions are deemed to be associated with rational beliefs, and unhealthy negative emotions with irrational beliefs. For example, concern is an emotion that is associated with the belief "I hope that this threat does not happen, but if it does, it would be unfortunate." Anxiety occurs when a person believes "This threat must not happen, and it would be awful if it does." Healthy anger (sometimes known as annoyance) occurs when another person disregards an individual's rule of living. Such a person tends to believe "I wish the other person did not do that, and I don't like what he or she did, but it does not follow that he or she must not break my own rule of conduct." In unhealthy anger, however, the person does believe that the other absolutely must not break this rule, and thus damns the other for doing so (Ellis, 1977c). It should be noted that REBT therapists do not target healthy negative emotions (sadness as opposed to depression; remorse vs. guilt; disappointment vs. shame) for change during therapy, since they are deemed to be consequences of rational thinking.

If ego disturbance and discomfort disturbance are cornerstones of the REBT view of human psychological problems, self-acceptance and a high level of discomfort tolerance are the two cornerstones of psychological health and are implicit in a philosophy of nondevout desire. Ellis (1979a) has outlined nine other criteria of positive mental health: (1) enlightened self-interest, (2) social interest, (3) self-direction, (4) acceptance of ambiguity and uncertainty, (5) scientific thinking, (6) commitment and being vitally absorbed in important projects, (7) flexibility, (8) calculated risk taking, and (9) acceptance of reality.

Acquisition and Perpetuation of Psychological Disturbance

REBT theory does not advance an elaborate view concerning the acquisition of psychological disturbance. This partly follows from Ellis's (1976a) hypothesis that humans have a distinct biological tendency to think and act irrationally, but it also reflects the REBT viewpoint that theories of acquisition do not necessarily suggest therapeutic interventions. Although Ellis argues that humans' tendencies toward irrational thinking are biologically rooted, he does acknowledge that environmental variables contribute to psychological disturbance and thus encourage people to make their biologically based demands (Ellis, 1979a). Thus Ellis (1984c) has said that "parents and culture usually teach children which superstitions, taboos, and prejudices to abide by, but they do not originate their basic tendency to superstitiousness, ritualism and bigotry" (p. 209).

REBT theory also posits that humans vary in their disturbability. Some people emerge relatively unscathed psychologically from being raised by uncaring or overprotective parents, while others emerge emotionally damaged from more "healthy" child-rearing approaches (Werner & Smith, 1982). In this respect, Ellis (1984c) claims that "individuals with serious aberrations are more innately predisposed to have rigid and crooked thinking than those with lesser aberrations, and consequently they are likely to make lesser advances" (p. 223). Thus, the REBT theory of acquisition can be summed up in the view that, as humans, we are not made disturbed simply by our experiences; rather, we bring our ability to disturb ourselves to our experiences.

Although REBT theory does not put forward an elaborate view to explain the acquisition of psychological disturbance, it does deal more extensively with how such disturbance is perpetuated. First, people tend to maintain their psychological problems by their own "naive" theories concerning the nature of these problems and to what they can be attributed. They lack what Ellis (1979a) calls REBT's "Insight Number 1": that psychological disturbance is primarily determined by the absolutistic beliefs that people hold about negative life events (B determines C). Rather, they consider that their disturbances are caused by these situations (A causes C). Since people make incorrect hypotheses about the major determinants of their problems, they consequently attempt to change A rather than B. Second, people may have Insight Number 1 but lack REBT's "Insight Number 2": that people remain disturbed by reindoctrinating themselves *in the present* with their absolutistic beliefs. Although they may see that their problems are determined by their beliefs, they may distract themselves and thus perpetuate their problems by searching for the historical antecedents of these beliefs instead of directing themselves to change them as currently held. Third, people may have Insight Numbers 1 and 2 but still sustain their disturbance because they lack REBT's "Insight Number 3": that only if people diligently work and practice in the present as well as in the future to think, feel, and act against their irrational beliefs are they likely to change them and make themselves significantly less disturbed. People who have all three insights clearly see that they would do better to persistently and strongly challenge their beliefs cognitively, emotively, and behaviorally, in order to break the perpetuation of the disturbance cycle. Merely acknowledging that a belief is irrational is usually insufficient to effect change.

Ellis (1979a) has argued that the major reason why people perpetuate their psychological problems is because they adhere to a philosophy of LFT. Such people believe that they must be "comfortable," and thus do not work to effect change because such work involves experiencing discomfort. They are short-range hedonists because they are motivated to avoid short-term discomfort, even though accepting and working against their temporary uncomfortable feelings would probably help them to reach their long-range goals. Such people rate cognitive and behavioral therapeutic tasks as "too painful," and as even more painful than the psychological disturbance for which they have achieved some measure of tolerance. They prefer to remain with their "comfortable" discomfort rather than face the change-related discomfort that they believe they must not experience. Maultsby (1975) has argued that people often back away from change because they are afraid that they will not feel right about it. He calls this the "neurotic fear of feeling a phony," and actively shows clients that these feelings of "unnaturalness" are natural concomitants of relearning. Another prevalent form of LFT is anxiety about anxiety. In this case, individuals believe that they must not be anxious and thus do not expose themselves to anxiety-provoking situations because they are anxious that they might become anxious if they did so—an experience they would rate as "awful." As such, they perpetuate their problems and overly restrict their lives to avoid experiencing anxiety.

Anxiety about anxiety constitutes an example of the clinical fact that people often make themselves disturbed about their disturbances. Having created secondary disturbances about their original disturbance, they become preoccupied with these metaproblems and thus find it difficult to get back to solving the original problem. Humans are often very inventive in this respect. They can make themselves depressed about their depression, guilty about being angry, anxious about their anxiety, and so on. Consequently, people often need to tackle their disturbances about their disturbances before they can successfully solve their original problems.

A major way in which people perpetuate their psychological problems is by acting in ways that are consistent with their irrational beliefs. For example, if a man is anxious about making new friends because he believes that he must not be rejected, this irrational belief influences him to act in a variety of dysfunctional ways. If he actually acts in these ways, he strengthens his conviction in his irrational beliefs and makes it harder for him to overcome his fear of rejection. Thus, in therapy, when the clinician helping this man to dispute his irrational beliefs, it is very important to encourage him to act in ways that are consistent with his newly developed rational beliefs. If he challenges his irrational beliefs cognitively, but continues to act in dysfunctional ways, he will easily go back to his irrational beliefs.

REBT theory endorses the Freudian view of human defensiveness in explaining how people perpetuate their psychological problems (Freud, 1937). Thus people maintain their problems by employing various defense mechanisms (e.g., rationalization, avoidance) that are designed to help deny the existence of these problems or to minimize their severity. The REBT view is that these defenses are used to ward off self-damnation tendencies, and that under such circumstances, if these people were to honestly take responsibility for their problems, they would severely denigrate themselves for having them. In addition, these defense mechanisms are employed to ward off discomfort anxiety, since (again) if such people admitted their problems, they would rate them as "too hard to bear" or "too difficult to overcome."

Ellis (1979a) has noted that people sometimes experience a form of perceived payoff for their psychological problems other than the avoidance of discomfort. The existence of these payoffs serves to perpetuate the problems. Thus, for instance, a woman who claims to want to overcome her procrastination may avoid tackling the problem because she is afraid that should she become successful, she might then be criticized by others as being "too masculine"—a situation she would evaluate as "awful." Her procrastination serves to protect her (in her mind) from this "terrible" state of affairs (Dryden, 1984b). Finally, the well-documented "self-fulfilling prophecy" phenomenon helps to explain why people perpetuate their psychological problems (Jones, 1977; Wachtel, 1977). Here people act according to their evaluations and consequent predictions, and thus often elicit from themselves or from others responses that they then interpret in a manner confirming their initial hypotheses. Thus, for example, a socially anxious man may believe that other people will not want to get to know "so worthless an individual as I truly am." He then attends a social function and acts as if he were worthless, avoiding eye contact and keeping away from others. Unsurprisingly, such social behavior does not invite approaches from others. He interprets this lack of response thus: "You see, I was right; other people don't want to know me. I really am no good."

In conclusion, REBT theory holds that people "naturally tend to perpetuate their problems and have a strong innate tendency to cling to self-defeating, habitual patterns and thereby resist basic change. Helping clients change, then, poses quite a challenge for RE[B]T practitioners" (Dryden, 1984b, pp. 244–245).

Theory of Therapeutic Change

The REBT view of the person is basically an optimistic one: Although it posits that humans have a distinct biological tendency to think irrationally, REBT also holds that humans have the capacity to choose to work toward changing this irrational thinking and its self-defeating effects, and that the most elegant and long-lasting changes humans can effect are ones that involve the philosophical restructuring of irrational beliefs. Change at this level can be specific or general. Specific philosophical change means that individuals change their irrational absolutistic demands ("musts," "shoulds") about given situations to rational relative preferences. General philosophical change involves people adopting a nondevout attitude toward life events in general. Ellis has distinguished between "superelegant" and "semielegant" philosophical change at the general level. Discussing these changes, Ellis has said:

> By superelegant I mean that practically under all conditions for the rest of their life they would not upset themselves about anything. Very few will ever do this because it is against the human condition and people fall back to *must*urbating and thereby disturbing themselves. Some will effect a semielegant solution, meaning that in most instances they will call up a new rational–emotive philosophy that will enable them to feel sad or annoyed but not anxious, depressed, or angry when poor conditions occur. (Quoted in Weinrach, 1980, p. 156)

To effect a philosophical change at either the specific or the general level, people need to do the following:

1. Realize that to a large degree they create their own psychological disturbances, and that while environmental conditions can contribute to their problems, they are in general secondary considerations in the change process.
2. Recognize that they do have the ability to significantly change these disturbances.

3. Understand that emotional and behavioral disturbances stem largely from irrational, absolutistic dogmatic beliefs.
4. Detect their irrational beliefs and discriminate between them and their rational alternatives.
5. Dispute these irrational beliefs using the logico-empirical methods of science.
6. Work toward the internalization of their new rational beliefs by employing cognitive, emotive, and behavioral methods of change—in particular, ensuring their behavior is consistent with their rational beliefs.
7. Continue this process of challenging irrational beliefs and using multimodal methods of change for the rest of their lives.

When people effect a philosophical change at B in the ABC model, they often are able to correct spontaneously their distorted inferences of reality (overgeneralizations, faulty attributions, etc.) that can be viewed as cognitions (Wessler & Wessler, 1980). However, they often need to challenge these distorted inferences more directly, as REBT has always emphasized (Ellis, 1962, 1971a, 1973; Ellis & Harper, 1961a, 1961b; see also Beck et al., 1979).

Although REBT theory argues that irrational beliefs are the breeding grounds for the development and maintenance of inferential distortions, it is possible for people to effect inferentially based changes without making a profound philosophical change. Thus, they may regard their inferences as hunches about reality rather than facts, may generate alternative hypotheses, and may seek evidence and/or carry out experiments that test out each hypothesis. They may then accept the hypothesis that represents the "best bet" of those available. Consider a man who thinks that his coworkers view him as a fool. To test this hypothesis, he may first specify their negative reactions to him. These constitute the data from which he quickly draws the conclusion "They think I'm a fool." He could then realize that what he has interpreted to be negative responses to him may not be negative. If they seem to be negative, he could then carry out an experiment to test out the meaning he attributes to their responses. Thus he could enlist the help of a trusted colleague to carry out a "secret ballot" of others' opinions of him. Or, he could test his hunch more explicitly by directly asking others for their view of him. As a result of these strategies, this person may conclude that his coworkers find some of his actions foolish, rather than considering him to be a complete fool. His mood may lift because his inference of A (i.e., the situation) has changed, but he may still believe at B "If others think I'm a fool, they're right I am a fool, and that would be awful." Thus he has made an inferential change, but not a philosophical one. If this person were to attempt to make a philosophical change, he would *first* assume that his inference were true, then address himself to his evaluations about this inference and hence challenge these if they were discovered to be irrational. Thus he might conclude, "Even if I act foolishly, that makes me a person with foolish behavior, not a foolish person. And even if they deem me a total idiot, that is simply *their* view, with which I can choose to disagree." REBT therapists hypothesize that people are more likely to make a profound philosophical change if they first assume that their inferences are true and then challenge their irrational beliefs, rather than if they first correct their inferential distortions and then challenge their underlying irrational beliefs. However, this hypothesis awaits full empirical inquiry.

People can also make direct changes of the situation at A. Thus, in the example quoted above, the man could leave his job or distract himself from the reactions of his colleagues by taking on extra work and devoting himself to it. Or he could carry out relaxation exercises whenever he comes in contact with his coworkers and thus distract himself once again from their perceived reactions. In addition, the man could have a word with his supervisor, who might then instruct the other workers to change their behavior toward the man.

When we use this model to consider behavioral change, it is apparent that a person can change his or her behavior to effect inferential and/or philosophical change. Thus, again in the example above, the man whose coworkers view him as a fool might change his own behavior towards them and thus elicit a different set of responses from them, which would lead him to reinterpret his previous inference (i.e., behavior change to effect inferential change). However, if it could be determined that they did indeed consider him to be a fool, then the man could actively seek them out and show himself that he could stand the situation and that just because they think him a fool doesn't make him one. Thus he would learn to accept himself in the face of their views while exposing himself to their negative reactions (i.e., behavior change to effect philosophical change).

Although REBT therapists prefer to help their clients make profound philosophical changes at B, they do not dogmatically insist that their clients make such changes. If it becomes apparent that clients are not able at any given time to change their irrational beliefs, then REBT therapists will endeavor to help them either to change A directly (by avoiding the troublesome situation, or by behaving differently) or to change their distorted inferences about the situation.

Differences from Other Forms of CBT[1]

Ellis (1980b) has distinguished between "specialized" REBT and "general" REBT. He argues that general REBT is synonymous with broad-based CBT. He further argues that specialized REBT differs from CBT in a number of important respects:

1. REBT has a distinct philosophical emphasis that is one of its central features and that other forms of CBT appear to omit. It stresses that humans appraise themselves, others, and the world in terms of (a) rational, preferential, flexible, and tolerant philosophies, and in terms of (b) irrational, "musturbatory," rigid, intolerant, and absolutistic philosophies.

2. REBT has an existential–humanistic outlook that is intrinsic to it and that is omitted by most other CBT approaches. Thus it sees people "as holistic, goal-directed individuals who have importance in the world just because they are human and alive; it unconditionally accepts them with their limitations, and it particularly focuses upon their experiences and values, including their self-actualizing potentialities" (Ellis, 1980b, p. 327). It also shares the views of ethical humanism by encouraging people to emphasize human interest (self and social) over the interests of deities, material objects, and lower animals.

3. REBT favors striving for pervasive and long-lasting (philosophically based) change, rather than symptomatic change.

4. REBT attempts to help humans eliminate all self-ratings, and views self-esteem as a self-defeating concept that encourages them to make conditional evaluations of self. Instead, it teaches people unconditional self-acceptance (Dryden, 1998; Ellis, 1972b, 1976b, 1983b, 1996c; Ellis & Harper, 1997).

5. REBT sees psychological disturbance as resulting in part from taking life too seriously. It advocates the appropriate use of various humorous therapeutic methods (Ellis, 1977a, 1977b, 1981b).

6. REBT stresses the use of "antimusturbatory" rather than antiempirical disputing methods. It favors going to the philosophical core of emotional disturbance and disputing the irrational beliefs at this core, rather than merely disputing antiempirical inferences, which are more peripheral. Also, specialized REBT teaches clients how to become their own scientists and favors the use of forceful logico-empirical disputing of irrational beliefs, rather than only stressing the employment of rationally oriented, coping self-statements whenever possible.

7. REBT employs, but only mildly encourages, the use of palliative cognitive methods that serve to distract people from their disturbed philosophies (e.g., relaxation methods). Specialized REBT holds that such techniques may help clients better in the short term, but do not encourage them to identify, challenge, and change the devout philosophies that underpin their psychological problems in the long term. REBT also employs problem-solving and skill training methods, along with, but not instead of, teaching people to work at understanding and changing their irrational beliefs.

8. REBT gives a more central explanatory role to the concept of discomfort anxiety in psychological disturbance than do other forms of CBT.

Discomfort anxiety is defined as "emotional hypertension that arises when people feel (1) that their life or comfort is threatened, (2) that they must not feel uncomfortable and have to feel at ease and (3) that it is awful or catastrophic (rather than merely inconvenient or disadvantageous) when they don't get what they supposedly must" (Ellis, 1980b, p. 331). Although other forms of CBT recognize specific instances of discomfort anxieties (e.g., "fear of fear"; Mackay, 1984), they tend not to regard discomfort disturbance to be as centrally implicated in psychological problems as does specialized REBT.

9. REBT emphasizes more than other approaches to CBT that humans frequently make themselves disturbed about their original disturbances. Thus in specialized REBT, therapists actively look for secondary and tertiary symptoms of disturbances, and encourage clients to work on overcoming these before addressing themselves to the primary disturbances.

10. REBT has clear-cut theories of disturbance and its treatment, but is eclectic or multimodal in its techniques (see the section on therapeutic techniques). It favors some techniques (e.g., active disputing) over others (e.g., cognitive distraction), and strives for profound or elegant philosophical change where feasible.

11. REBT discriminates between healthy and unhealthy negative emotions. Specialized REBT considers negative emotions as constructive affective responses to thwarted desires, when based on a nondevout philosophy of desire, and when they do not needlessly interfere with people's goals and purposes. However, unconstructive emotions are based on absolutistic demands about thwarted desires. REBT considers these latter feelings as symptoms of disturbance, because they very frequently sabotage people's attempts to pursue constructively their goals and purposes. Other CBT approaches do not make such fine discriminations between healthy and unhealthy negative emotions.

12. REBT advocates that therapists give unconditional acceptance, rather than giving warmth or approval, to clients. Other forms if CBT tend not to make this distinction. Specialized REBT holds that therapist warmth and approval have their distinct dangers, in that they may unwittingly encourage clients to strengthen their dire needs for love and approval. REBT therapists who unconditionally accept their clients also serve as good role models, in that they also help clients to accept themselves unconditionally.

13. REBT stresses the importance of the use of vigor and force in counteracting irrational philosophies and behaviors (Dryden, 1984a; Ellis, 1979d, 1994b, 1996d). Specialized REBT stresses that humans are, for the most part, biologically predisposed to originate and perpetuate their disturbances, and thus often experience great difficulty in changing the ideological roots of these problems. Since it holds this view, it urges both therapists

and clients to use considerable force and vigor in interrupting clients' irrationalities.

14. REBT is more selective than most other forms of CBT in choosing behavioral change methods. Thus it sometimes favors the use of penalization in encouraging resistant clients to change. Often these clients won't change to obtain positive reinforcements, but may be encouraged to change to avoid stiff penalties, such as burning a $100 bill when they fail to stop smoking or fail to come to work on time. Furthermore, specialized REBT has reservations concerning the use of social reinforcement in therapy. It considers that humans are too reinforceable and that they often do the right thing for the wrong reason. Specialized REBT therapists aim to help clients become maximally nonconformist, nondependent, and individualistic, and thus use social reinforcement techniques sparingly. Finally, specialized REBT favors the use of *in vivo* desensitization and flooding methods rather than the use of gradual desensitization techniques, since it argues that the former procedures best help clients to raise their level of frustration tolerance (Ellis, 1962, 1983c).

15. Although REBT therapists prefer to use specialized REBT wherever feasible, they do not dogmatically insist that it be employed. When, on pragmatic grounds, they employ general REBT, their therapeutic practice is frequently indistinguishable from that of therapists employing other types of CBT (Ellis, 1996d).

CLINICAL APPLICATIONS

In this section, we discuss the major clinical applications of REBT. First, we use the therapeutic modality of individual therapy to consider (1) the therapeutic bonds that REBT therapists endeavor to establish with their clients, (2) the clinical process of REBT from inception to termination, and (3) the major therapeutic techniques employed in REBT. Second, we outline the application of REBT to a case of anxiety and a case of depression.

Individual Therapy

THERAPEUTIC BONDS

Many psychotherapy systems regard the therapeutic relationship as the major vehicle of change in effective therapy. REBT considers that the establishment of effective therapeutic bonds between clients and therapists to be an important ingredient but not a necessary component of successful therapy. Ellis (1979c) has argued that effective REBT is best done in a highly active, directive manner, although he has also acknowledged that it can be success-fully practiced using a more passive therapeutic style (Ellis, 1984a). Since the major goals of REBT therapists are to teach clients to think more ratio-nally and ultimately to help them to use its methods for themselves, they see themselves as educators and thus strive to establish the most appropri-ate learning climate for each client.

Given the major goals of REBT, REBT therapists strive to accept their clients unconditionally as fallible human beings who cannot be given a le-gitimate global rating. Therapists acknowledge that their clients often act self-defeatingly, but no matter how badly clients behave inside or outside therapy, therapists show their clients that they accept them but do not nec-essarily go along with their negative behaviors. Although accepting of their clients, most REBT therapists do not interact with their clients in a very warm fashion for two main reasons. First, undue therapist warmth may lead to the entrenchment of clients' needs for love and approval—two qual-ities irrationally believed to be necessary for happiness. This belief lies at the core of much human disturbance. Clients of warm therapists may ap-pear to improve and certainly feel better, because they come to believe that they must be worthy, since their therapists like them. However, their self-acceptance is still dependent upon outside approval, and they may never have the opportunity to challenge this philosophy of conditional self-accep-tance with their warm, loving therapists, who may themselves have dire needs for their clients' approval. Second, undue therapist warmth may rein-force clients' philosophies of LFT (Ellis, 1982a). However, there may be oc-casions (e.g., with severely depressed clients) when therapist warmth is ap-propriate for a restricted period of time, and since REBT therapists are not dogmatically against interacting warmly with their clients, they may do so under such conditions.

Most REBT therapists tend to interact in an open manner with their clients and do not hesitate to give personal information about themselves if clients ask for it, except when it is judged that clients may use such infor-mation against themselves. REBT therapists often disclose to their clients whether they have experienced similar problems, and, if so, how they solved these problems using REBT. They thus serve as good role models for their clients, as well as inspiring their clients with the hope that it is possible to overcome emotional and behavioral problems.

REBT therapists would agree with Carl Rogers (1957) concerning the importance of therapist empathy in helping clients. However. REBT thera-pists offer their clients not only affective empathy (i.e., showing their clients that they know how they feel), but also philosophical empathy (i.e., show-ing their clients that they understand the underlying philosophies upon which their emotions are based).

REBT therapists often favor an informal style of interacting with their clients. They employ humor when appropriate, because, as mentioned earlier, they believe that emotional disturbance can be viewed as a result of taking things too seriously. Thus they hypothesize that their humorous style will loosen up their clients and encourage them to stand back and laugh at their dysfunctional thinking and behavior, but not at themselves. This latter point is in keeping with the REBT perspective of the self as composed of a myriad of different, ever-changing aspects rather than as one rateable whole. Consequently, REBT therapists direct their own humor at aspects of a client's dysfunctioning and not at the client as a person. Indeed, REBT therapists often direct their humor against some of their own irrationalities, and show by so doing that they do not take themselves too seriously (Ellis, 1983b).

Although REBT therapists tend to favor an informal, humorous, active, and directive style of therapeutic participation, they are flexible in this respect and are mindful of the important question "Which therapeutic style is most effective with which kind of client?" (Eschenroeder, 1979, p. 5). Thus some clients learn better if their therapists assume a more formal, more serious, and less self-disclosing style. In such cases, REBT therapists will not hesitate to emphasize these aspects of themselves for therapeutic purposes. The issue of appropriate therapeutic styles in REBT warrants more formal research. Varying one's therapeutic style in REBT, however, does not mean departing from the theoretical principles on which the content of therapy is based (Beutler, 1983; Dryden & Ellis, 1986).

THERAPEUTIC PROCESS[2]

When clients seek help from REBT therapists, they vary concerning how much they already know about the type of therapeutic process they are likely to encounter. Some may approach a particular therapist because they know he or she is a practitioner of REBT, while others may know nothing about this therapeutic method. In any event, it is often beneficial to explore clients' expectations for therapy at the outset of the process. Duckro, Beal, and George (1979) have argued that it is important to distinguish between "preferences" and "anticipations" when expectations are assessed. Clients' preferences for therapy concern what kind of experience they want, while their anticipations concern what service they think they will receive. Clients who have realistic anticipations for the REBT therapeutic process and have a preference for this process in general require far less induction into REBT therapy than clients who have unrealistic anticipations of the process and/ or preferences for a different type of therapeutic experience.

Induction procedures generally involve showing clients that REBT is an active, directive, structured therapy oriented to discussion about clients' present and future problems, and one that requires clients to play an active role in the change process (Dryden, 1999). Induction can take a number of different forms. First, therapists may develop and use a number of pre-therapy role induction procedures, in which a typical course of REBT is outlined and productive client behaviors are demonstrated (Macaskill & Macaskill, 1983). Second, therapists may give a short lecture at the outset of therapy concerning the nature and process of REBT. Third, therapists may employ induction-related explanations in the initial therapy sessions, using client problem material to illustrate how these problems may be tackled in REBT and to outline the respective roles of client and therapist.

REBT therapists in general spend little time gathering background information on their clients, although they may ask them to fill out forms designed to assess which irrational ideas they spontaneously endorse at the outset of therapy (see Figure 9.2). Rather, they are likely to ask clients for a description of their major problem(s). As clients describe their problem(s), REBT therapists intervene fairly early to break these down into their ABC components. If clients begin by describing A (the inferred event), then the therapists ask for C (their emotional and/or behavioral reactions). However, if clients begin by outlining C, therapists ask for a brief description of A.

When A is assessed, some REBT therapists prefer to fully assess the client's inferences in search of the most relevant inference that the client then evaluates at B. This is known as "inference chaining" (Moore, 1983). An example of this procedure is described below:

THERAPIST: So what was your major feeling here?

CLIENT: I guess I was angry.

THERAPIST: Angry about what? [The therapist has obtained C and is probing for A.]

CLIENT: I was angry that he did not send me a birthday card. [The client provides A.]

THERAPIST: And what was anger-provoking in your mind about that? [Probing to see whether A is most relevant in the inference chain.]

CLIENT: Well . . . he promised me he would remember. [A2.]

THERAPIST: And because he broke his promise? [Probing for relevance of A2.]

CLIENT: I felt that he didn't care enough about me. [A3.]

THERAPIST: But let's assume that for a moment. What would be disturbing about that for you? [Probing for relevance of A3.]

CLIENT: Well, he might leave me. [A4.]

THERAPIST: And if he did? [Probing for relevance of A4.]

Albert Ellis Institute
46 East 65th Street New York, NY 10021
Personality Data Form

Instructions: Read each of the following items and circle after each one the word STRONGLY, MODERATELY, or WEAKLY to indicate how much you believe in the statement described in the item. Thus, if you strongly believe that it is awful to make a mistake when people are watching, circle the word STRONGLY in item 1; and if you weakly believe that it is intolerable to be disapproved by others circle the word WEAKLY in item 2. DO NOT SKIP ANY ITEMS. Be as honest as you possibly can be.

Acceptance

1. I believe that it is awful to make a mistake when other people are watching. STRONGLY MODERATELY WEAKLY
2. I believe that it is intolerable to be disapproved of by others. STRONGLY MODERATELY WEAKLY
3. I believe that it is awful for people to know certain undesirable things about one's family or one's background. STRONGLY MODERATELY WEAKLY
4. I believe that it is shameful to be looked down upon by people for having less than they have. STRONGLY MODERATELY WEAKLY
5. I believe that it is horrible to be the center of attention of others who may be highly critical. STRONGLY MODERATELY WEAKLY
6. I believe it is terribly painful when one is criticized by a person one respects. STRONGLY MODERATELY WEAKLY
7. I believe that it is awful to have people disapprove of the way one looks or dresses. STRONGLY MODERATELY WEAKLY
8. I believe that it is very embarrassing if people discover what one really is like. STRONGLY MODERATELY WEAKLY
9. I believe that it is awful to be alone. STRONGLY MODERATELY WEAKLY
10. I believe that it is horrible if one does not have the love or approval of certain special people who are important to one. STRONGLY MODERATELY WEAKLY
11. I believe that one must have others on whom one can always depend for help. STRONGLY MODERATELY WEAKLY

Frustration

12. I believe that it is intolerable to have things go along slowly and not be settled quickly. STRONGLY MODERATELY WEAKLY
13. I believe that it is too hard to get down to work at things it often would be better for one to do. STRONGLY MODERATELY WEAKLY
14. I believe that it is terrible that life is so full of inconveniences and frustrations. STRONGLY MODERATELY WEAKLY
15. I believe that people who keep one waiting frequently are pretty worthless and deserve to be boycotted. STRONGLY MODERATELY WEAKLY

FIGURE 9.2. Personality Data Form. Adapted from Ellis (1968). Copyright 1968 by the Institute for Rational–Emotive Therapy. Adapted with permission of the Albert Ellis Institute for Rational Emotive Behavior Therapy.

16. I believe that it is terrible if one lacks desirable traits that other people possess.　STRONGLY　MODERATELY　WEAKLY

17. I believe that it is intolerable when other people do not do one's bidding or give one what one wants.　STRONGLY　MODERATELY　WEAKLY

18. I believe that some people are unbearably stupid or nasty, and that one must get them to change.　STRONGLY　MODERATELY　WEAKLY

19. I believe that it is too hard for one to accept serious responsibility.　STRONGLY　MODERATELY　WEAKLY

20. I believe that it is dreadful that one cannot get what one wants without making real effort to get it.　STRONGLY　MODERATELY　WEAKLY

21. I believe that things are too rough in this world, and that therefore it is legitimate for one to feel sorry for oneself.　STRONGLY　MODERATELY　WEAKLY

22. I believe that it is too hard to persist at many of the things one starts, especially when the going gets rough.　STRONGLY　MODERATELY　WEAKLY

23. I believe that it is terrible that life is so unexciting and boring.　STRONGLY　MODERATELY　WEAKLY

24. I believe that it is awful for one to have to discipline oneself.　STRONGLY　MODERATELY　WEAKLY

Injustice

25. I believe that people who do wrong things should suffer strong revenge for their acts.　STRONGLY　MODERATELY　WEAKLY

26. I believe that wrongdoers and immoral people should be severely condemned.　STRONGLY　MODERATELY　WEAKLY

27. I believe that people who commit unjust acts are bastards, and that they should be severely punished.　STRONGLY　MODERATELY　WEAKLY

Achievement

28. I believe that it is horrible for one to perform poorly.　STRONGLY　MODERATELY　WEAKLY

29. I believe that it is awful if one fails at important things.　STRONGLY　MODERATELY　WEAKLY

30. I believe that it is terrible for one to make a mistake when one has to make important decisions.　STRONGLY　MODERATELY　WEAKLY

31. I believe that it is terrifying for one to take risks or to try new things.　STRONGLY　MODERATELY　WEAKLY

Worth

32. I believe that some of one's thoughts or actions are unforgivable.　STRONGLY　MODERATELY　WEAKLY

33. I believe that if one keeps failing at things, one is a pretty worthless person.　STRONGLY　MODERATELY　WEAKLY

(cont.)

FIGURE 9.2. *(cont.)*

34. I believe that killing oneself is preferable to a miserable life of failure.	STRONGLY	MODERATELY	WEAKLY
35. I believe that things are so ghastly that one cannot help feel like crying much of the time.	STRONGLY	MODERATELY	WEAKLY
36. I believe that it is frightfully hard for one to stand up for oneself and not give in too easily to others.	STRONGLY	MODERATELY	WEAKLY
37. I believe that when one has shown poor personality traits for a long time, it is hopeless for one to change.	STRONGLY	MODERATELY	WEAKLY
38. I believe that if one does not usually see things clearly and act well on them, one is hopelessly stupid.	STRONGLY	MODERATELY	WEAKLY
39. I believe that it is awful to have no good meaning or purpose in life.	STRONGLY	MODERATELY	WEAKLY

Control

40. I believe that one cannot enjoy oneself today because of one's early life.	STRONGLY	MODERATELY	WEAKLY
41. I believe that if one kept failing at important things in the past, one must inevitably keep failing in the future.	STRONGLY	MODERATELY	WEAKLY
42. I believe that once one's parents train one to act and feel in certain ways, there is little one can do to act or feel better.	STRONGLY	MODERATELY	WEAKLY
43. I believe that strong emotions like anxiety and rage are caused by external conditions and events, and that one has little or no control over them.	STRONGLY	MODERATELY	WEAKLY

Certainty

44. I believe it would be terrible if there were no higher being or purpose on which to rely.	STRONGLY	MODERATELY	WEAKLY
45. I believe that if one does not keep doing certain things over and over again, something bad will happen if one stops.	STRONGLY	MODERATELY	WEAKLY
46. I believe that things must be in good order for one to be comfortable.	STRONGLY	MODERATELY	WEAKLY

Catastrophizing

47. I believe that it is awful if one's future is not guaranteed.	STRONGLY	MODERATELY	WEAKLY
48. I believe that it is frightening that there are no guarantees that accidents and serious illnesses will not occur.	STRONGLY	MODERATELY	WEAKLY
49. I believe that it is terrifying for one to go to new places or meet a new group of people.	STRONGLY	MODERATELY	WEAKLY
50. I believe that it is ghastly for one to be faced with the possibility of dying.	STRONGLY	MODERATELY	WEAKLY

FIGURE 9.2. *(cont.)*

CLIENT: I'd be left alone. [A5.]

THERAPIST: And if you were alone? [Probing for relevance of A5.]

CLIENT: I couldn't stand that. [Irrational belief.]

THERAPIST: Okay, so let's back up a minute. What would be most disturbing for you—the birthday card incident, the broken promise, the fact that he didn't care, being left by your husband, or being alone? [The therapist checks to see which A is most relevant in a chain.]

CLIENT: Definitely being alone.

This example shows not only that inferences are linked together, but that emotions are too. Here anger was linked to anxiety about being alone. Although this REBT therapist chose then to dispute the client's irrational belief underlying her anxiety, he would still have to deal with her anger-creating belief. Other REBT therapists might have chosen to take the first element in the chain (anger about the missing birthday card) and disputed the irrational belief related to anger. Skillful REBT therapists do succeed in discovering the hidden issues underlying the presenting problem during the disputing process. It is important for REBT therapists to assess correctly *all* relevant issues related to a presenting problem.

Although C is assessed mainly by the client's verbal report, occasionally clients experience difficulty in accurately reporting their emotional and behavioral problems. REBT therapists may use a variety of emotive (e.g., Gestalt two-chair dialogue, psychodrama), imagery-based, and other techniques (e.g., keeping an emotion/behavior diary) to facilitate this part of the assessment process (Dryden, 1999). If the assessment has revealed unhealthy negative emotions and/or dysfunctional behaviors at C, the therapist proceeds to help the client identify relevant irrational beliefs at B. An important step here is to help clients see the link between their irrational beliefs and their unhealthy affective and behavioral consequences at C. Some REBT therapists like to give a short lecture at this point on the role of the "musts" in emotional disturbance and how they can be distinguished from preferences. Ellis, for example, often gives the following account:

ELLIS: Imagine that you prefer to have a minimum of $11.00 in your pocket at all times, and you discover you only have $10.00. It's not essential, only preferable, that you have $11.00. How will you feel?

CLIENT: Frustrated.

ELLIS: Right. Or you'd feel concerned or sad, but you wouldn't kill yourself. Right?

CLIENT: Right.

ELLIS: Okay. Now this time imagine that you absolutely *have to* have a minimum of $11.00 in your pocket at all times. You must have it; it is a *necessity*. You must, you must, you must have a minimum of $11.00, and again you look and you find you only have $10.00. How will you feel?

CLIENT: Very anxious.

ELLIS: Right, or depressed. Now remember it's the same $11.00 but a different belief. Okay, now this time you still have that same belief. You *have to* have a minimum of $11.00 at all times, you must. It's absolutely *essential.* But this time you look in your pocket and find that you've got $12.00. How will you feel?

CLIENT: Relieved, content.

ELLIS: Right. But with that same belief you *have to* have a minimum of $11.00 at all times, something will soon occur to you that you would feel very anxious about. What do you think that would be?

CLIENT: What if I lose $2.00?

ELLIS: Right. What if you lose $2.00, what if you spend $2.00, what if you get robbed? That's right. Now the moral of this model—which applies to all humans, rich or poor, black or white, male or female, young or old, in the past or in the future, assuming that humans are still human—is that people make themselves disturbed if they don't get what they think they *must*, but they are also panicked when they do because of the must. For even if they have what they think they must, they could always lose it.

CLIENT: So I have no chance to be happy when I don't have what I think I must, and little chance of remaining unanxious when I do have it?

ELLIS: Right! Your *must*urbation will get you nowhere except depressed or panicked!

An important goal of the assessment stage of REBT is to help clients distinguish between their original problems (e.g., depression, anxiety, withdrawal, addiction) and their metaproblems—that is, their problems about their primary problems (e.g., depression about depression, anxiety about anxiety, shame about withdrawal, or guilt about addiction). REBT therapists often assess metaproblems before their clients' original problems, because these often require prior therapeutic attention. For example, clients frequently find it difficult to focus on their original problem of anxiety when they are severely blaming themselves for being anxious. Metaproblems are assessed in the same manner as original problems.

When particular problems have been adequately assessed according to the ABC model, and clients clearly see the link between their irrational beliefs and their dysfunctional emotional and behavioral consequences, then therapists can proceed to the disputing stage. The initial purpose of disputing is to help clients gain intellectual insight into the fact that there is no evidence in support of the existence of their absolutistic demands, or the irrational derivatives of these demands (awfulizing, LFT, and depreciation). There exists only evidence that if they stay with their nonabsolutistic preferences and if these are not fulfilled, they will get unfortunate or "bad" results, whereas if they are fulfilled, they will get desirable or "good" results. Intellectual insight in REBT is defined as an acknowledgment that an irrational belief frequently leads to emotional disturbance and dysfunctional behavior, and that a rational belief almost always abets emotional health. But when people lightly and occasionally see and hold rational beliefs, they have intellectual insights that may not help them change (Ellis, 1963, 1985a, 1985b, 1994b). So REBT does not stop with intellectual insight, but uses it as a springboard for the working-through phase of REBT. In this phase, clients are encouraged to use a large variety of cognitive, emotive, and behavioral techniques designed to help them achieve emotional insight. "Emotional insight" in REBT is defined as a very strong and frequently held belief that an irrational idea is dysfunctional and that a rational idea is helpful (Ellis, 1963). When a person has achieved emotional insight, he or she thinks, feels, and behaves according to the rational belief.

It is mainly in the working-through phase of REBT that therapists frequently encounter obstacles to client progress. Three major forms of such obstacles are deemed to occur in REBT: (1) relationship obstacles, (2) client obstacles, and (3) therapist obstacles.

Relationship obstacles to client progress basically take two forms. First, therapists and clients may be poorly matched and thus fail to develop productive working relationships. Early referral to a more suitable therapist is indicated in such situations. Second, therapists and clients may get on *too* well, with the results that (1) they collude to avoid dealing with uncomfortable issues, and (2) the therapists fail to encourage their clients to push themselves to change irrational beliefs in their life situation. In this case, therapy can become merely an enjoyable experience for both, with the result that client improvement would threaten the existence of this happy relationship. Here therapists would do better to remind themselves and their clients that the major purpose of their relationship is to help the clients overcome their psychological problems and to pursue their goals *outside* of the therapeutic situation. Consequently, therapists need to strive to raise their own level of frustration tolerance and that of their clients, thus working toward this end.

Therapist obstacles to client progress also take two basic forms. First, therapists may have a number of skill deficits and therefore conduct REBT in an ineffective manner. If this occurs, close supervision and further training are called for. Second, therapists may bring their own dire needs for approval, success, and comfort to the therapeutic situation, interfering with client progress in the process. In this situation, therapists would do better either to use REBT on themselves or to seek personal therapy (Ellis, 1983b, 1985b).

Ellis (1983d) found that clients' own extreme level of disturbance is a significant obstacle to their own progress. He replicated a frequent finding in the psychotherapy literature that the clients who benefit most from therapy are precisely those who need it least (i.e., those who are less disturbed at the outset). Ellis (1983e, 1983f, 1984d, 1985b) has outlined a large variety of therapeutic strategies for use with resistant clients. First, therapists need to maintain an unusually accepting attitude toward resistant clients. Second, they should preferably strive to consistently encourage such clients to change. Third, they should persist in showing their clients the negative consequences that undoubtedly follow their refusal to work on their problems. Fourth, much therapeutic flexibility, innovation, and experimentation are called for in work with resistant clients (Dryden & Ellis, 1986).

Termination preferably takes place in REBT when clients have made some significant progress and when they have become proficient in REBT's self-change techniques. Thus terminating clients should preferably be able to (1) acknowledge that they experience unhealthy negative emotions, and act dysfunctionally when they do; (2) detect the irrational beliefs that underpin these experiences; (3) discriminate between their irrational beliefs and their rational alternatives; (4) challenge these irrational beliefs; and (5) counteract them by using cognitive, emotive, and behavioral self-change methods. In addition, it is often helpful for therapists to arrange for their clients to attend a series of follow-up sessions after termination, to monitor their progress and deal with any remaining obstacles to sustained improvement.

MAJOR THERAPEUTIC TECHNIQUES

We now consider the major therapeutic techniques employed in REBT. Because our purpose is to highlight the unique features of REBT, we emphasize the technical aspects of specialized REBT, in which the goal is to effect profound philosophical change. When general REBT is conducted, therapists employ a variety of additional techniques that are adequately covered elsewhere in this handbook. Although we outline the most commonly employed techniques, it is important to note at the outset that REBT therapists freely employ techniques derived from other schools of therapy. However, we want to stress that REBT "is based on a clear-cut theory of emotional health and disturbance: The many techniques it employs are used in the light of that theory" (Ellis, 1984c, p. 234). Because REBT therapists adhere to the theory's emphasis on long-range hedonism, they will rarely employ a technique that has beneficial short-range but deleterious long-range effects. While we list techniques under "cognitive," "emotive," and "behavioral" headings, it should be noted that this is to emphasize the major modality tapped by each techniques. However, in keeping with the REBT viewpoint that cognition, emotion, and behavior are really interdependent processes, we note that probably all of the following techniques include cognitive, emotive, and behavioral elements.

Cognitive Techniques. The most commonly employed technique in REBT is probably the disputing of irrational beliefs. Phadke (1982) has clearly shown that the disputing process consists of three steps. First, therapists help clients to *detect* their irrational beliefs that underpin their self-defeating emotions and behaviors. Second, they *debate* with their clients concerning the truth or falsehood of their irrational beliefs. During the process, they help their clients to *discriminate* between their irrational and rational beliefs. Debating is usually conducted according to the Socratic method of asking questions such as "Where is the evidence that you must do this?" and "How does it follow that because you want this you must get it?" But skillful REBT therapists use a variety of different debating styles with their clients (DiGiuseppe, 1991; Dryden, 1984a; Ellis, 1985b; Wessler & Wessler, 1980; Young, 1984a, 1984b, 1984c).

There are a number of cognitive written homework forms available to assist clients in disputing their irrational beliefs between sessions (see Figure 9.3). Clients can also listen to audiotapes of therapy sessions and dispute their own irrational beliefs on tape. Here they initiate and sustain a dialogue between the rational and irrational parts of themselves. Clients who find the disputing process too difficult are encouraged to develop rational self-statements that they can write on small cards and repeat to themselves at various times between therapy sessions. An example of such a statement might be "I want my boyfriend's love, but I don't need it."

Three cognitive methods that therapists often suggest to their clients to help them reinforce this new rational philosophy are (1) bibliotherapy, in which clients are given self-help books and materials to read (e.g., Ellis & Becker, 1982; Ellis & Harper, 1997; Young, 1974); (2) listening to audiocassettes of REBT lectures on various themes (e.g., Ellis, 1971b, 1972a); and (3) using REBT with others, in which clients use REBT to help friends and relatives with their problems so that the clients can gain practice at using rational arguments.

A number of semantic methods are also employed in REBT. Thus defining techniques are sometimes employed, the purpose of which is to help clients use language in a less self-defeating manner. For example, instead of

REBT Self-Help Form

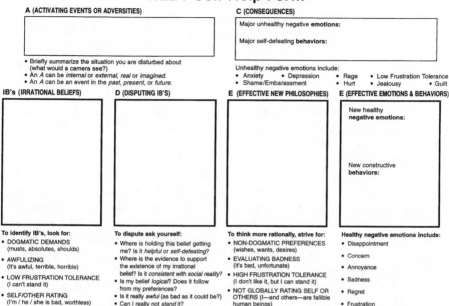

A (ACTIVATING EVENTS OR ADVERSITIES)

- Briefly summarize the situation you are disturbed about (what would a camera see?)
- An *A* can be *internal* or *external, real* or *imagined.*
- An *A* can be an event in the *past, present,* or *future.*

C (CONSEQUENCES)

Major unhealthy negative **emotions:**

Major self-defeating **behaviors:**

Unhealthy negative emotions include:
- Anxiety
- Depression
- Rage
- Low Frustration Tolerance
- Shame/Embarrassment
- Hurt
- Jealousy
- Guilt

IB's (IRRATIONAL BELIEFS)

D (DISPUTING IB'S)

E (EFFECTIVE NEW PHILOSOPHIES)

E (EFFECTIVE EMOTIONS & BEHAVIORS)

New healthy **negative emotions:**

New constructive **behaviors:**

To identify IB's, look for:
- DOGMATIC DEMANDS (musts, absolutes, shoulds)
- AWFULIZING (It's awful, terrible, horrible)
- LOW FRUSTRATION TOLERANCE (I can't stand it)
- SELF/OTHER RATING (I'm / he / she is bad, worthless)

To dispute ask yourself:
- Where is holding this belief getting me? Is it *helpful* or *self-defeating?*
- Where is the evidence to support the existence of my irrational belief? Is it *consistent with social reality?*
- Is my belief *logical?* Does it follow from my preferences?
- Is it really *awful* (as bad as it could be?)
- Can I really not *stand* it?

To think more rationally, strive for:
- NON-DOGMATIC PREFERENCES (wishes, wants, desires)
- EVALUATING BADNESS (it's bad, unfortunate)
- HIGH FRUSTRATION TOLERANCE (I don't like it, but I can stand it)
- NOT GLOBALLY RATING SELF OR OTHERS (I—and others—are fallible human beings)

Healthy negative emotions include:
- Disappointment
- Concern
- Annoyance
- Sadness
- Regret
- Frustration

FIGURE 9.3. REBT Self-Help Form. From Dryden and Walker (1996). Copyright 1996 by the Institute for Rational–Emotive Therapy. Reprinted with permission of the Albert Ellis Institute for Rational Emotive Behavior Therapy.

saying "I can't," clients are urged to use "I haven't yet." Referenting techniques are also employed (Danysh, 1974). Here clients are encouraged to list both the negative and positive referents of a particular concept such as smoking. This method is employed to counteract clients' tendencies to focus on the positive aspects of a harmful habit and to neglect its negative aspects.

REBT therapists also employ a number of imagery techniques. Rational emotive imagery (Ellis, 1993c; Maultsby & Ellis, 1974) is often employed, in which clients gain practice at changing their unhealthy negative emotions to healthy ones (C) while maintaining a vivid image of the negative event at A. Time projection imagery methods are also employed in REBT (Lazarus, 1984). For instance, a client may say that a particular event would be "awful" if it occurred. Rather than directly challenging this irrational belief at this stage, the therapist may temporarily go along with this, but may help the client to picture what life might be like at regular intervals after the "awful" event has occurred. In this way the client is indirectly helped to change the irrational belief, because the client comes to see that life goes on after the "awful" event, that he or she will usually recover from it, and that he or she can continue to pursue the original goals or develop new ones. Such realizations encourage the client to reevaluate his or her irrational belief. Finally, a number of therapists have successfully employed REBT in a hypnosis paradigm (e.g., Boutin & Tosi, 1983; Golden, 1983).

Emotive Techniques. REBT therapy has often been falsely criticized for neglecting the emotive aspects of psychotherapy. However, this is far from the truth; REBT therapists frequently employ a number of emotive techniques. REBT therapists use a variety of emotive techniques that are designed to help the client challenge his or her irrational beliefs but avoiding appearing to challenge the client as a person. First, a number of humorous methods are employed to encourage clients to think rationally by not taking themselves too seriously (Ellis, 1977a, 1977b). Second, REBT therapists do not hesitate to model a rational philosophy through self-disclosure. They honestly admit that they have had similar problems and show that they overcame them by using REBT. Thus one of us (W. D.) frequently tells clients, "I used to feel ashamed of my stammer." She then relates how she accepted herself with her speech impediment, and how she forced herself to tolerate the discomfort of speaking in public whenever the opportunity arose. Third, REBT therapists frequently use a number of stories, mottos, parables, witticisms, poems, and aphorisms as adjuncts to cognitive disputing techniques (Wessler & Wessler, 1980). Fourth, both of us (see, e.g., Ellis, 1977a, 1977b, 1981b) have written rational humorous songs that are designed to present rational philosophies in an amusing and memorable format. The following is such a song, written by Dryden to the tune of "God Save the Queen":

> God save my precious spleen
> Send me a life serene
> God save my spleen!
>
> Protect me from things odious
> Give me a life melodious
> And if things get too onerous
> I'll whine, bawl, and scream!

Ellis (1979d) has advocated the use of force and energy in the practice of psychotherapy, and has emphasized the employment of such interventions that fully involve clients' emotions. REBT therapists suggest that clients can move from intellectual to emotional insight by vigorously disputing their irrational beliefs (Ellis, 1993g). Vigor is often employed by clients in rational role reversal, where they forcefully and dramatically adopt the role of their rational self, whose goal is to successfully dispute self-defeating beliefs as articulated by their irrational self. Force and energy also play a significant part in REBT's now famous shame-attacking exercises (Ellis, 1969, 1995; Ellis & Becker, 1982). Here clients deliberately seek to act "shamefully" in public in order to accept themselves and to tolerate the ensuing discomfort. Since clients do best to harm neither themselves nor other people, minor infractions of social rules often serve as suitable shame-attacking exercises (e.g., calling out the time in a crowded department store, wearing bizarre clothes designed to attract public attention, and going into a hardware store and asking the clerks whether they sell tobacco). Risk-taking exercises come into the same category. Here clients deliberately force themselves to take calculated risks in areas where they wish to make changes. While disputing relevant irrational beliefs, one of us (A. E.) overcame his anxiety about approaching women by deliberately forcing himself to speak to 100 women in the Bronx Botanical Gardens. The other (W. D.) pushed himself to speak on national and local radio as part of a campaign to overcome his public speaking anxiety. Both of us took these risks while showing ourselves that nothing "awful" would result from such experiences. Repeating rational self-statements in a passionate and forceful manner is also often used in conjunction with such exercises (Ellis, 1985b).

Behavioral Techniques. REBT has advocated the use of behavioral techniques from its inception in 1955, since it is realized that cognitive change is very often facilitated by behavioral change (Emmelkamp, Kuipers, & Eggeraat, 1978). Since REBT therapists are concerned about helping clients raise their level of frustration tolerance, they encourage them to carry out homework assignments based on *in vivo* desensitization and flooding paradigms rather than those that are based on the gradual desensitization paradigm (Ellis, 1979e; Ellis & Abrahms, 1978; Ellis & Becker, 1982; Ellis & Grieger, 1977). However, pragmatic considerations do have to be taken into account, and some clients refuse to carry out such assignments. REBT therapists negotiate a compromise, encouraging such clients to undertake tasks that are sufficiently challenging for them but that are not overwhelming, given their present status (Dryden, 1985).

Other behavioral methods are frequently or occasionally employed in REBT:

1. "Stay in there" activities (Grieger & Boyd, 1980) present clients with opportunities to tolerate chronic discomfort while remaining in uncomfortable situations for a long period of time.
2. Antiprocrastination exercises encourage clients to push themselves to start tasks sooner rather than later, while again tolerating the discomfort of breaking the "*mañana*" habit.
3. Rewards and penalties are employed to encourage clients to under-

take uncomfortable assignments in the pursuit of their long-range goals (Ellis, 1979c); as mentioned earlier, stiff penalties are found to be particularly helpful with chronically resistant clients (Ellis, 1985b).

4. Kelly's (1955) fixed-role therapy is sometimes employed in REBT; here clients are encouraged to act as if they already think rationally, to enable them to experience the fact that change is possible.

A number of other behavioral methods are employed in both specialized and general REBT (e.g., various forms of skills training methods). When these are used in specialized REBT, they are done to encourage philosophical change, whereas in general REBT they are employed to teach clients skills that are absent from their repertoire. When skills training is the goal in specialized REBT, it is employed *along with* the disputing of irrational beliefs and *after* some measure of philosophical change has been effected.

Techniques That Are Avoided in REBT. By now it should be clear that REBT is a multimodal form of therapy that advocates the employment of techniques in the cognitive, emotive, and behavioral modalities. However, because the choice of therapeutic techniques is inspired by REBT theory, the following available therapeutic techniques are avoided or used sparingly in the practice of REBT (Ellis, 1979c, 1983c, 1984c). REBT therapists do not absolutistically avoid using the following methods, however. They may on certain occasions and with certain clients utilize such techniques particularly for pragmatic purposes (Ellis, 1985b).

1. Techniques that help people become more dependent (e.g., undue therapist warmth as a strong reinforcement, the creation and analysis of a transference neurosis).

2. Techniques that encourage people to become more gullible and suggestible (e.g., Pollyanna-like positive thinking).

3. Techniques that are long-winded and inefficient (e.g., psychoanalytic methods in general and free association in particular, encouraging clients to give lengthy descriptions of activating experiences at A).

4. Methods that help people feel better in the short term, rather than get better in the long term (Ellis, 1972b—e.g., some experiential techniques such as fully expressing one's feelings in a dramatic or cathartic manner, some Gestalt methods and primal techniques).

5. Techniques that distract clients from working on their irrational philosophies (e.g., relaxation methods, yoga, and other cognitive distraction methods). These methods may be employed, however,

along with cognitive disputing designed to yield some philosophical change.

6. Methods that may unwittingly reinforce clients' philosophy of LFT (e.g., gradual desensitization).

7. Techniques that include an antiscientific philosophy (e.g., faith healing and mysticism; Ellis, 1985b; Ellis & Yeager, 1989).

8. Techniques that attempt to change activating events (A) before or without showing clients how to change their irrational beliefs (B) (e.g., some strategic family systems techniques).

9. Techniques that have dubious validity (e.g., neurolinguistic programming).

Case Examples

FREDA: A CASE OF ANXIETY

Freda was a 40-year-old divorced woman with two grown-up children, both of whom lived with her. She consulted one of us (W. D.—"I" in this and the following case) because she suffered from severe anxiety about driving. She had been involved in a car accident 18 months previously in which she was a passenger. Although not seriously hurt, she had experienced anxiety when driving ever since that time. Freda's anxiety was experienced on two levels. First, she became anxious whenever a large truck approached her from the rear. Second, she became enormously anxious about her anxiety and felt intense panic. I first worked with her on this metaproblem. Her irrational belief here was "I must not be anxious, and it is horrible when I am." I disputed this belief and helped her to see that anxiety is uncomfortable, but not dangerous (Low, 1952). Her original anxiety problem was tackled next. I used "inference chaining" (Moore, 1983) to reveal that she was terrified about (1) dying "before her time" and (2) what would happen to her two sons in the event of her death. First, I helped her see that there was no law of the universe declaring that she must not die in a car crash and that she must live longer than she will live. Second, I asked her what was the worst fate she could imagine for her sons. She was particularly anxious about her elder son, who seemed somewhat vulnerable. She was also anxious that he might not be able to cope on his own and might become a vagrant, which she evaluated as "terrible." I disputed this irrational belief as well and helped her to see that if he did become a vagrant, that would be very bad or tragic but hardly terrible, since there was no law of the universe that said that he must not become a vagrant. I pointed out further that if he did become a vagrant, he might still obtain some happiness. Behaviorally, I first encouraged her to drive even though she was anxious, and to tolerate this experience as "bad" but not "awful." After this brought about some improvement, I urged her to seek out actively big trucks and tolerate the discomfort of being "hemmed in." In addition, I helped her to see that her irrational beliefs at B led to her overestimating the likelihood of (1) her dying and (2) her son's becoming a vagrant in the event of her death, both of which were cognitive consequences (3) of her irrational beliefs.

The disclosure of the theme of being "hemmed in" revealed further problems. She was at that same time being romantically pursued by a man in whom she felt no interest. She felt trapped because he was not discouraged by her polite requests for him to leave her alone. I asked her what would stop her from being firm and back this assertion up with a refusal to talk to him. She thought that this approach would discourage him, but said that she would feel guilty if he were hurt by such a direct approach. I helped her to see that her guilt stemmed from the belief "I would be a bad person for causing him pain." First I disputed this belief and showed her that even if she did directly cause the man pain, she could accept herself as a fallible human being for acting badly. I then helped her see that she would be responsible for depriving him rather than for cruelly hurting him, since if he felt hurt or denigrated by her rejections, he would create these feelings by irrationally downing himself. In the next session, she claimed success at asserting herself with the man and reported further alleviation of her anxiety about driving. She spontaneously reported that feeling less hemmed in her personal relationships helped her feel less hemmed in while driving.

In subsequent sessions, Freda discussed further problems concerning lack of assertion, guilt, and embarrassment. I helped her to see that there were links between these problems, and she became increasingly proficient at detecting and disputing her irrational beliefs. Most noteworthy was the way she counteracted some of her irrational philosophies through dramatic action. I explained to her the concept of shame-attacking exercises, and in the next session she reported undertaking one. For years she had been anxious about bringing men home to meet her two sons. On this occasion she met a much younger man at a dance and took him home that night. She did so to dispute her shame-inducing belief "My sons would look down on me as a cradle snatcher, and that would prove that I am a shit." She felt this was very beneficial. Her sons did make several negative comments that she did not like. She reported that she had told them that she was going to live her life her way, and that she would like their approval; however, if they chose to regard her as "a desperate old woman," that was unfortunate but hardly the end of the world.

At the end of 12 weekly sessions, Freda had made significant progress in disputing her dire needs for approval and comfort. More importantly, she had learned to internalize the scientific method of disputing and saw clearly the benefits of actively working to counteract her irrational philosophies.

A 6-month follow-up revealed that she had maintained her progress. She was able to drive quite comfortably, although she still did not like having big trucks behind her. However, she was no longer anxious about encountering this situation. Interpersonally, she felt much freer about saying what she thought and acting more in her own interests, even though others might view her in a negative light. She reported that her sons had changed their attitude toward her, saying, "They seem to respect the 'new me' more than the old one."

BOB: A CASE OF DEPRESSION

Bob, a 50-year-old man, was severely depressed after losing his job and as a result was experiencing sex problems. He was referred to me (W. D.) after his general practitioner had discovered that he was feeling suicidal. In our first session, I learned that he was feeling hopeless about his future because he considered that he was "finished as a man." I very persistently showed him that he could accept himself as a man who had temporarily lost employment and erectile sufficiency, rather than damn himself as being less of a man for these two losses. His mood lifted appreciably by the end of the session, but I told him that he could telephone me between sessions if he became suicidal again.

In our second session, I discovered that Bob was also ashamed about being depressed and about seeking psychotherapeutic help. Again I helped him to dispute his irrational belief—in this case, "I must be able to solve my problems on my own"—and also encouraged him to counteract his shame by telling his best friend about his problems.

Bob reported feeling much better in our third session. He did not feel ashamed about telling his friend about his problems and had received a sympathetic response from the friend, who in turn confided that he had had similar problems the previous year. This actually had a profound effect on Bob, because it helped him to see that he could gain happiness by changing some of his priorities. He began to see that friendship was as important as achievement, and that it was possible for him to redefine what it meant to be a man.

In our fourth session, I disputed his anxiety-creating belief about his sexual performance: "I must get it up to be a man." Even by the fourth session, it was apparent that Bob clearly understood the difference between rational and irrational beliefs. He went home and enjoyed several sexual experiences with his wife when he resolved to act on the belief that "an erection and orgasm would be nice, but sex can be enjoyed without them." In addition, Bob decided to do some voluntary work in a local hospital and enjoyed it, even though he predicted he would gain no satisfaction from doing so.

Bob began to show increasing interest in the area of gender identity and read several books on the pressures of being a male in today's society. He began taking a more active role doing domestic chores, and by the seventh session no longer regarded it as "women's work." In the eighth session, however, he relapsed and reported feeling depressed again. Interestingly, when this was explored, it transpired that he was condemning himself for being "an erstwhile male chauvinist." I showed him again that he was a fallible human being and that he could accept himself as such, even if he had adhered to a male chauvinistic philosophy in the past and even if he still retained some of this philosophy today. We had a full discussion of the concept of unconditional self-acceptance, and he resolved to act on this philosophy.

In our final two sessions, we discussed several career-related issues. Bob decided as a result of this discussion to attend a university and study for a degree in social work. At our final session, he considered that he had changed some fundamental attitudes: "Looking back, I can realize that I had believed in the concept of the two-dimensional man. I was okay as long as I was in a good job and my cock functioned well. Now I can see that there is much more to being a man than that. I feel you have helped me widen my horizons, and I now view myself as being considerably more complex than before. I have an increased enjoyment of friendship, and sex with my wife is incredibly more enriching."

A 6-month follow-up revealed that Bob was enjoying his university course and was free from depression. At his initial therapy session, his Beck Depression Inventory score had been in the severe range (42). At his 10th and final session of regular therapy his score had gone down to 3, and at the 6-month follow-up it was 1.

ADDITIONAL CONSIDERATIONS

In this section we discuss additional considerations about REBT, including assessment technology and the kind of research that has been done with REBT assessment; the empirical status of the REBT approach, especially in regard to experimental investigation of the validity of its main treatment methods; and directions for future development in REBT.

Assessment Technology of REBT

Assessment of the kind and degree of emotional disturbance of clients is held to be important in REBT for several reasons:

1. To determine how seriously disturbed clients are, so that therapists can see how likely they are to benefit from any form of therapy (including REBT), and so that they can decide which REBT techniques of the many possible ones that are available may be most suitably employed and which avoided with each particular client.
2. To assess with a fair degree of accuracy how difficult clients are likely to be, how they will probably take to the main REBT procedures, and how long psychotherapy will take.
3. To discover which type of therapist involvement (e.g., a more or less active or a more or less passive and supportive kind) is likely to help an individual client.
4. To discover what types of skill deficiencies clients have and what kinds of training they might best undertake to remedy some of their skill deficiencies. On the basis of this assessment, certain kinds of skill training (such as assertiveness, social skills, communication, or vocational training) may be recommended for specific clients.

REBT practitioners are at liberty to use all kinds of assessment procedures, but generally favor the types of cognitive-behavioral interventions described in Kendall and Hollon (1980). They tend to take a dimmer view of diagnostic procedures such as the Rorschach and other projective techniques than they do of more objective personality questionnaires and behavioral tests, largely because the former often have dubious validity, incorporate questionable psychoanalytic and psychodynamic interpretations, and usually are not particularly relatable to effective treatment processes.

Ellis and many other REBT practitioners take the view that although assessment interviews and some standard diagnostic tests may at times be useful in exploring clients' disturbances, perhaps the best form of assessment consists of having several REBT sessions with the client. Some of the advantages of this kind of therapy-oriented assessment include the following:

1. Clients get to work on their problems almost immediately; can gain therapeutically while being assessed; and can be helped to suffer less pain, hardship, and expense while undergoing treatment.
2. The preferable techniques to be used with different clients are often best determined mainly through experimenting with some of these techniques in the course of the therapeutic process. By actually experimenting with certain specific methods, the REBT therapist can see how the client reacts to them, and consequently how they should be continued or discontinued.

3. Assessment procedures divorced from ongoing psychotherapy (such as giving a whole battery of tests prior to beginning therapy) may be iatrogenic for a number of clients. Especially if the assessment procedures take some time to complete, clients may imagine "horrors" about themselves that lead them astray and make it more difficult for them to benefit from therapy.

4. Certain conventional assessment procedures (e.g., the Rorschach and Thematic Apperception Test) may wrongly predict problems, symptoms, and dynamics that many clients do not really have, and they may help lead their therapists away from more scientifically based evaluations.

5. Clients sometimes take diagnoses obtained from complicated assessment procedures as the gospel truth, feel that they have thereby received a valid "explanation" of what ails them, and wrongly conclude that they have been helped by this "explanation." REBT assessment procedures—including using therapy itself as an integral part of the assessment process—primarily focus on what clients can do to change, rather than on clever diagnostic "explanations" of what ails them.

Because REBT is strongly cognitive, emotive, and behavioral, it assesses not only clients' irrational beliefs, but also their unhealthy feelings and self-defeating behaviors. As we have noted in previous sections of this chapter, the usual REBT assessment process almost always includes the following:

1. Clients are helped to acknowledge and describe their unhealthy feelings, and these are clearly differentiated from their negative healthy feelings.
2. Clients are led to acknowledge and delineate their self-defeating behaviors, rather than to overemphasize idiosyncratic but nondeleterious behaviors.
3. Clients are asked to point out specific activating events or adversities in their lives that tend to occur just prior to their experienced disturbed feelings and behaviors.
4. Clients' rational beliefs that accompany their activating events and that lead to undisturbed consequences are assessed and discussed.
5. Clients' irrational beliefs that accompany their activating events and that lead to disturbed consequences are assessed and discussed.
6. Clients' irrational beliefs that involve absolutistic "musts" and grandiose demands on themselves, others, and the universe are particularly determined.
7. Clients' second-level irrational beliefs that tend to be derived from their absolutistic "shoulds" and "musts" (e.g., awfulizing; LFT; depreciation of the self, others, and the world; and unrealistic overgeneralizations) are revealed.

8. Clients' irrational beliefs that lead to their disturbances about their disturbances (e.g., anxiety about anxiety, depression about being depressed) are revealed and discussed in particular.

As these specialized REBT assessment and diagnostic procedures are instituted, specific treatment plans are made—normally in close collaboration with clients—in order to work first on the most important and self-sabotaging emotional and behavioral symptoms that they present, and later on related and possibly less important symptoms. REBT practitioners, however, always try to maintain an exceptionally open-minded, skeptical, and experimental attitude toward clients and their problems, so that what at first seem to be their crucial and most debilitating ideas, feelings, and actions may later be seen in a different light, and emphasis may be changed to working on other equally or more pernicious irrationalities that might not be evident during the clients' early sessions.

Research on REBT Tests of Irrational Beliefs

When Ellis hypothesized in his early writings on REBT (Ellis, 1957a, 1957b, 1958, 1962) that emotional and behavioral disturbance stems largely from irrational beliefs, he at first outlined from 10–12 basic irrationalities. His hypothesized irrational beliefs seemed to have such obvious face validity that they have been widely quoted in literally hundreds of articles and books on human personality and psychotherapy. Researchers soon began systematic investigations of Ellis's basic disturbance-creating irrationalities and made them the source of about 50 standardized tests. Specific REBT tests of irrational beliefs have been devised and popularly used in many research studies, including tests by DiGiuseppe, Tafrate, and Eckhard (1994), Jones (1968), Kassinove, Crisci, and Tiegerman (1977), and Shorkey and Sutton-Simon (1983).

Literally hundreds of controlled studies have been done using these and similar tests of dysfunctional beliefs, and in almost all of these studies the tests have been shown to distinguish reliably between various kinds of disturbed individuals and control groups (Clark, 1997; Glass & Arnkoff, 1997).

Empirical Status of REBT

The first controlled study of REBT was published in 1957 and consisted of Ellis's comparing the results he had obtained from using classical psychoanalysis, psychoanalytically oriented psychotherapy, and RET (Ellis, 1957b). It was hardly an unbiased study, and its positive results are not to be taken too seriously. However, starting in the 1960s and continuing into the 1980s, more than 1,000 outcome studies were done on REBT and on closely related forms of CBT. The great majority of these controlled studies have shown that, when compared to a control group, clients treated with REBT or with a form of CBT that is an essential part of REBT fare significantly better than those who are not so treated. Outcome studies have been reviewed by Hajzler and Bernard (1991), Hollon and Beck (1994), and Lyons and Woods (1991). Outcome studies testing the use of REBT and of types of CBT derived from REBT continue to proliferate, most of them continuing to indicate that treatment methods consisting of REBT procedures help clients or subjects significantly more than control groups.

In addition to empirical studies that tend to back the main therapeutic hypotheses of REBT, literally hundreds of other controlled experiments have been published that tend to indicate that many of the main theoretical hypotheses of REBT—especially its ABC theory of human disturbance—now have considerable experimental backing. Also, hundreds more research studies present evidence that many of the REBT-favored therapeutic techniques—such as active, directive therapy; direct disputing of irrational ideas; the use of rational or coping statements; and the employment of psychoeducational methods—have distinct effectiveness. Ellis (1979g) cited hundreds of these studies in his comprehensive review of the REBT-oriented literature at that time. If his review were brought up to date, it would now include hundreds of additional studies that present empirical confirmation of many of the most important REBT theories and therapeutic applications.

This is not to claim that REBT has undisputed evidence of the validity of its theories or the effectiveness of its practice. Like all other major systems of psychotherapy, it is still exceptionally wanting in these respects; considerable further research needs to be done to check on its major hypotheses. Although its treatment methods have been tested many times against the methods of other kinds of psychotherapy and against non-treated control groups, and they have usually been proven adequate, they have not as yet often been compared to the procedures of other popular forms of CBT. Considerable experimental studies could be done in this area.

REBT has had many applications to various aspects of psychotherapy, including child and adolescent therapy (Bernard & Joyce, 1984), marriage and family therapy (Ellis, 1991, 1993d; Ellis & Dryden, 1997; Ellis, Sichel, Yeager, DiMattia, & DiGiuseppe, 1989), sex and relationship therapy (Ellis, 1976c, 1979f; Ellis & Lange, 1994; Ellis & Tafrate, 1997; Wolfe, 1992), brief therapy (Dryden, 1996; Ellis, 1996a, 1996b), treatment of personality disorders (Ellis, 1994a, 1994c), hypnosis (Ellis, 1993e, 1996e), constructivist therapy (Ellis, 1997b), group therapy (Ellis, 1997c), treatment of eating disorders (Ellis, Abrams, & Dengelegi, 1992), addiction treatment (Ellis & DiGiuseppe, 1994; Ellis & Velten, 1992), stress counseling (Ellis, Gordon, Neenan, & Palmer, 1997), geriatric therapy (Ellis & Velten, 1998), treatment of obsessive–compulsive disorder (Ellis, 1997d), and thanatology (Ellis & Abrams, 1994).

Directions for the Future Development of REBT

The future of REBT obviously cannot be predicted with complete accuracy, because psychotherapy in general and REBT in particular may take any number of likely and unlikely turns in the next century or two. Judging by recent trends, however, we would like to make the following predictions.

REBT may or may not be immensely popular under its present name in the future, but many of its most important and pioneering aspects are likely to be incorporated into almost all effective forms of therapy. Its famous ABC theory of personality and emotional disturbance is more or less acknowledged and distinctly employed by most of today's professional therapists. Most therapists now pay considerable attention to their clients' unrealistic and irrational beliefs, and will probably continue to do so in years to come, though perhaps not as actively and forcefully as do REBT practitioners. CBT, pioneered by REBT, is now one of the most popular forms of psychological treatment. It and REBT will probably continue to grow and eventually perhaps be the basic therapy method that includes the most effective elements of other systems.

Although REBT is a comprehensive system of therapy that normally uses a large number of cognitive, emotive, and behavioral methods, there is good reason to believe that many more effective techniques will be invented and researched and will be added to the REBT armamentarium.

REBT was originally created as a one-on-one therapy and then adapted to regular group therapy (Ellis, 1962, 1982b). But, as has been stated, over the years it has been very widely used with large groups, classroom courses, workshops and seminars, intensives, and other mass applications (Dryden, 1998; Ellis & Bernard, 1985). It is also popular in the form of REBT pamphlets, books, audiocassettes, videocassettes, and programmed material. In its mass media presentations, it has already reached and affected literally millions of people, including many who are not seriously disturbed but who have used its principles to enhance and actualize their lives.

Because REBT is, more than most other therapies, a psychoeducational process that involves teaching people how to look for and uproot their irrationalities; because it shows them how to keep doing REBT self-help homework as a major part of the therapeutic process; and because it can be stated in simple, self-help terms and made available to large numbers of people (Ellis & Harper, 1997; Ellis & Knaus, 1977; Young, 1974), we believe that the future of REBT is likely to reside more in its mass applications and its educational procedures than in its use for individual and group psychotherapy. We hope that its popular media applications will grow enormously over the coming years, thus fulfilling one of the fondest hopes of its originator.

REBT has had many lay applications and has been found useful in a number of fields, such as politics, business, education, parenting, communication, sports, religion, and assertion training (Barrish & Barrish, 1989; Bernard & DiGiuseppe, 1994; Dryden, 1998; Ellis, 1972c, 1993b, 1993f; Johnson, 1993; Vernon, 1989). Many additional applications of REBT in these and other aspects of human life can be confidently expected.

NOTES

1. We have chosen here to focus on the distinctiveness of specialized REBT as compared with other forms of CBT in general. Other theorists have outlined the differences between REBT and other specific schools of CBT. Thus Wessler and Wessler (1980) have outlined the differences between REBT and Maultsby's rational behavior therapy, and Haaga and Davison (1991) have compared and contrasted REBT with Beck's cognitive therapy.

2. In this section, we focus primarily on the process of specialized REBT. When general REBT is employed, the process of therapy is almost indistinguishable from the process of other systems of CBT covered in this handbook.

REFERENCES

Adler, A. (1927). *Understanding human nature*. New York: Garden City.

Adler, A. (1964). *Social interest: A challenge to mankind*. New York: Capricorn.

Bandura, A. (1969). *Principles of behavior modification*. New York: Holt, Rinehart & Winston.

Bandura, A. (1977). *Social learning theory*. Englewood Cliffs, NJ: Prentice-Hall.

Bard, J. (1980). *Rational–emotive therapy in practice*. Champaign, IL: Research Press.

Barrish, I. J., & Barrish, H. H. (1989). *Surviving and enjoying your adolescent*. Kansas City, MO: Wesport.

Beck, A. T. (1967). *Depression*. New York: Hoeber.

Beck, A. T. (1976). *Cognitive therapy and the emotional disorders*. New York: International Universities Press.

Beck, A. T., Rush, A. J., Shaw, B. F., & Emery, G. (1979). *Cognitive therapy of depression*. New York: Guilford Press.

Bernard, M. E., & DiGiuseppe, R. (Eds.). (1994). *Rational–emotive consultation in applied settings*. Hillsdale, NJ: Erlbaum.

Bernard, M. E., & Joyce, M. R. (1984). *Rational-emotive therapy with children and adolescents: Theory, treatment strategies, preventative methods.* New York: Wiley.

Beutler, L. E. (1983). *Eclectic psychotherapy: A systematic approach.* New York: Pergamon Press.

Boutin, G. E., & Tosi, D. J. (1983). Modification of irrational ideas and test anxiety through rational stage directed hypnotherapy (RSDH). *Journal of Clinical Psychology, 39,* 382–391.

Burns, D. D. (1980). *Feeling good: The new mood therapy.* New York: William Morrow.

Clark, D. A. (1997). Twenty years of cognitive assessment: Current status and future directions. *Journal of Consulting and Clinical Psychology, 65,* 996–1000.

Corsini, R. J. (Ed.). (1977). *Current personality theories.* Itasca, IL: Peacock.

Danysh, J. (1974). *Stop without quitting.* San Francisco: International Society for General Semantics.

DiGiuseppe, R. (1991). Comprehensive cognitive disputing in RET. In M. E. Bernard (Ed.), *Using rational–emotive therapy effectively* (pp. 173–195). New York: Plenum Press.

DiGiuseppe, R., Tafrate, R., & Eckhard, C. (1994). Critical issues in the treatment of anger. *Cognitive and Behavioral Practice, 1,* 111–132.

Dryden, W. (1984a). *Rational–emotive therapy: Fundamentals and innovations.* London: Croom Helm.

Dryden, W. (1984b). Rational–emotive therapy. In W. Dryden (Ed.), *Individual therapy in Britain* (pp. 235–263). London: Harper & Row.

Dryden, W. (1985). Challenging but not overwhelming: A compromise in negotiating homework assignments. *British Journal of Cognitive Psychotherapy, 3*(1), 77–80.

Dryden, W. (1996). *Brief rational emotive behaviour therapy.* Chichester, England: Wiley.

Dryden, W. (1998). *Developing self-acceptance.* Chichester, England: Wiley.

Dryden, W. (1999). *Rational emotive behaviour therapy: A personal view.* Bicester, England: Winslow Press.

Dryden, W., & Ellis, A. (1986). Rational–emotive therapy. In W. Dryden & W. L. Golden (Eds.), *Cognitive-behavioural approaches to psychotherapy* (pp. 129–168). London: Harper & Row.

Dryden, W., & Walker, J. (1996). *REBT Self-Help Form* (rev. by A. Ellis). New York: Albert Ellis Institute for REBT.

Duckro, P., Beal, D., & George, C. (1979). Research on the effects of disconfirmed role expectations in psychotherapy: A critical review. *Psychological Bulletin, 86,* 260–275.

Dunlap, K. (1932). *Habits: Their making and unmaking.* New York: Liveright.

Ellis, A. (1957a). *How to live with a "neurotic"* (rev. ed.). New York: Crown.

Ellis, A. (1957b). Outcome of employing three techniques of psychotherapy. *Journal of Clinical Psychology, 13,* 334–350.

Ellis, A. (1958). Rational psychotherapy. *Journal of General Psychology, 59,* 245–253.

Ellis, A. (1962). *Reason and emotion in psychotherapy.* New York: Stuart.

Ellis, A. (1963). Toward a more precise definition of "emotional" and "intellectual" insight. *Psychological Reports, 13,* 125–126.

Ellis, A. (1968). *Personality Data Form.* New York: Institute for Rational–Emotive Therapy.

Ellis, A. (1969). A weekend of rational encounter. *Rational Living, 4*(2), 1–8.

Ellis, A. (1971a). *Growth through reason.* North Hollywood, CA: Wilshire Books.

Ellis, A. (Speaker). (1971b). *How to stubbornly refuse to be ashamed of anything* (Cassette recording). New York: Institute for Rational–Emotive Therapy.

Ellis, A. (Speaker). (1972a). *Solving emotional problems* (Cassette recording). New York: Institute for Rational–Emotive Therapy.

Ellis, A. (1972b). Helping people get better: Rather than merely feel better. *Rational Living, 7*(2), 2–9.

Ellis, A. (1972c). *Executive leadership: The rational–emotive approach.* New York: Institute for Rational–Emotive Therapy.

Ellis, A. (1973). *Humanistic psychotherapy: The rational–emotive approach.* New York: McGraw-Hill.

Ellis, A. (1976a). The biological basis of human irrationality. *Journal of Individual Psychology, 32,* 145–168.

Ellis, A. (1976b). RET abolishes most of the human ego. *Psychotherapy: Theory, Research and Practice, 13,* 343–348.

Ellis, A. (1976c). *Sex and the liberated man.* New York: Stuart.

Ellis, A. (1977a). Fun as psychotherapy. *Rational Living, 12*(1), 2–6.

Ellis, A. (Speaker). (1977b). *A garland of rational humorous songs* (Cassette recording). New York: Institute for Rational–Emotive Therapy.

Ellis, A. (1977c). *Anger—how to live with and without it.* Secaucus, NJ: Citadel Press.

Ellis, A. (1979a). The theory of rational–emotive therapy. In A. Ellis & J. M. Whiteley (Eds.), *Theoretical and empirical foundations of rational–emotive therapy* (pp. 33–60). Monterey, CA: Brooks/Cole.

Ellis, A. (1979b). Discomfort anxiety: A new cognitive behavioral construct. Part 1. *Rational Living, 14*(2), 3–8.

Ellis, A. (1979c). The practice of rational–emotive therapy. In A. Ellis & J. M. Whiteley (Eds.), *Theoretical and empirical foundations of rational–emotive therapy* (pp. 61–100). Monterey, CA: Brooks/Cole.

Ellis, A. (1979d). The issue of force and energy in behavioral change. *Journal of Contemporary Psychotherapy, 10*(2), 83–97.

Ellis, A. (1979e). A note on the treatment of agoraphobics with cognitive modification versus prolonged exposure in vivo. *Behaviour Research and Therapy, 17,* 162–164.

Ellis, A. (1979f). *The intelligent woman's guide to dating and mating* (rev. ed.). Secaucus, NJ: Stuart.

Ellis, A. (1979g). Rational–emotive therapy: Research data that support the clinical and personal hypotheses of RET and other modes of cognitive-behavior therapy. In A. Ellis & J. M. Whiteley (Eds.), *Theoretical and empirical foundations of rational–emotive therapy* (pp. 101–173). Monterey, CA: Brooks/Cole.

Ellis, A. (1980a). Discomfort anxiety: A new cognitive behavioral construct. Part 2. *Rational Living, 15*(l), 25–30.

Ellis, A. (1980b). Rational–emotive therapy and cognitive behavior therapy: Similarities and differences. *Cognitive Therapy and Research, 4,* 325–340.

Ellis, A. (1981a). The place of Immanuel Kant in cognitive psychotherapy. *Rational Living, 16*(2), 13–16.

Ellis, A. (1981b). The use of rational humorous songs in psychotherapy. *Voices, 16*(4), 29–36.

Ellis, A. (1982a). Intimacy in rational–emotive therapy. In M. Fisher & G. Striker (Eds.), *Intimacy* (pp. 203–217). New York: Plenum Press.

Ellis, A. (1982b). Rational–emotive group therapy. In G. M. Gazda (Ed.), *Basic approaches to group psychotherapy and group counseling* (pp. 381–412). Springfield, IL: Thomas.

Ellis, A. (1983a). *The case against religiosity.* New York: Institute for Rational–Emotive Therapy.

Ellis, A. (1983b). How to deal with your most difficult client: You. *Journal of Rational-Emotive Therapy, 1*(1), 3–8.

Ellis, A. (1983c). The philosophic implications and dangers of some popular behavior therapy techniques. In M. Rosenbaum, C. M. Franks, & Y. Jaffe (Eds.), *Perspectives in behavior therapy in the eighties* (pp. 138–151). New York: Springer.

Ellis, A. (1983d). Failures in rational–emotive therapy. In E. B. Foa & P. M. G. Emmelkamp (Eds.), *Failures in behavior therapy* (pp. 159–171). New York: Wiley.

Ellis, A. (1983e). Rational–emotive therapy (RET) approaches to overcoming resistance: I. Common forms of resistance. *British Journal of Cognitive Psychotherapy, 1*(1), 28–38.

Ellis, A. (1983f). Rational–emotive therapy (RET) approaches to overcoming resistance: II. How RET disputes clients' irrational resistance-creating beliefs. *British Journal of Cognitive Psychotherapy, 1*(2), 1–16.

Ellis, A. (1984a). The essence of RET. 1984. *Journal of Rational–Emotive Therapy, 2*(1), 19–25.

Ellis, A. (1984b, August). *Rational–emotive therapy and transpersonal psychology.* Paper presented at the 92nd Annual Convention of the American Psychological Association, Toronto.

Ellis, A. (1984c). Rational–emotive therapy. In R. J. Corsini (Ed.), *Current psychotherapies* (3rd ed., pp. 196–238). Itasca, IL: Peacock.

Ellis, A. (1984d). Rational–emotive therapy (RET) approaches to overcoming resistance: III. Using emotive and behavioural techniques of overcoming resistance. *British Journal of Cognitive Psychotherapy, 2*(1), 11–26.

Ellis, A. (1985a). Expanding the ABCs of rational–emotive therapy. In M. J. Mahoney & A. Freeman (Eds.), *Cognition and psychotherapy* (pp. 313–323). New York: Plenum Press.

Ellis, A. (1985b). Rational–emotive therapy (RET) approaches to overcoming resistance: IV. Handling special kinds of clients. *British Journal of Cognitive Psychotherapy, 3*(1), 26–42.

Ellis, A. (1991). Rational–emotive family therapy. In A. M. Horne & J. L. Passmore (Eds.), *Family counseling and therapy* (2nd ed., pp. 403–434). Itasca, IL: Peacock.

Ellis, A. (1993a). Changing rational–emotive therapy (RET) to rational emotive behavior therapy (REBT). *Behavior Therapist, 16,* 257–258.

Ellis, A. (1993b). General semantics and rational emotive behavior therapy. *Bulletin of General Semantics, 58,* 12–28.

Ellis, A. (1993c). Rational emotive imagery: RET version. In M. E. Bernard & J. L. Wolfe (Eds.), *The RET source book for practitioners* (pp. II,8–II,10). New York: Institute for Rational–Emotive Therapy.

Ellis, A. (1993d). The rational–emotive therapy (RET) approach to marriage and family therapy. *Family Journal: Counseling and Therapy for Couples and Families, 1,* 292–307.

Ellis, A. (1993e). Rational–emotive therapy and hypnosis. In J. W. Rhue, S. J. Lynn, & I. Kirsch (Eds.), *Handbook of clinical hypnosis* (pp. 173–186). Washington, DC: American Psychological Association.

Ellis, A. (Speaker). (1993f). *The sport of avoiding sports and exercise* (Cassette recording). Aurora, CO: Sound & Images.

Ellis, A. (1993g). Vigorous RET disputing. In M. E. Bernard & J. L. Wolfe (Eds.), *The RET resource book for practitioners* (pp. II,7). New York: Institute for Rational–Emotive Therapy.

Ellis, A. (1994a). Rational emotive behavior therapy approaches to obsessive–compulsive disorder (OCD). *Journal of Rational–Emotive and Cognitive-Behavior Therapy, 12,* 121–141.

Ellis, A. (1994b). *Reason and emotion in psychotherapy* (rev. ed.). Secaucus, NJ: Birch Lane.

Ellis, A. (1994c). The treatment of borderline personalities with rational emotive behavior therapy. *Journal of Rational–Emotive and Cognitive-Behavior Therapy, 12,* 101–119.

Ellis, A. (1995). Rational emotive behavior therapy. In R. Corsini & D. Wedding (Eds.), *Current psychotherapies* (5th ed., pp. 162–196). Itasca, IL: Peacock.

Ellis, A. (1996a). *Better, deeper, and more enduring brief therapy.* New York: Brunner/Mazel.

Ellis, A. (Speaker). (1996b). *Demonstration of brief rational emotive behavior therapy* (Videotape). Phoenix, AZ: Milton A. Erickson Foundation.

Ellis, A. (1996c). *REBT diminishes much of the human ego* (rev. ed.). New York: Institute for Rational–Emotive Therapy.

Ellis, A. (1996d). Responses to criticisms of rational emotive behavior therapy (REBT) by Ray DiGiuseppe, Frank Bond, Windy Dryden, Steve Weinrach, and Richard Wessler. *Journal of Rational–Emotive and Cognitive-Behavior Therapy, 14,* 97–121.

Ellis, A. (1996e). Using hypnosis in rational–emotive behavior therapy in the case of Ellen. In S. J. Lynn, I. Kirsch, & J. W. Rhue (Eds.), *Casebook of clinical hypnosis* (pp. 335–347). Washington, DC: American Psychological Association.

Ellis, A. (1997a). The evolution of Albert Ellis and rational emotive behavior therapy. In J. K. Zeig (Ed.), *The evolution of psychotherapy: The third conference* (pp. 69–82). New York: Brunner/Mazel.

Ellis, A. (1997b). Postmodern ethics for active–directive counseling and psychotherapy. *Journal of Mental Health Counseling, 18,* 211–225.

Ellis, A. (1997c). REBT and its application to group therapy. In J. Yankura & W.

Dryden (Eds.), *Special applications of REBT: A therapist's casebook* (pp. 131–161). New York: Springer.

Ellis, A. (1997d). REBT with obsessive–compulsive disorder. In J. Yankura & W. Dryden (Eds.), *Using REBT with common psychological problems: A therapist's casebook* (pp. 197–239). New York: Springer.

Ellis, A. (1998). *How to control your anxiety before it controls you*. Secaucus, NJ: Carol.

Ellis, A., & Abrahms, E. (1978). *Brief psychotherapy in medical and health practice*. New York: Springer.

Ellis, A., & Abrams, M. (1994). *How to cope with a fatal illness*. New York: Barricade Books.

Ellis, A., Abrams, M., & Dengelegi, L. (1992). *The art and science of rational eating*. New York: Barricade Books.

Ellis, A., & Becker, I. (1982). *A guide to personal happiness*. North Hollywood, CA: Wilshire Books.

Ellis, A., & Bernard, M. E. (Eds.). (1985). *Clinical applications of rational–emotive therapy*. New York: Plenum Press.

Ellis, A., & DiGiuseppe, R. (Speakers). (1994). *Dealing with addictions* (Videotape). New York: Institute for Rational–Emotive Therapy.

Ellis, A., & Dryden, W. (1997). *The practice of rational emotive behavior therapy* (rev. ed.). New York: Springer.

Ellis, A., Gordon, J., Neenan, M., & Palmer, S. (1997). *Stress counseling: A rational emotive behaviour approach*. London: Cassell.

Ellis, A., & Grieger, R. (Eds.). (1977). *Handbook of rational–emotive therapy*. New York: Springer.

Ellis, A., & Harper, R. A. (1961a). *A guide to rational living*. Englewood Cliffs, NJ: Prentice-Hall.

Ellis, A., & Harper, R. A. (1961b). *A guide to successful marriage*. North Hollywood, CA: Wilshire Books.

Ellis, A., & Harper, R. A. (1975). *A new guide to rational living*. North Hollywood, CA: Wilshire Books.

Ellis, A., & Harper, R. A. (1997). *A guide to rational living* (3rd rev. ed.). North Hollywood, CA: Melvin Powers.

Ellis, A., & Knaus, W. (1977). *Overcoming procrastination*. New York: New American Library.

Ellis, A., & Lange, A. (1994). *How to keep people from pushing your buttons*. New York: Carol.

Ellis, A., Sichel, J. L., Yeager, R. J., DiMattia, D. J., & DiGiuseppe, R. A. (1989). *Rational–emotive couples therapy*. Needham, MA: Allyn & Bacon.

Ellis, A., & Tafrate, R. C. (1997). *How to control anger before it controls you*. Secaucus, NJ: Birch Lane.

Ellis, A., & Velten, E. (1992). *When AA doesn't work for you: Rational steps for quitting alcohol*. New York: Barricade Books.

Ellis, A., & Velten, E. (1998). *Optimal aging: How to get over growing older*. Chicago: Open Court.

Ellis, A., & Yeager, R. (1989). *Why some therapies don't work: The dangers of transpersonal psychology*. Buffalo, NY: Prometheus.

Emmelkamp, P. M. G., Kuipers, A. C. M., & Eggeraat, J. B. (1978). Cognitive modification versus prolonged exposure *in vivo*: A comparison with agoraphobics as subjects. *Behaviour Research and Therapy, 16,* 33–41.

Eschenroeder, C. (1979). Different therapeutic styles in rational–emotive therapy. *Rational Living, 14*(1), 3–7.

Freud, A. (1937). *The ego and the mechanisms of defense.* London: Hogarth Press.

Glass, C. R., & Arnkoff, D. B. (1997). Questionnaire methods of cognitive self-statement assessment. *Journal of Consulting and Clinical Psychology, 65,* 911–927.

Golden, W. L. (1983). Rational–emotive hypnotherapy: Principles and practice. *British Journal of Cognitive Therapy, 1*(1), 47–56.

Goldfried, M., & Davison, G. (1976). *Clinical behavior therapy.* New York: Holt, Rinehart & Winston.

Grieger, R., & Boyd, J. (1980). *Rational–emotive therapy: A skills-based approach.* New York: Van Nostrand Reinhold.

Grieger, R., & Grieger, I. (Eds.). (1982). *Cognition and emotional disturbance.* New York: Human Sciences Press.

Haaga, D. A. F., & Davison, G. C. (1991). Disappearing differences do not always reflect healthy integration: An analysis of cognitive therapy and rational–emotive therapy. *Journal of Psychotherapy Integration, 1*(4), 287–303.

Hajzler, D., & Barnard, M. E. (1991). A review of rational–emotive outcome studies. *School Psychology Quarterly, 6*(1), 27–49.

Hauck, P. A. (1972). *Reason in pastoral counseling.* Philadelphia: Westminster.

Heidegger, M. (1949). *Existence and being.* Chicago: Henry Regnery.

Herzberg, A. (1945). *Active psychotherapy.* New York: Grune & Stratton.

Hollon, S. D., & Beck, A. T. (1994). Cognitive and cognitive-behavioral therapies. In A. E. Bergin & S. L. Garfield (Eds.), *Handbook of psychotherapy and behavior change* (4th ed., pp. 428–466). New York: Wiley.

Horney, K. (1950). *Neurosis and human growth.* New York: Norton.

Janis, I. L. (1983). *Short-term counseling.* New Haven, CT: Yale University Press.

Johnson, W. B. (1993). Christian rational–emotive therapy: A treatment protocol. *Journal of Psychology and Christianity, 12,* 254–261.

Jones, M. C. (1924). A laboratory study of fear: The case of Peter. *Journal of Genetic Psychology, 31,* 308–315.

Jones, R. A. (1977). *Self-fulfilling prophecies: Social, psychological and physiological effects of expectancies.* Hillsdale, NJ: Erlbaum.

Jones, R. G. (1968). *A factored measure of Ellis' irrational belief system, with personality and maladjustment correlates.* Unpublished doctoral dissertation, Texas Technological College.

Kassinove, H., Crisci, R., & Tiegerman, S. (1977). Developmental trends in rational thinking: Implications for rational–emotive school mental health programs. *Journal of Community Psychology, 5,* 266–274.

Kelly, G. (1955). *The psychology of personal constructs* (2 vols.). New York: Norton.

Kendall, P., & Hollon, S. (1980). *Assessment strategies for cognitive-behavioral interventions.* New York: Academic Press.

Korzybski, A. (1933). *Science and sanity.* San Francisco: International Society of General Semantics.

Lazarus, A. A. (1981). *The practice of multimodal therapy.* New York: McGraw-Hill.

Lazarus, A. A. (1984). *In the mind's eye.* New York: Guilford Press.

Lazarus, R. (1966). *Psychological stress and the coping process.* New York: McGraw-Hill.

Low, A. A. (1952). *Mental health through will-training.* West Hanover, MA: Christopher.

Lyons, L. C., & Woods, P. J. (1991). The efficacy of rational–emotive therapy: A quantitative review of the outcome research. *Clinical Psychology Review, 11,* 357–369.

Macaskill, N. D., & Macaskill, A. (1983). Preparing patients for psychotherapy. *British Journal of Clinical and Social Psychiatry, 2,* 80–84.

Mackay, D. (1984). Behavioural psychotherapy. In W. Dryden (Ed.), *Individual therapy in Britain.* London: Harper & Row.

Mahoney, M. J. (1977). Personal science: A cognitive learning theory. In A. Ellis & R. Grieger (Eds.), *Handbook of rational–emotive therapy* (pp. 352–366). New York: Springer.

Maultsby, M. C., Jr. (1975). *Help yourself to happiness: Through rational self-counseling.* New York: Institute for Rational–Emotive Therapy.

Maultsby, M. C., Jr. (1984). *Rational behavior therapy.* Englewood Cliffs, NJ: Prentice-Hall.

Maultsby, M. C., Jr., & Ellis, A. (1974). *Technique for using rational–emotive imagery.* New York: Institute for Rational–Emotive Therapy.

Meichenbaum, D. (1977). *Cognitive-behavior modification.* New York: Plenum Press.

Moore, R. H. (1983). Inference as "A" in RET. *British Journal of Cognitive Psychotherapy, 1*(2), 17–23.

Phadke, K. M. (1982). Some innovations in RET theory and practice. *Rational Living, 17*(2), 25–30.

Popper, K. R. (1959). *The logic of scientific discovery.* New York: Harper.

Popper, K. R. (1963). *Conjectures and refutations.* New York: Harper.

Powell, J. (1976). *Fully human, fully alive.* Niles, IL: Argus.

Reichenbach, H. (1953). *The rise of scientific philosophy.* Berkeley: University of California Press.

Rogers, C. R. (1957). The necessary and sufficient conditions of therapeutic personality change. *Journal of Consulting Psychology, 21,* 95–103.

Russell, B. (1930). *The conquest of happiness.* New York: New American Library.

Russell, B. (1965). *The basic writings of Bertrand Russell.* New York: Simon & Schuster.

Shorkey, C. T., & Sutton-Simon, K. (1983). Reliability and validity of the Rational Behavior Inventory with a clinical population. *Journal of Clinical Psychology, 39,* 34–38.

Shorkey, C. T., & Whiteman, V. L. (1974). *Rational Behavior Inventory: Test booklet.* Austin, TX: Authors.

Shorkey, C. T., & Whiteman, V. L. (1977). Development of the Rational Behavior Inventory: Initial validity and reliability. *Educational and Psychological Measurement, 37,* 527–534.

Tillich, P. (1953). *The courage to be.* New Haven, CT: Yale University Press.

Vernon, A. (1989). *Thinking, feeling, behaving: An emotional education curriculum for children.* Champaign, IL: Research Press.

Wachtel, P. L. (1977). *Psychoanalysis and behavior therapy: Toward an integration.* New York: Basic Books.

Walen, S. R., DiGiuseppe, R., & Wessler, R. L. (1980). *A practitioner's guide to rational–emotive therapy.* New York: Oxford University Press.

Watson, J. B., & Rayner, R. (1920). Conditioned emotional reactions. *Journal of Experimental Psychology, 3,* 1–14.

Weinrach, S. G. (1980). Unconventional therapist: Albert Ellis. *Personnel and Guidance Journal, 59*(2), 152–160.

Werner, E. E., & Smith, R. S. (1982). *Vulnerable but invincible: A study of resilient children.* New York: McGraw-Hill.

Wessler, R. A., & Wessler, R. L. (1980). *The principles and practice of rational–emotive therapy.* San Francisco: Jossey-Bass.

Wessler, R. L. (1984). Alternative conceptions of rational–emotive therapy: Toward a philosophically neutral psychotherapy. In M. A. Reda & M. J. Mahoney (Eds.), *Cognitive psychotherapies: Recent developments in theory, research, and practice* (pp. 65–79). Cambridge, MA: Ballinger.

Wolfe, J. L. (1992). *What to do when he has a headache.* New York: Hyperion.

Young, H. S. (1974). *A rational counseling primer.* New York: Institute for Rational–Emotive Therapy.

Young, H. S. (1984a). Practising RET with lower-class clients. *British Journal of Cognitive Psychotherapy, 2*(2), 33–59.

Young, H. S. (1984b). Practising RET with Bible-belt Christians. *British Journal of Cognitive Psychotherapy, 2*(2), 60–76.

Young, H. S. (1984c). Teaching rational self-value concepts to tough customers. *British Journal of Cognitive Psychotherapy, 2*(2), 77–97.

10

Cognitive Therapy

ROBERT J. DeRUBEIS
TONY Z. TANG
AARON T. BECK

BASIC THEORY OF COGNITIVE THERAPY

Historical Background

The rationale and procedures of cognitive therapy have evolved over the last four decades, their initial impetus having come from Beck's early interviews with depressed patients (Beck, 1963). While operating initially from a classically Freudian perspective, he found, following several systematic studies (Beck, 1961; Beck & Hurvich, 1959; Beck & Ward, 1961), that Freud's (1917/1957) formulations of the depressive syndrome (melancholia) missed the mark in several respects. Beck eschewed an anger-turned-inward model and saw that, clinically, a more satisfying formulation would be one focused on the *content* of the depressed person's negative thinking. His early descriptions emphasized the negative biases and distortions that he found common among depressed patients. These descriptions led to hypotheses about the content and processes of cognitions that are relatively distinctive to depression. More importantly, he argued that these cognitive aspects are more central to depression and more verifiable than the dynamic (motivational) processes posited in work to that time. Early studies were generally supportive of this view; they have been reviewed elsewhere (see Hollon & Beck, 1979).

In this chapter, we first outline the theory of psychopathology that cognitive therapy is based upon. Next, we describe clinical techniques and treatment procedures that follow from the theory. We then consider the evidence for the efficacy of the treatment approach, as well as evidence concerning the critical elements of cognitive therapy. Finally, we discuss future directions for cognitive therapy and for research about cognitive therapy.

Basic Theory

Beck posits that the depressed person exhibits distorted information processing, which results in a consistently negative view of him- or herself, the future, and the world. These cognitive contents and processes are presumed to underlie the behavioral, affective, and motivational symptoms of depression.

Beck's cognitive model of emotional disorders states that in order to understand the nature of an emotional episode or disturbance, one must focus on the cognitive content of one's reaction to the upsetting event or stream of thought. The heuristic and therapeutic value of the cognitive model lies in its emphasis on the relatively easily accessed (preconscious or conscious) mental events that patients can be trained to report. It does not depend on "unconscious" motivations, the nature of which it is the therapist's duty to ascertain in psychoanalytic therapies.

During the treatment of depression, the beliefs reported by the patient are examined as they pertain to the patient's views of him- or herself, the future, and the world. This trio of domains has been labeled the "cognitive triad" (Beck, Rush, Shaw, & Emery, 1979) and is used to help the therapist and patient identify areas of concern that are involved in emotional distress. The assumption is that sadness, loss of motivation, suicidal wishes, and so on are related to concerns in one (or more) of these three domains. Similar relations between overt symptoms and beliefs are assumed to operate in other disorders as well. In anxious patients, the cognitive aspects of the anxious state are of the greatest interest. As is the case in depression, common themes are found in the cognitions of anxious patients, typically focused on future disaster or discomfort.

TREATMENT MECHANISMS

Cognitive therapy focuses on beliefs of various kinds: the patient's expectations, evaluations (or ascriptions), and attributions of causality or responsibility (Hollon & Kriss, 1984). Once the patient has attended to the content of his or her cognitive reaction, he or she is encouraged to view it as a hypothesis (rather than as a fact)—that is, as a possible but not necessarily true proposition. Framing a belief as a hypothesis has been called "distancing," to emphasize the way in which one can dissociate oneself from a belief in order to allow a more objective examination of it (see Hollon, 1999).

Through careful scrutiny and consideration of the belief, the patient can gradually arrive at a different view. By virtue of changing the relevant belief, change in the emotional reaction should follow. That is, with the attenuation of the cognitive basis for an emotionally upsetting reaction to an event or problem, the emotional reaction will subside.

Through repeated attempts to identify and question the content of the patient's reactions to events, several outcomes are expected to follow. First, concern over troubling events in the recent past diminishes, since the initially troubling aspects of the beliefs about them are no longer held. This reduced concern has the effect of limiting the negative affect that would normally occur during ruminations about, or recollections of, these events. The result is a less negative "basal" level of emotion or mood

Second, the "foreign" or unexplainable quality that emotional reactions have for many patients becomes understandable. This sense of control, hopefulness, and comfort that follows the adoption of the cognitive model is said to be common to many forms of psychotherapy (Frank, 1973). Simply by adopting a set of organizing principles or a coherent world view, the patient comes to see a "light at the end of the tunnel." The simple, common-sense model that the patient learns in cognitive therapy is particularly useful in achieving this effect.

Third, as a result of experience with the successful use of the methods employed in cognitive therapy, the patient begins to use them when confronted with day-to-day difficulties. When used properly, these methods should have the effect of ameliorating many of the concerns that would otherwise lead to emotional distress. Since cognitive therapy is largely a skills-based therapy, it is expected that the patient will eventually come to employ the approach on his or her own, tackling more and more of the problems that confront him or her. In successful cases, it is assumed that the patient continues to employ the cognitive model and its methods in the face of difficult circumstances long after formal therapy is terminated.

Since people are often careless when they make inferences about interpersonal and self-relevant matters (see Nisbett & Ross, 1980), the thinking skills taught in cognitive therapy are applicable even after the depressive episode remits. Indeed, many of these skills are probably used quite often by people who never experience episodes of depression. In addition, the risk of relapse is quite high in most disorders for which cognitive therapy is used. The patient who is ready to apply the thinking skills learned during therapy is assumed to be at a lower risk for subsequent relapse. As reviewed below, several studies have pointed to a prophylactic effect of cognitive therapy.

SCHEMA WORK

Cognitive therapy also aims to work on another, "deeper" level. Through the analysis of many instances of negative emotional experiences, the patient and therapist come to see that the patient has certain patterns of thinking, or "schemata" (Beck, 1964, 1972; J. S. Beck, 1995; Hollon & Kriss, 1984; Persons, 1989). Schemata are the underlying cognitive structures that organize the patient's experience and that can form the basis for the individual instances of bias or distortion. These schemata are thought to represent the core of the cognitive disturbance, and can be called "core beliefs." When identified, schemata can usually be stated in the form of "if–then" propositions, and are similar in breadth to Ellis's irrational beliefs (e.g., "If I am not competent in every way, then I'm a failure"; see, e.g., Ellis & Harper, 1975). Though not as readily accessible as the individual instances of thought (often called "automatic thoughts"), these schemata become apparent to the patient and therapist as they identify the consistencies or themes that run through the individual instances of emotional upset.

When these themes are identified, their utility (the balance of the pros and cons of holding them) or validity (their fit with available evidence) can be examined. If these inquiries help to change the patient's schemata, he or she can begin to recognize situations in which these core beliefs are implicit in his or her reactions to potentially disturbing events; the patient can then consider alternative inferences. In addition, the extent to which the patient holds these core beliefs and their corollaries will diminish over time, as the patient's commitment to them is weakened. Presumably, new schemata replace the old. So, for example, the patient may replace the aforementioned schema with something like this: "If I've given a task the effort it's due, I can be satisfied with it."

COGNITIVE ERRORS

During the course of therapy, yet another perspective on the patient's thinking is given to him or her. The patient is taught that we are all subject to several "types" of thinking errors, and that these occur more frequently during affective episodes. These are the "cognitive errors" that Beck and others have written about (Beck et al., 1979; see Table 10.1). They can be easily memorized by the motivated patient, who can then look for instances of them in his or her own thinking. The labels given to these errors serve a heuristic function, reminding the patient of the ways in which his or her thinking in any given instance may be in error. When an error is identified, the patient can then either simply discount the inference that involved the error, or use more general analytic techniques to question the validity of the inference.

TABLE 10.1. Definitions of 11 Common Cognitive Errors

All-or-nothing thinking: Placing experiences in one of two opposite categories—for example, flawless or defective, immaculate or filthy, saint or sinner.

Overgeneralizing: Drawing sweeping inferences (e.g., "I can't control my temper") from a single instance.

Discounting the positives: Deciding that if a good thing has happened, it couldn't have been very important.

Jumping to conclusions: Focusing on one aspect of a situation in deciding how to understand it (e.g., "The reason I haven't received a phone call from the job I applied to is that they have decided not to offer it to me").

Mind reading: Believing one knows what another person is thinking, with very little evidence.

Fortunetelling: Believing one knows what the future holds, while ignoring other possibilities.

Magnifying/minimizing: Evaluating the importance of a negative event, or the lack of importance of a positive event, in a distorted manner.

Emotional reasoning: Believing that something must be true, because it feels like it is true.

Making "should" statements: Telling oneself one should do (or should have done) something, when it is more accurate to say that one would like to do (or wishes one had done) the preferred thing.

Labeling: Using a label ("bad mother," "idiot") to describe a behavior, and then imputing all the meanings the label carries.

Inappropriate blaming: Using hindsight to determine what one "should have done," even if one could not have known the best thing to do at the time; ignoring mitigating factors; or ignoring the roles played by others in determining a negative outcome.

THE NATURE OF THE THERAPEUTIC INTERACTION

Much of what distinguishes cognitive therapy from other cognitive-behavioral therapies lies in the role assumed by the therapist and the role that he or she recommends to the patient. The relationship is clearly meant to be one of collaboration, in which the therapist and patient assume an equal share of the responsibility for solving the patient's problems. The patient is assumed to be the expert on his or her own experience and on the meanings he or she attaches to events. That is, the cognitive therapist does not assume that he or she knows why the patient reacted a certain way in a certain situation; the therapist asks for the patient's recollection of ongoing thoughts and images. Furthermore, the cognitive therapist does not assume knowledge of the reason why a certain thought was upsetting, but asks the patient why this was so.

The reliance on the patient's report of the meaning of his or her thoughts distinguishes cognitive therapy from Ellis's rational emotive behavior therapy (REBT; Ellis, 1984; Dryden & Ellis, Chapter 9, this volume) on the one hand, and from a Meichenbaum-type cognitive-behavior modification (CBM; Meichenbaum, 1977) on the other. REBT employs a deductive approach in which the therapist more readily infers the nature of a patient's thinking errors, on the basis of experience with other patients and of knowledge of REBT theory. In this theory can be found rules for determining the underlying or basic beliefs implied by the reactions that patients report for upsetting events. Ellis recommends that the therapist be "a step ahead" of the patient, supplying the patient with the meanings of his or her reported thoughts (see, e.g., Ellis, 1984, p. 221). In a learning-theory-derived system such as Meichenbaum's CBM, thoughts are treated more as behaviors, so that one thought can replace another or can be differentially reinforced; there is less emphasis on the *meaning of* the thoughts involved. Though a cognitive therapist may on occasion encourage the patient to view an automatic thought as a habit, and therapy may aim to eliminate the habit or replace it with a new (less distressing) one, these strategies would not be employed before the patient has thoroughly explored the meanings or implications of the thought, and has decided that the meaning of the habitual thought is not true.

The assumption in cognitive therapy is that the meaning system of each patient is idiosyncratic. For this reason the patient must take a very active role in his or her treatment. He or she is taught to be prepared to question his or her thoughts during a distressing event or shortly thereafter. By contrast, in Meichenbaum's self-instructional training (SIT; Meichenbaum, 1977), the therapist helps the patient to prepare to make specific coping statements to him- or herself when the patient is confronted with difficulties. A simple way to refer to this difference between cognitive therapy and SIT is that in cognitive therapy the therapist teaches the patient to question his or her inferences, whereas in SIT the therapist teaches the patient to change them.

The focus on questioning in cognitive therapy leads advocates to believe that it is a more general approach that can be readily applied by the patient to new situations or to new reactions in familiar situations. Insofar as this distinction captures a major difference between cognitive therapy and SIT, it also implies that in cognitive therapy more responsibility is placed on the shoulders of the patient.

When new data are to be gathered, or when experiments that address an idiosyncratic belief of the patient are attempted, the cognitive therapist tries very hard to involve the patient in planning the data collection or the experiment. The therapist's goal is to help the patient devise tests whose results would be convincing to the *patient*, rather than to the therapist, to another patient, or to a logician. Thus the patient is actively involved in his or her treatment, and again is the expert on his or her own case.

The cognitive therapist, of course, is the expert on the cognitive model and, especially at the beginning of therapy, is responsible for teaching the patient the principles that underlie the therapy. He or she is also the expert on the analytic methods used to test the beliefs reported by the patient.

As in any intense relationship, problems between therapist and patient may arise. In cognitive therapy, concerns that the patient has about the therapy or the therapist are actively discussed. The therapist seeks feedback, and responds to it in ways that are consistent with the model. Thus the therapist helps the patient attend to his or her thoughts about the therapy itself, and together they examine them.

CLINICAL APPLICATIONS

Behavioral Methods

Cognitive therapy borrows some procedures originated in other active, directive schools of therapy, and often adapts behavioral methods to suit the goals of cognitive change. In this section, the more prominent behavioral methods used in cognitive therapy are highlighted. Although at times these methods are used to increase activity or to provide experiences of pleasure or mastery, the cognitive therapist will always focus on changes in beliefs that may result from the use of these methods. The cognitive therapist will often explain the assignment of behavioral tasks in this way, indicating that the patient's attempts to engage in the assigned task will serve either to test a hypothesis that the patient holds, or to provide a setting that will provoke the formation of new hypotheses that can be tested subsequently. Jacobson et al. (1996) reported that a 12-week course of treatment with only behavioral methods achieved outcomes comparable to those produced by a 12-week course of cognitive therapy. Thus, while these methods have traditionally been considered auxiliary in cognitive therapy, their potential therapeutic impact should not be underestimated.

SELF-MONITORING

Most patients who begin a course of cognitive therapy are asked to keep, for at least 1 week, a careful hour-by-hour record of their activities and associated moods or other pertinent phenomena. One useful variant is to have the patient record his or her mood on a 0–100 scale, where 0 is the worst he or she has ever felt, and 100 is the best. As suggested in Beck et al. (1979), the patient can also record the degree of mastery or pleasure associated with each recorded activity.

This record can serve several functions, the most obvious of which is to acquaint the therapist with the ways the patient is spending his or her time. In the process, the patient is often surprised by some aspect of the record, such as how much time he or she spends watching television. It can also serve as a baseline against which later records can be compared.

A number of hypotheses can be tested via self-monitoring, such as "It doesn't do any good for me to get out of bed," "I'm always miserable; it never lets up," and "My schedule is too full for me to accomplish what I must." A careful examination of the completed record is a far better basis for judging such hypotheses than is the patient's memory of recent events, since his or her memory will often be selective.

Another common use of the self-monitoring record is to obtain a record of particularly bad or particularly good events that can be discussed in the next session. The therapist can then ask the patient to recall the thoughts that occurred at the time in question.

Finally, if there are consistencies in the record—such that certain kinds of events are associated with good or bad moods, or with mastery or pleasure—these activities can be identified, and then sought out or avoided, through the scheduling or structuring of activities.

SCHEDULING ACTIVITIES

The purpose of scheduling activities in cognitive therapy is twofold: (1) to increase the probability that the patient will engage in activities that he or she has been unwisely avoiding, and (2) to remove decision making as an obstacle in the initiation of an activity. Since the decision has been made in the therapist's office, or in advance by the patient him- or herself, the patient need only carry out that which he or she has agreed (or decided) to do.

When the patient does not carry out the agreed-upon activities, grist is provided for the therapeutic mill. Homework nonadherence may simply be a result of the therapist's being overly ambitious in assigning tasks, in which case the therapist will assume responsibility. However, most often such "failures" are quite similar in character to what has been troubling the patient generally, in that they are often caused by unrealistic negative beliefs as well. A thorough analysis of the cognitive obstacles is then indicated. For example, a cognitive therapist will work through the pessimistic thoughts that prevented the patient from initiating a task, pointing out that, given that the patient fully believed the proposition (e.g., "I am not capable of writing this letter") at the time, it made perfect sense that he or she did not follow through on it. Then work can be done on the hypothesis itself (i.e., "I am not capable of writing this letter").

Activities that are scheduled can come from three domains: (1) those that were associated with mastery, pleasure, or good mood during self-monitoring; (2) those that had been rewarding in the past, but that the patient has been avoiding during the disorder (depression, anxiety, etc.); and (3) new activities agreed upon by the patient and therapist that may be rewarding or informative. When scheduling activities, the cognitive therapist tries to help the patient anticipate the environmental or cognitive obstacles that are likely to interfere with the scheduled activities. These obstacles can then be discussed in the session, or the schedule can be altered in order to avoid them.

A test of a hypothesis discussed in the session may be embedded in the schedule. For example, television watching can be scheduled for some evenings, reading for others, and visiting with friends for others. The patient can then monitor his or her mood, or the degree of mastery and pleasure he or she experiences in each activity, to provide a test of beliefs about the utility of these activities. An added benefit of such a suggestion is that the patient is often more willing to carry out an activity if it is couched in terms of an experiment, perhaps because he or she is not at the same time making a commitment to the activity beyond the time of the experiment.

OTHER BEHAVIORAL STRATEGIES

Since tasks that have been avoided by the patient are often exactly those that have been difficult to do, modifying the structure of these tasks is often appropriate. Large tasks (e.g., finding a job, giving a speech) are explicitly broken down into their smaller units (circling want ads, outlining the main points of the speech, etc.) in order to make the task more concrete and less overwhelming. This intervention has been termed "chunking."

"Graded tasks" can also be constructed, such that easier tasks or simpler aspects of larger tasks are explicitly set out as the first to be attempted. This process is also referred to as "success therapy," as it is assumed that success on the earlier, easier tasks provides an impetus to move on to the more difficult ones. Though chunking and graded task assignments may seem simplistic, it is often surprising to both the patient and the therapist how these simple alterations in the structure of a task will change the patient's view of the task, and subsequently the likelihood of accomplishment.

This overview of common behavioral aspects of cognitive therapy is intended to show how behavioral assignments can be incorporated into cognitive therapy, and how the focus on the cognitive aspects of these assignments can produce therapeutic effects. Variations on these simple procedures, suited to the goals of a particular case, are often desirable and can provide a solid foundation for the cognitive change that is the focus of the therapy.

Cognitive Methods

Whereas the aims of the behavioral procedures are primarily to create alterations in the actions of the patient, many of the cognitive therapy procedures aim expressly at change in cognition, since cognitive theory considers that change in affect and behavior comes chiefly as a result of cognitive changes. An overview of the basic concepts employed in procedures that are explicitly aimed at cognitive change is presented below.

DAILY RECORD OF DYSFUNCTIONAL THOUGHTS

Much of the work in cognitive therapy centers around the use of a device called the Daily Record of Dysfunctional Thoughts (DRDT; see Beck et al., 1979), which is presented here to illustrate several of the principles and options embedded in the cognitive therapy approach. The four most important columns in the DRDT (see Figure 10.1) correspond to the three points in the cognitive model of emotion (situation, belief, emotional consequence), plus the alternative responses or counterresponses to the beliefs (i.e., the more "rational" or functional beliefs). Patients are typically first taught to use the DRDT by noting those times when they experience an unpleasant or puzzling affective state. Thus the cognitive therapist first must be certain that the patient understands what the therapist means by "feelings," "emotions," or "moods"; that the patient can differentiate among different feelings; and that he or she can offer a judgment of the intensity of these states. The therapist also asks the patient to note the situation or stream of thoughts during which the feelings occurred. For many patients, the situation and the emotional state are the two aspects of their experience that they most readily attend to at times of emotional disturbance (e.g., "I was hurt because he didn't answer me"). It is also true that many patients view situations as directly causing emotional responses, considering in addition that there is "something" wrong with themselves that results in maladaptive or upsetting emotional reactions. The job of the cognitive therapist is thus to teach the patient to attend to his or her thoughts and images at these times. At least initially, thoughts often must be reported retrospectively in response to the in-session queries of the therapist.

Once the patient is able to report situations, thoughts, and emotional reactions (preferably at the time of the event and on paper), intervention can begin. Though entries in the "Alternative Responses" column of the DRDT (see Figure 10.1) have sometimes been termed "rational responses," it is not necessary to assume that patients' original beliefs are always irrational, or even incorrect. To say that the work of cognitive therapy involves coming up with "rational responses" to "automatic thoughts" is only a rough approximation to the actual intent of cognitive therapy. More pre-

DAILY RECORD OF DYSFUNCTIONAL THOUGHTS

Directions: When you notice your mood getting worse, ask yourself, "What's going through my mind right now?" and as soon as possible, jot down the thought or mental image in the Automatic Thoughts column. Then consider how accurate or realistic those thoughts are.

Date	Situation Where were you— and what was going on—when you got upset?	Emotions What emotions (sad, anxious, angry, etc.) did you feel at the time? Rate the intensity of each (0–100%).	Automatic Thoughts What thoughts and/or images went through your mind? Rate your belief in each (0–100%).	Alternative Responses Use the questions at the bottom to compose responses to the automatic thoughts. Rate your belief in each (0–100%). Also, consult the list of possible distortions.	Outcome Rerate your belief in your automatic thoughts (0–100%) and in the intensity of your emotions (0–100%).

(1) What is the **evidence** that the automatic thought is true? What is the evidence that it is not true?
(2) Are there **alternative explanations** for that event, or **alternative ways** to view the situation?
(3) What are the **implications** if the thought is true? What's the most upsetting thing about it? What's the most realistic view? What can I do about it?

Possible distortions: All-or-nothing thinking; overgeneralizing; discounting the positives; jumping to conclusions; mind reading; fortunetelling; magnifying/minimizing; emotional reasoning; making "should" statements; labeling; inappropriate blaming.

FIGURE 10.1. The Daily Record of Dysfunctional Thoughts (DRDT). Adapted from Beck, Rush, Shaw, and Emery (1979). Copyright 1979 by The Guilford Press. Adapted by permission.

cisely, it involves the examination of inferences that are made when the patient is emotionally distressed, and that may be considered the cause of the distress. Thus, whether the responses to the initial thoughts are called "rational," "adaptive," "alternative," or some other term, the intervention focuses upon helping the patient learn to question and examine his or her inferences.

Many useful secondary features of the DRDT are worth mentioning. Patients can record the degree of their belief in each "automatic thought," both before and after it is examined. This re-rating allows for a check on the effect of the questioning. When a high degree of belief in the automatic thought remains, it indicates that as elegant or thorough as the questioning may have seemed, it has not resolved the initial concern. Either a key meaning has been missed, or the patient has actually made a thorough and accurate characterization of the situation. In the latter case, the therapist may then help the patient examine the significance or meaning of his or her characterization (see the discussion of the downward arrow technique, below).

Similarly, the degree of the affective response can be recorded both before and after an analysis of the thoughts. Little or no change in affect tells the cognitive therapist that something important is still missing from the analysis, such that the patient still holds relevant beliefs that have not been touched by it. Further exploration is suggested.

Finally, there is a space where the degree of belief in the alternative response can be recorded. If the response is trite (e.g., "Things will get better soon") or in any way not convincing to the patient, they can be picked up and worked with here.

The DRDT can be worked on in the session; especially as therapy progresses, it can also be used independently by the patient, with the therapist checking it over during the session. Though patients eventually do the work of the DRDT without paper and pen, it is quite useful for them to save the records they have filled out, since many of the concerns and responses worked through during therapy are relevant later in the therapy and after therapy has ended. When cognitive therapy has a prophylactic effect, it is assumed that, in part, it is because the patient has retained the ability to attend to and question his or her thinking, as was the case during therapy.

THREE QUESTIONS

Although there are many ways to classify the questions that can be asked of inferences, one classification serves a heuristic function for patients while they learn the methods of cognitive therapy. The three basic questions patients are taught are (1) "What is the evidence for and against the belief?"

(2) "What are alternative interpretations of the event or situation?" and (3) "What are the real implications, if the belief is correct?" Each of the questions is stated here in a general form, and can of course be modified to suit the patient's situation or style.

DOWNWARD ARROW TECHNIQUE

The thought reported initially by a patient is often in a form that would yield little if analyzed for its validity. For instance, a patient may think, in response to a perceived snub by someone at a party, "She doesn't think I'm exciting enough." Though any therapist can imagine a number of reasons why this thought may be upsetting to the patient, presumably the patient extracts some implications or meanings from this inference that are particularly important to him or her. Thus, rather than first asking questions about how reasonable the inference is (e.g., "Did she give any other indications of her interest or disinterest?" "Could there be other reasons why she acted that way?"), the therapist would do well to ask a question of this form: "And what would it mean (regarding you or your future) if it were true that she sees you as not exciting enough for her?" Though basically a variant of the third of the three questions listed above, this way of approaching a reported belief has been termed the "downward arrow" technique. "Downward arrow" refers to a series of questions that can be asked of almost any inference, where each answer calls for another question. They are of the form "What if it is true that . . . ?" or "What about that bothers you?" The aim of each question is to probe for the personal meaning of the inference to the patient, until an inference is brought out that will profit from the work of cognitive therapy. So, in the example above, the downward arrow technique might yield "I'm basically an uninteresting person," "I'll never attract that sort of person," or some other meaning that the original inference implies for the patient. It is important for the therapist to realize that the meanings are idiosyncratic and often difficult to predict, even after the therapist has come to know the patient well. Furthermore, though a therapist may choose to ask the first two of the three questions immediately, there are times when it is clearly more productive first to follow the downward arrow.

These efforts are not mutually exclusive, however. In many instances it is worthwhile both to proceed "downward" to discover the meanings of the inference, and to use the first two of the three questions at more than one level during the inquiry. So, in the preceding example, the therapist may encourage the patient both to question the belief that the fellow partygoer finds the patient uninteresting, as well as the idea that even if this belief were true, it follows that the patient is uninteresting or doomed to loneliness.

COGNITIVE ERRORS

An alternative and often complementary approach to the three questions involves the therapist's teaching the patient to learn to recognize when his or her thinking falls into one of the categories of cognitive errors (see Table 10.1). These labels are used to remind the patient that he or she, as a member of the human race, is prone to various forms of exaggeration and other biased thinking. At these times the patient can discount the improbable or illogical inference, reframe it in a less extreme form, or analyze the inference using the three questions. For example, a patient who teaches may conclude that he or she has given a poor lecture, since 3 of the 40 students in the class were inattentive from time to time during the lecture. The patient may then notice that he or she has "personalized," particularly if another reason can be readily given for the inattentiveness that does not involve the quality of the lecture (e.g., the temperature was 80 degrees in the lecture hall, the students are apathetic, etc.). Alternatively, the patient may decide that he or she has "overgeneralized," if on reflection he or she recalls that most of the students seemed quite interested during the lecture, and that several students came to him or her after class with thoughtful questions.

IDENTIFYING SCHEMATA

After a therapist and patient have been working together for several sessions, they often notice a certain consistency in the kinds of beliefs that are involved in emotional disturbance for the patient. This consistency will not be found at the "surface" level, but rather at the level of personal meaning. For example, the therapist and patient may note that many of the patient's entries in the DRDT include beliefs of this form: "If I am not the best X, then it is not worth pursuing, and I am worthless as an X."

The Dysfunctional Attitude Scale (DAS; Weissman & Beck, 1978) is an assessment device that can be used to tap these underlying assumptions or schemata, and to track change during and following treatment. The DAS consists of a series of attitudinal statements that the patient is asked to consider. The patient rates the degree to which he or she agrees with each statement. The DAS has been factor-analyzed and found to contain nine interpretable factors (Beck, Brown, Steer, & Weissman, 1991). The nine factors, along with sample items, are as follows: (1) vulnerability ("Whenever I take a chance or risk, I am only looking for trouble"); (2) approval ("My value as a person depends greatly on what others think of me"); (3) perfectionism ("My life is wasted unless I am a success"); (4) need to please others ("It is best to give up your own interests in order to please other people"); (5) imperatives ("I should be happy all the time"); (6) need to impress others ("I should try to impress people if I want them to like me"); (7) avoidance of weakness ("If a person asks for help, it is a sign of weakness"); (8) control over emotions ("Criticism need not upset the person who receives the criticism"); and (9) disapproval ("It is awful to be disapproved of by people important to you"). (Note that all factors except the eighth have names that reflect cognitive vulnerability, as do the items chosen to exemplify them. The name given to the eighth factor, as well as its exemplar, reflects more resilient attitudes.) Scores on these factors can point to the most troublesome clusters of attitudes or schemata, or the patient and therapist can look for more idiosyncratic patterns.

SOCRATIC QUESTIONING AND GUIDED DISCOVERY

Perhaps the most distinctive stylistic feature of cognitive therapy, as well as the most difficult for therapists in training to master, is the judicious and persistent use of the "Socratic" method of questioning. The term "guided discovery" also refers to the process, through the use of leading questions, of helping patients to arrive at new perspectives that challenge their faulty conclusions. The art of Socratic questioning as it is used in cognitive therapy is for the therapist to walk the line between leading the patient where the therapist would like him or her to go on the one hand, and allowing the patient to "free-associate" on the other. The most common error made by an inexperienced cognitive therapist is to be in such a hurry, or to be so certain of a conclusion the patient should come to, that he or she either lectures the patient or asks such obviously leading questions that there can be but one set of answers. As a matter of fact, the use of questions by Socrates himself as recorded in the *Socratic Dialogues* (Cooper, 1997; see especially *Euthypro* and *Crito*) was often quite like the latter, in that Socrates tended to know exactly where he was going with his line of questions. Therefore, good "Socratic" questions of the cognitive therapy sort are much more open-ended and theory-free than were those asked by the method's originator (see Overholser, 1993a, 1993b, for a discussion of Socratic questioning in therapy). A good exercise for practicing Socratic questions is for the therapist to listen to an audiotape recording of a session; to stop the tape each time he or she has uttered a declarative statement or asked a closed-ended question; and then to generate a Socratic question that would have made the same point, but in a potentially more fruitful manner. One reason such questioning is believed to be especially productive in therapy is that the patient is maximally engaged to think about the problem under discussion, as well as its solution. Moreover, good Socratic questioning will prevent a common problem in nonoptimal cognitive therapy, which is that the therapist can become quite convinced that the patient's thoughts are in error, but the patient is left with idiosyncratic doubts and concerns that were not addressed in the discussion between patient and therapist.

TREATMENT PROCEDURES

Depression

BEGINNING OF TREATMENT

The cognitive therapist has several complementary goals at the beginning of treatment for depression. They can be categorized as (1) assessment, (2) socializing the patient into the cognitive model, and (3) dealing with the patient's pessimism (about treatment and in general).

Assessment efforts can include administration and scoring of the self-report Beck Depression Inventory—II (BDI-II; Beck, Steer, & Brown, 1996), which can then be used as a session-to-session measure of depression level. Though its validity as a depression severity measure has been well demonstrated (see Beck & Beamesderfer, 1974, for a review), it is of greatest use during the course of therapy as a within-patient change measure.

It is important in the beginning of cognitive therapy that the patient and therapist have a common understanding of the model that will be used during treatment. To this end, patients are asked to read the booklet *Coping with Depression* (Beck & Greenberg, 1974), or a similar description of the cognitive model of depression and its treatment. The therapist and patient can discuss the patient's reaction to the booklet, and a recent experience can be framed in the cognitive model. Though this early "socialization" of the patient into the cognitive model of treatment often involves intensive didactic explanation, it serves a greater purpose than merely that of preparing the patient for treatment. It has the added benefit of giving the patient an account of his or her difficulties that leaves room for understanding and improvement. Thus the patient's hopelessness, a common feature of depression, is dealt with thoroughly and directly.

At the beginning of treatment, additional interventions are often directed toward the patient's pessimism or hopelessness. These interventions can take the form of working through a task that the patient has not been able to tackle, or that the patient believes he or she does not have the resources to overcome. The therapist first elicits and records the patient's expectations for his or her performance on the task, and then guides the patient through the anticipated obstacles to its completion. When the patient is able to accomplish more than he or she expected, the success is used as a foundation upon which further attempts can be built.

THE MIDDLE PHASE

Although work on cognitive coping skills has already begun in the early phase of treatment, it is in the middle phase that the therapist and patient work to solidify these skills. The patient works between sessions to identify the situations and thoughts that bring about negative affect. Ideally, he or she uses the DRDT to keep written records, and is beginning to question his or her thinking either at the time of or shortly following the disturbance. The therapist helps the patient "fine-tune" his or her responses to initial thoughts, often by using the downward arrow technique described above. That is, the therapist reviews the patient's DRDT with him or her, and helps the patient to see where he or she could attempt alternative analyses of his or her automatic thoughts.

It is also during the middle phase that patterns associated with schemata or underlying assumptions are identified. The developmental histories of these schemata are also discussed, so as to help the patient make sense of the patterns that have been identified. Without such an inquiry, the patient is apt to view his or her idiosyncratic way of interpreting events in the world as coming "out of the blue." Not surprisingly, unexplained negative affect can leave the patient feeling helpless and, worse yet, believing he or she is fundamentally flawed in some way. In this respect, cognitive therapy is similar to the "depth" approaches to psychotherapy, in that it aims to understand the influence of early experience upon subsequent attitudes and concerns. These aspects of cognitive therapy have been especially well described by J. S. Beck (1995) and Persons (1989).

THE FINAL PHASE

During the final phase of therapy, gains are reviewed, and therapy is focused on the prevention of relapse. The therapist and patient anticipate difficult situations or problems that may arise in the future and would tax the patient's coping skills. This is an important aspect of the therapy, since it is easy for patients to be unclear about the importance of the skills they have learned. Many patients attribute their recovery to changes in their environment, even if it has been through their own effort that these changes have come about. Since by this time the patient is feeling better, it is vital for his or her skills to be tested and demonstrated, so that he or she becomes likely to call upon them when difficult situations inevitably arise.

It is also during this phase that the patient's beliefs about his or her ability to leave therapy must be addressed. The patient may believe that he or she will be fine so long as therapy continues, but that it will be impossible to handle problems on his or her own. If a collaborative working relationship has already been developed, the therapist will need to place more responsibility for the treatment on the shoulders of the patient over time, so that the therapist becomes more a consultant than an active therapist. This gradual shift can serve as the context for a test of the patient's ability to work problems out on his or her own.

Finally, the therapist and patient may agree to schedule "booster sessions" to follow up the work that has been done. Jarrett et al. (1998) describe evidence that such sessions, scheduled at monthly intervals during the period following response to cognitive therapy for depression, reduce the rate of relapse and recurrence. Clinicians and patients report that even less frequent booster sessions (e.g., three times per year) can be beneficial for maintaining the patient's focus on gains that were made during the more intensive weekly (or twice-weekly) sessions during treatment of acute depression.

Panic Disorder and Agoraphobia

Cognitive therapies have been developed for many other disorders, such as generalized anxiety disorder (GAD), obsessive–compulsive disorder (OCD), and hypochondriasis. These other approaches all follow a form similar to that described above for depression (see Salkovskis, 1996). Each population requires somewhat different treatment emphases, however, based on the phenomenology that defines the disorder. The phenomenology and treatment of panic disorder, in particular, have been well developed (see Beck, Emery, & Greenberg, 1985; Clark, 1996). In what follows, we describe the phenomenology and treatment of panic disorder from a cognitive therapy perspective.

The symptomatology in the development of a panic attack follows an almost stereotyped sequence. First, the patient experiences some type of sensation that is usually unpleasant and that he or she cannot discount as nonpathological. If the patient has had one or more previous panic attacks, he or she may "recognize" this symptom as a prelude to such a reaction, and indeed may anticipate that another panic attack is coming on. In any event, the progression will continue if the patient ascribes some pathological significance to the particular sensation or symptom and is unable to dismiss it as not dangerous. The meaning or interpretation given by the patient will "make sense" to the therapist, in that it will bear a relation to the sensation(s). Thus a pain in the chest is likely to be interpreted as a heart attack; tightness or shortness of breath may be viewed as a sign that one will stop breathing. Lightheadedness is often viewed as signaling impending loss of consciousness, numbness or tingling in the extremities as having a stroke, some mental confusion as a sign that one is going crazy, and so on.

There are often precipitating factors of which the patient is unaware that can readily explain the onset of these physiological or psychological experiences. For instance, an individual may feel faint if he or she gets up suddenly from a chair, has gone for a long time without eating, or is looking down from a high place. He or she may become generally aroused by hearing unpleasant (or even pleasant) news. Each of these sensations may be interpreted by the individual as a sign of an impending disaster.

A large proportion of patients subject to panic attacks also seem to experience hyperventilation. A person who is upset or who experiences shortness of breath, for example, may start to breathe rapidly and as a result of "blowing off" carbon dioxide may experience symptoms of alkalosis (numbness and tingling in the extremities, generalized discomfort).

A patient who has had a certain amount of "cognitive strain" may have a sudden lapse of memory or difficulty in reasoning that he or she attributes to a serious mental disorder. A father experiencing a burst of emotion during a quarrel with his children may interpret the accompanying bodily feelings as a sign that he is out of control and may assault them.

As the panic attack develops, the individual's attention becomes fixed on the symptoms. He or she is now quite aware of a pounding heartbeat, faintness, dizziness, or shortness of breath. The individual then begins to focus on a catastrophic consequence of having the symptoms, and may fear that if the symptoms continue any longer, he or she will die. Some patients report vivid visual images such as falling down, being surrounded by people, and then being placed in an ambulance and taken to the hospital. Occasionally a patient, particularly one who also has a high level of depression, may have an image of him- or herself lying dead in a coffin and feeling extremely lonely because he or she is isolated from other people.

One of the most striking aspects of the panic attack is the patient's loss of ability during the attack to view his or her sensations objectively and to apply an appropriate label to them. Even though the patient may have agreed a few minutes previously that the symptoms do not represent any serious threat to life or mental stability, he or she may lose the ability to apply this information once the attack has started. It is not clear whether there is an actual suppression of the higher evaluative functions, or whether the individual's attention is so focused on the symptoms and their (inappropriate) meanings that he or she does not have the cognitive capacity left to evaluate these interpretations. In any event, the loss of capacity to apply reason and medical knowledge to the interpretation of the symptoms seems to be a necessary component of the disorder. A patient may have all the features of intense anxiety without having a panic attack, if he or she retains the ability to regard his or her symptoms objectively.

The next stage in the development of the panic disorder takes the form of a vicious cycle. As the individual begins to interpret his or her symptoms (e.g., rapid heart rate, shortness of breath) as pathological, his or her sense of danger increases. This increased fear in turn produces an increased intensity of the symptoms. With the increased focus on the symptoms and their imagined consequences, the patient becomes even less able to apply reason to his or her understanding of the symptomatology. Thus the symptoms continue to escalate. A special feature of this progression is the patient's recognition that his or her usual attempts to ward off fear, such as walking around or trying to divert his or her own attention, do not seem to quell the disturbance. The symptoms appear to be uncontrollable, and the patient begins to believe that they will continue to escalate until a disaster occurs. In contrast to panic attacks associated with phobias of specific environmental situations (e.g., acrophobia, claustrophobia), the spontaneous "attack" represents a "phobia" (fear) of a set of internal conditions.

GENERAL TREATMENT APPROACH

The cognitive treatment of panic disorder has undergone an important change since the first edition of this chapter, following the growing recognition of the insidious role played by "safety behaviors" in the maintenance of anxiety disorders (see Salkovskis, 1996), including panic disorder. In the first edition of this chapter, following the writings of Beck, Clark, and their colleagues (Beck et al., 1985; Clark, Salkovskis, & Chalkley, 1985), we recommended that patients be taught to use relaxation procedures, controlled breathing, and distraction as means of diminishing or blunting incipient panic attacks. It is now clear that these procedures, while helpful in some cases, can prevent the full benefit of the treatment in other cases. This paradoxical effect occurs because patients with panic disorder can come to believe that they *must* engage in these practices, lest the feared consequence come about. Whereas the original recommendations of these methods stemmed from the observation that patients could use them to learn that panic attacks are controllable and thus essentially harmless, many patients learn something rather different: that the panic-blunting procedures are essential for their well-being. For example, a patient who has learned controlled breathing may become convinced that if in the beginning of a panic attack he or she does not gain control of breathing, he or she will faint. This belief is then reinforced (via negative reinforcement) each time he or she engages in the controlled breathing, because indeed he or she does not faint. Thus, instead of encouraging these potentially ameliorative efforts, cognitive therapists now actively discourage them. More than that, it is now seen as important for the therapist and patient to identify and cease any safety behaviors the patient has already been employing during panic attacks. These behaviors can include calling a friend for support, going to the emergency room, leaning against a wall (to prevent falling), or monitoring one's heart rate. It is impossible to provide a comprehensive list of safety behaviors, because patients can be rather creative in their use of thoughts or behaviors they believe to be safety-enhancing. For this reason, patients must be thoroughly educated about the concept of safety behaviors. Some of these behaviors will have become so automatic that patients will not be able to report about them retrospectively, so that they will need to be on the lookout for them.

The current version of cognitive therapy for panic disorder, the Oxford-based Cognitive Therapy Package (Clark, 1996), can be summarized as including four cognitive methods and two behavioral methods. The cognitive methods are the following:

1. The therapist and patient together map out the sequence of a recent panic attack, using the "vicious cycle" model.

2. Within this sequence, the patient's beliefs (e.g., "The fact that my heart is pounding means I am having a heart attack") are identified and challenged. One means of testing the patient's beliefs is to show the patient that if during an attack he or she gains control of breathing, or uses a distraction procedure, the symptoms decrease. Most patients will see that heart attacks and other life-threatening events (e.g., stroke) cannot be controlled by distraction or measured breathing, so this can serve as a disconfirmation of their belief. However, as noted above, this procedure is now used only to test beliefs, and not as a means of preventing panic attacks.

3. More realistic beliefs are identified and considered (e.g., "I am anxious, and therefore my heart is pounding more than usual").

4. The images experienced by the patient (e.g., of being placed in an emergency vehicle and taken to a hospital) are altered, so that the next time the patient begins to have such an image, he or she can correct it to an image that befits the circumstance, such as the image of a gradual resolution of the anxiety attack.

The behavioral methods in the Cognitive Therapy Package are as follows:

1. Procedures are engaged to induce the feared sensations. Patients are taught to hyperventilate, to focus attention on their body, or to read pairs of words or phrases in which one member of the pair represents a feared sensation (e.g., heart pounding) and the other a feared catastrophe (e.g., heart attack). The purpose of these procedures is for patients to see that the symptoms can be readily brought about by measures that do not cause the feared catastrophe. Patients learn, as a consequence, that these sensations are by no means reliable signals of impending danger.

2. Patients are encouraged to expose themselves to and remain in feared situations they have either avoided or fled. For some patients, this exposure is primarily to situations that involve physical exertion, such as exercise or sexual activity. For others, it may involve anxiety-arousing situations, such as crowded shopping malls, or simply those situations in which panic attacks have occurred in the past.

ADDITIONAL CONSIDERATIONS

Empirical Status of the Approach

EFFICACY OF COGNITIVE THERAPY FOR DEPRESSION

Acute Treatment. In 1977, Rush, Beck, Kovacs, and Hollon reported their landmark study of cognitive therapy versus medication in the treatment of depression. Using a two-group design, Rush and his colleagues found that patients treated with cognitive therapy experienced greater symptom remission by the end of the 12-week active treatment period than did those treated with imipramine (a tricyclic antidepressant). This was not only the first study that demonstrated the efficacy of cognitive therapy, but it was also the first published account of a randomized trial that found a psychotherapeutic approach to be superior to a pharmacological one in the treatment of depression.

Following Rush et al. (1977), Blackburn, Bishop, Glen, Whalley, and Christie (1981) and Murphy, Simons, Wetzel, and Lustman (1984) also compared cognitive therapy against tricyclic antidepressants. Although in neither of these studies was cognitive therapy found to be significantly more effective than antidepressants, in both studies cognitive therapy performed as well as the respective antidepressant drugs. The decade of the 1980s concluded with Dobson's (1989) meta-analysis of outcome research on cognitive therapy for depression, in which he concluded that the results from efficacy studies "document a greater degree of change for cognitive therapy compared with a waiting list or no-treatment control, pharmacotherapy, behavior therapy, and other psychotherapies" (p. 414). His conclusion supported what many experts in the field had by that time come to believe: that cognitive therapy for depression was the best example of an empirically validated psychological treatment for a serious mental disorder.

This emerging consensus began to break down with publication of a series of findings from the Treatment of Depression Collaborative Research Program (TDCRP; Elkin et al., 1989). This study received a great deal of attention in part because it included a placebo control group, which allowed direct comparisons between the treatment conditions and a bona fide control condition. Like Blackburn et al. (1981) and Murphy et al. (1984), Elkin et al. reported no significant differences in outcome between cognitive therapy and antidepressant medication. However, among the more severely depressed patients, cognitive therapy did not perform significantly better than the placebo control, whereas medications did. Moreover, in a later report in which more sensitive analytic procedures were used, on one of the primary depression outcome measures (the Hamilton Rating Scale for Depression; Hamilton, 1960), cognitive therapy performed significantly worse than medications among the more severely depressed patients

(Elkin, Gibbons, Shea, & Sotsky, 1995). (The same analytic procedures did not reveal a difference between cognitive therapy and medications on the other primary outcome measure, the BDI.) These findings generated a great deal of controversy (see the *Journal of Consulting and Clinical Psychology* special issue on the TDCRP, which includes papers by Elkin, Gibbons, Shea, & Shaw, 1996; Jacobson & Hollon, 1996a, 1996b; and Klein, 1996). They also led many observers to conclude that medication is clearly superior to cognitive therapy for severely depressed patients, and they led to the development of treatment guidelines based solely on the TDCRP findings with the Hamilton Rating Scale for Depression (see American Psychiatric Association, 1993).

While the field was digesting the series of papers from the TDCRP, Hollon et al. (1992) reported on another comparison study of cognitive therapy versus medications, in which, once again, cognitive therapy was as effective as an antidepressant medication. Moreover, they found that cognitive therapy performed as well as antidepressants even among the more severely depressed patients in their sample.

DeRubeis, Gelfand, Tang, and Simons (1999) recently reanalyzed data from the more severely depressed patients from the Rush et al. (1977) and Murphy et al. (1984) studies, and found that cognitive therapy performed at least as well as medication. They then pooled the individual patient data from the Rush et al., Murphy et al., Hollon et al. (1992), and Elkin et al. (1989) studies, and performed a "mega-analysis" (a type of meta-analysis that employs raw data from studies rather than means). Taking data from all four of these studies into account, DeRubeis et al. found cognitive therapy to be just as effective as medication in the treatment of severely depressed patients.

Jarrett et al. (1999) reported findings from the only major placebo-controlled randomized trial other than the TDCRP in which cognitive therapy has been compared with medications in adults with major depressive disorder. Their sample consisted of patients with atypical major depression. Jarrett et al. found that, unlike in the TDCRP, cognitive therapy outperformed the placebo control condition. And like most research in which the acute effects of cognitive therapy have been compared to antidepressant medication, the two treatments performed about equally well.

Several conclusions can now be drawn from studies conducted thus far of the acute treatment effects of cognitive therapy for depression. First, because almost all studies have found cognitive therapy to be as effective as medication in the treatment of depression, it is fair to say that even in the short run, cognitive therapy is a potent alternative to antidepressant medications. Second, for more severely depressed patients, only one study (the TDCRP) has found medication to be superior to cognitive therapy, on one depression severity measure (the Hamilton Rating Scale for Depression);

moreover, this finding is contradicted by data from three other major studies. Thus cognitive therapy also appears to be as effective as medication in the treatment of severe depression. Third, the ability of cognitive therapy to outperform a control condition, challenged by the TDCRP findings, has been supported by Jarrett et al.'s (1999) result. Future studies employing a placebo control group will help us reach a more definitive answer to this question. Given cognitive therapy's demonstrated equivalence with medication, along with the demonstrated superiority of medications over placebo treatments, it will be surprising if well-conducted studies do not generally find cognitive therapy to be superior to placebo controls.

Relapse Prevention. Most of the studies described above have included, in addition to tests of the acute effects of cognitive therapy for depression, examinations of its relapse prevention effects. In most studies this examination has taken the form of a comparison of symptom severity or relapse rates evidenced during follow-up by patients who have responded to cognitive therapy, relative to patients who have responded to antidepressant medication. In both groups, treatment would have terminated at the end of the acute period (3 to 4 months), and follow-ups have typically been for 1 to 2 years. A 1-year naturalistic follow-up of the Rush et al. (1977) study revealed that the cognitive therapy group scored significantly lower on depression severity measures than the antidepressant medication group at the 12-month (but not the 6-month) follow-up point (Kovacs, Rush, Beck, & Hollon, 1981). In a follow-up of the Murphy et al. (1984) study, Simons, Murphy, Levine, and Wetzel (1986) reported that patients who received cognitive therapy during the acute treatment phase were less likely than drug-treated patients to have relapsed in the year following acute treatment. A 2-year follow-up of the Hollon et al. (1992) study (Evans et al., 1992) also reported that patients who had responded to cognitive therapy during the acute phase evidenced a significantly lower relapse rate than did patients who had responded to antidepressant medication, and whose medications were discontinued at the end of the acute phase. Once again, however, findings from the TDCRP were somewhat inconsistent with those of the other major studies. In the follow-up phase of that study, even though the cognitive therapy group fared better than the medication group by most criteria, the differences were not large and were not statistically significant (Shea et al., 1992).

Cognitive therapy's potential as a relapse prevention treatment is further bolstered by evidence from studies of the effects of brief cognitive therapy following successful pharmacotherapy. Several studies have found that a relatively brief course of cognitive therapy (about 10 sessions) following a successful course of pharmacotherapy is as effective in preventing relapse as is the continuation of active medication, and it has been significantly more effective than clinical management without active medication (Blackburn & Moore, 1997; Fava, Grandi, Zielezny, Canestrari, & Morphy, 1994; Fava, Grandi, Zielezny, Rafanelli, & Canestrari, 1996; Fava, Rafanelli, Grandi, Conti, & Belluardo, 1998).

EFFICACY OF COGNITIVE THERAPY FOR OTHER FORMS OF PSYCHOPATHOLOGY

Encouraged by the demonstrated successes of cognitive therapy in the treatment of depression, researchers and clinicians have adapted cognitive therapy's core principles to the treatments of other forms of psychopathology. We have already described the Oxford-based Cognitive Therapy Package. Evidence concerning its efficacy has been reviewed by Clark (1996), who showed that across five separate studies, between 74% and 94% of patients assigned to cognitive therapy became panic-free and maintained this status through the respective follow-up periods, which ranged from 6 months to 15 months. Moreover, results from these outcome studies indicate that cognitive therapy not only outperformed waiting-list control conditions, but that it was superior in efficacy to applied relaxation, pharmacotherapy, and exposure therapy.

In 1985, Beck et al. outlined a cognitive therapy treatment for GAD. Chambless and Gillis (1993) have reviewed nine clinical trials evaluating this treatment's efficacy, and found that empirical evidence mostly supported cognitive therapy's efficacy in treating GAD (see also DeRubeis & Crits-Christoph, 1998). This conclusion has been bolstered by two additional studies (Barlow, Rapee, & Brown, 1992; Durham et al., 1994) published since the Chambless and Gillis review.

For OCD, Van Oppen et al. (1995) found cognitive therapy (based on Beck et al., 1985; and Salkovskis, 1985) to be equivalent to exposure and response prevention, an OCD treatment with established efficacy. A number of studies have also found cognitive therapy to be an effective treatment of bulimia nervosa (see Compas, Haaga, Keefe, & Leitenberg, 1998, for a review). Taken together, these results demonstrate that the principles of cognitive therapy and treatments based on them can be applied successfully to a variety of disorders.

Research on the Process of Cognitive Therapy

Over the past two decades, numerous devices that aim to measure cognitive constructs in depression have been constructed. Most measures have been born of an interest in theoretical questions about depression. In this section, we focus on therapist and patient measures that have been used specifically to address questions about cognitive therapy and its effects. For a more general treatment of cognitive assessment, the reader can turn to one of the recent reviews in the area (e.g., Blankstein & Segal, Chapter 2, this volume).

The measures and applications described below stem from an interest in such questions as these: Does it matter what the therapist does in cognitive therapy (i.e., how faithful he or she is to the procedures; how high the quality of his or her work is)? Do patients change in ways that are predicted by the model of therapy in cognitive therapy? Are these changes specific to cognitive therapy, or do similar changes occur in other effective treatments? Questions such as these guide the type of thorough analysis that should be performed on any successful form of treatment (see Hollon & Kriss, 1984, for a model of change in therapy that incorporates these questions). Several measures have been developed that may help to answer some of these questions. It is to these measures and the preliminary results obtained from them that we now turn.

THERAPIST BEHAVIOR

Two measures of therapist behavior, the Cognitive Therapy Scale (CTS; Young & Beck, 1980) and the Collaborative Study Psychotherapy Rating Scale (CSPRS; Hollon, Evans, Auerbach, et al., 1985) have been employed in research on cognitive therapy of depression. The CTS was developed as a measure of therapists' cognitive therapy "competence." It was designed to take into account not only whether the therapist adhered to the methods of cognitive therapy, but also whether the implementation was of good quality. The CTS has been used primarily as a means of determining whether therapists in outcome trials are "competent" to deliver cognitive therapy. Scores on each of the 11 items of the CTS can range from 0 to 6, so that total scores can range from 0 to 66. The CTS has been shown to be rated with good reliability when used by raters who train in the use of the instrument together and who consult one another periodically to prevent rater drift. For example, Hollon, Emerson, and Mandell (1982) obtained a very respectable interrater reliability coefficient of .86. However, ratings made by experts on tapes from the Jacobson et al. (1996) outcome study evidenced very disappointing reliability, in the range of .10—possibly because those experts did not train together in the use of the CTS, nor did they check with one another during the course of the rating study (Jacobson & Gortner, 2000). Future research will be needed to understand the puzzling lack of reliability reported in the Jacobson & Gortner article, and to explore the predictive validity of the scale (i.e., whether higher scores indicate more productive therapy).

The CSPRS does not focus on the quality of cognitive therapy, but rather on the extent or amount of the therapist behavior of interest. The distinction has been made between measures of competence, such as the CTS, and measures of "adherence," which is what the CSPRS is intended to be. Raters are instructed not to judge the quality of the interventions that they rate, but to focus instead on the amount of time and effort spent by the therapist in a certain domain, such as helping the patient attend to the thoughts experienced while in an unpleasant emotional state. Behavior relevant to cognitive therapy is covered by 28 of the 96 CSPRS items. The other 68 items are designed to assess behavior relevant to other forms of therapy, such as interpersonal therapy and pharmacotherapy, as well as aspects of therapist behavior that cut across schools of therapy (e.g., facilitative conditions). DeRubeis and Feeley (1990) factor-analyzed the 28 cognitive therapy items and found that they separated into two factors. One factor, Cognitive Therapy—Concrete, represents the symptom-focused, active methods of cognitive therapy. A prototypic item from this factor asks the rater to indicate the extent to which the therapist "asked the patient to record [his or her] thoughts." The other factor, Cognitive Therapy—Abstract, represents less focused discussions about therapy processes and the like (e.g., "Did the therapist explain the cognitive therapy rationale . . . ?" and "Did the therapist explore underlying assumptions . . . ?").

In two separate studies, DeRubeis and his colleagues examined the role of these two factors in cognitive therapy for depression (DeRubeis & Feeley, 1990; Feeley, DeRubeis, & Gelfand, 1999). In both studies they found that higher scores on Cognitive Therapy—Concrete observed in Session 2 were associated with greater changes in BDI scores from that point until the end of therapy (Feeley et al.) or until the 12th week of therapy (DeRubeis & Feeley). Scores on Cognitive Therapy—Abstract in Session 2, however, were not associated with subsequent changes in BDI scores. These findings suggest that it is critical for therapists to focus on the problem-focused, pragmatic aspects of cognitive therapy for depression, at least early in therapy.

PATIENT COGNITIONS

Measures of cognitive characteristics have been used to address questions regarding what changes cognitive therapy produces in the patient that reduce depressive symptoms and decrease risk for symptom return. Answers to these questions have both theoretical and pragmatic import. Theories of change that are meant to explain both the short- and long-term benefits of cognitive therapy can be examined by testing whether expected cognitive and behavioral changes occur during successful treatment, and whether these changes mediate symptom reduction and relapse (or recurrence) prevention. Pragmatically, findings that concern causal mechanisms can lead to further refinements in the therapy, by telling us what kinds of cognitive or behavioral change therapists should attempt to maximize in order to produce the greatest benefit.

Hollon, Evans, and DeRubeis (1988) proposed that three kinds of changes may occur in cognitive therapy and may account for symptom reduction during treatment (see also Barber & DeRubeis, 1989). The first two kinds of changes, "deactivation" and "accommodation," refer to changes that occur in the patients' schemata. Change in a depressive schema is said to occur when the patient comes to use a nondepressive schema in responding to potentially upsetting events. At the beginning of therapy, when he or she is depressed, a patient's depressive schemata are said to be activated. So, for example, he or she may respond to the rejection of a manuscript with the inference "I'll never be successful." An indication that the deactivation or accommodation of the schema has occurred would be that, upon receiving similar news following therapy, the patient concludes, "I'll have to submit the manuscript to a more appropriate journal." According to this view, the difference between deactivation and accommodation is that following deactivation the depressive schema is simply suppressed and thus liable to become active again, whereas following accommodation the change is in the schema itself and is thus more enduring.

The third kind of change described by Hollon, Evans, and DeRubeis (1985) is the development of "compensatory skills." Insofar as the acquisition and use of compensatory skills are responsible for change, one would expect to find that even after therapy patients are still liable to respond to potentially upsetting events by making depressive inferences immediately, but that they then apply the skills they have learned during cognitive therapy.

Each of these change processes is a candidate for a mechanism that accounts for the short- and long-term change produced by cognitive therapy. The difficulties lie in finding or developing measures that tap schematic versus compensatory processes, and in applying those measures in the relevant studies of therapy process. No study has been conducted that has tested these models of change unambiguously, but investigators in two separate studies have reported intriguing results that distinguished, on cognitive measures, patients who benefited from cognitive therapy from patients who improved during pharmacotherapy.

DeRubeis et al. (1990), studying patients from the aforementioned Hollon et al. (1992) outcome study, found that improvement on the Hopelessness Scale (HS; Beck, Weissman, Lester, & Trexler, 1974), the DAS (Weissman & Beck, 1978), and the Attributional Style Questionnaire (ASQ; Seligman, Abramson, Semmel, & von Baeyer, 1979) in the first half (6 weeks) of therapy predicted subsequent change in depressive symptoms for those patients who received cognitive therapy. This pattern was not observed among patients who received imipramine pharmacotherapy only.

That is, although patients in the medication condition improved on these same measures in the first 6 weeks of treatment, degree of improvement on these measures did not predict further gains in treatment. Thus evidence was obtained that the HS, DAS, and ASQ played a mediational role in the reduction of depressive symptoms in the cognitive therapy condition, but not in the pharmacotherapy-only condition.

At the end of treatment, an even more provocative set of findings was obtained. Greater change was observed on the ASQ and DAS among patients whose symptoms improved following cognitive therapy than among those patients who improved following pharmacotherapy (DeRubeis & Hollon, 1999; Hollon, DeRubeis, & Evans, 1996). Moreover, lower scores on the ASQ and DAS at posttreatment were associated with greater protection against relapse in the 2-year follow-up period. The pattern in their data fit most of the conditions laid out by Baron and Kenny (1986) for detection of a mediational relation, suggesting that attributional style and dysfunctional attitudes mediate the reduction of risk engendered by cognitive therapy. Relatively small sample sizes limited the power of the tests of mediation, but these preliminary findings suggest that whatever is measured by the ASQ and DAS is specifically improved in cognitive therapy, and that it is critical in preventing future episodes of depression.

Although Hollon et al. (1996) were able to find differences at the end of treatment between responders to cognitive therapy and responders to medication therapy on measures of cognition, other investigators have not found such differences. Miranda and Persons (1988) suggested that standard cognitive measures are not well suited to uncover schematic content in a person who has recovered from depression, because the depressive schemata may have become latent. With the goal of revealing latent schemata, Miranda and Persons developed a negative mood induction procedure prior to administering the DAS. Segal, Gemar, and Williams (1999) applied this method to two samples of patients who had been successfully treated for depression. Those who had received cognitive therapy obtained lower scores in this condition than did those treated with pharmacotherapy, suggesting that the pharmacotherapy-treated patients possessed more negative (depressive) schemata than did the cognitive-therapy-treated patients. Moreover, just as was found for the ASQ and DAS in the Hollon et al. (1996) study, Segal et al. found that scores on the mood-induced DAS at posttreatment predicted relapse (or recurrence) during the 30-month period when they followed these patients.

The contents of the ASQ and DAS appear to make them suitable as measures of schema change, but in the process of filling them out, it is possible that cognitive-therapy-treated patients censor their "automatic" (schematic) responses, recruit compensatory skills learned in cognitive therapy, and give answers that reflect these skills rather than the schemata that generate the automatic responses. In order to test for schema change more unambiguously, what is needed is an assessment device that taps automatic processes. One such device, a version of the Implicit Associations Test (IAT; Greenwald, McGhee, & Schwartz, 1998) adapted for the assessment of attitudes toward the self, may get at the contents of schemata about the self by requiring subjects to make rapid responses that do not allow time for the application of compensatory skills.

Gemar, Segal, and Sagrati (1999) have applied the IAT in the context of a negative mood induction procedure, and found that a negative mood induction produced a greater effect on the IAT among persons who had a history of depression than among the never-depressed control group. This result suggests that schematic depressive processes were revealed by the mood induction in those vulnerable to depression. Although this was only the first demonstration of the potential of the IAT for uncovering schematic processes in depression, it suggests the possibility of distinguishing explicit (or compensatory) from implicit (or schematic) change in cognitive therapy of depression.

Whereas the DAS, ASQ, and IAT (with or without mood induction) have been used or proposed as measures of schema change, measures of change in compensatory skills have been less plentiful. The construct of "coping" is very close to that of compensatory skills, and there exist several validated coping measures. However, most measures and studies of coping strategies have grown out of interests other than cognitive therapy. Lazarus and his colleagues have developed a series of measures that assess coping from their point of view (Folkman & Lazarus, 1980; Lazarus & Folkman, 1984). Pearlin and Schooler (1979) have also developed a measure of coping. Although these measures have not been obtained from depressed patients who have gone through a course of cognitive therapy, it would be expected, given the nature of cognitive therapy, that patients would change their manner of coping with both major stressful events and minor annoyances or "hassles" (DeLongis, Coyne, Dakof, Folkman, & Lazarus, 1982).

Standard coping measures have one characteristic, however, that makes them poor candidates for a measure of change during cognitive therapy: Patients are asked to rate the degree to which they have used a variety of coping strategies in response to recent stressful events. Patients can fairly easily recognize those coping skills that they "should" have implemented, especially if they have been through a course of cognitive therapy. For this reason, a method is needed that would require that the patient *produce*, rather than recognize, the cognitive coping skills that he or she would use in a given situation. Such measures would need to employ a free-response format and a system that turns these free responses into coping categories.

To address this need, Barber and DeRubeis (1992) developed the Ways of Responding (WOR). The WOR provides subjects with stressful events and initial negative thoughts, and then requires the subjects to write out how they would respond to such situations and thoughts. Thus the subjects are required to describe compensatory skills in order to produce good responses. In addition, the scale assesses many cognitive techniques specifically encouraged in cognitive therapy but not assessed in typical coping skill inventories, such as generating alternative explanations and evaluating negative beliefs based on evidence. The scale has been shown to have good internal consistency and high interrater reliability.

Measures such as the DAS, ASQ, IAT, and WOR all measure cognition at one time point. To access cognitive change, these scales can be given at two different time points, and difference scores can be calculated. But until recently, no measure had been developed to assess changes in beliefs as they occur in cognitive therapy sessions. To access cognitive change in sessions directly, Tang and DeRubeis (1999a) developed the Patient Cognitive Change Scale (PCCS). The scale is used by a rater who listens to (or reads transcripts from) a therapy session. The rater indicates how many times changes in belief were explicitly acknowledged by the patient during the session. The PCCS was first designed to be used with audio taperecordings, and it yielded moderate levels of interrater reliability. Tang, DeRubeis, and Beberman (1999) have since developed a version that requires raters to use the audiotape recordings alongside the transcripts of the therapy sessions. They found the new version to have an excellent interrater reliability of .85. The validity of the PCCS has been demonstrated by its ability to distinguish "critical sessions" of cognitive therapy (the session just before a large, sudden symptom improvement) from control sessions.

THE TIME COURSE OF CHANGE IN COGNITIVE THERAPY

Most outcome studies have reported the group mean time course of cognitive therapy as a smooth curve, with depression severity in a gradual and decelerating decline. Ilardi and Craighead (1994) observed that 60–70% of symptom improvement in cognitive therapy occurs in the first 4 weeks. They also assumed that cognitive modification techniques are not extensively applied in these weeks, which led them to the conclusion that Beck's cognitive mediation hypothesis of cognitive therapy cannot explain most of the improvement in such therapy.

However, as Tang and DeRubeis (1999b) have pointed out, studies have shown that cognitive modification techniques are applied extensively as early as the second session of cognitive therapy. Also, in most cognitive therapy studies there have been two sessions per week for the first 4 weeks and one session per week thereafter. Thus 40–60% of cognitive therapy sessions in studies occur in the first 4 weeks, which arguably is enough therapeutic time for cognitive techniques to have a substantial effect on symptoms. In addition, Ilardi and Craighead (1994) inferred mechanisms based on group mean time course, implicitly assuming that individual patients' time courses are similar to that of the group mean. However, individual patients' time courses tend to be quite different from that of the group mean, which calls into question inferences about therapeutic mechanisms that are based on group mean time courses.

In their further investigation of individual patients' time courses, Tang and DeRubeis (1999a) observed a remarkable pattern: In contrast to the mostly smooth group mean time courses, many individual patients' depression severity improved suddenly and substantially in a single between-session interval. They named these sudden and substantial symptom improvements "sudden gains," and developed a set of quantitative criteria to identify them. The sudden gains occurred among more than 50% of cognitive therapy responders, and the magnitude of these sudden gains accounted for more than 50% of these patients' total symptom improvements. Sudden gains also appeared to represent a stable short-term symptom improvement, since the depression severity of the patients only infrequently bounced back after the sudden gain. As a result, the patients who experienced sudden gains enjoyed superb treatment outcomes. Their outcomes were also significantly better than that of the patients who did not experience sudden gains, during two of the three assessments during the 18-month follow-up period.

Furthermore, Tang and DeRubeis (1999a) observed that patients experienced substantial cognitive changes (as assessed by the PCCS) in the therapy session preceding the sudden gains (the pregain session), but very few cognitive changes in sessions selected to control for depression severity. This finding suggests that the sudden gains are triggered by cognitive changes occurring in the pregain sessions, and they offer direct support for the idea that cognitive changes are responsible for symptom improvements in cognitive therapy.

THERAPIST–PATIENT ALLIANCE

The "therapeutic alliance" refers to the collaborative relationship between the therapist and patient. Research in the early 1980s showed that the therapeutic alliance was positively related to change in various types of psychotherapy (see Morgan, Luborsky, Crits-Christoph, Curtis, & Solomon, 1982). Recent research (Gaston, Marmar, Gallagher, & Thompson, 1991) has continued to show a positive relation between therapeutic alliance and outcome.

Although relatively fewer studies have explored alliance's contribution to cognitive therapy outcomes, the results of three such studies suggest that good therapeutic alliance is more likely to be the product than the cause of good outcome. Beckham (1989), DeRubeis and Feeley (1990), and Feeley et al. (1999) all found that therapeutic alliance measured in the early therapy session did not predict subsequent symptom improvement, whereas, as described above, therapists' adherence to concrete cognitive therapy techniques did predict subsequent symptom improvement in both the DeRubeis and Feeley (1990) and Feeley et al. (1999) studies. In addition, DeRubeis and Feeley (1990), and Feeley et al. (1999) found that in the latter half of therapy, the level of therapeutic alliance was predicted by the amount of prior symptom improvement. In other words, these two studies found that a good therapeutic alliance early on did not predict good outcome, but that good outcome early on predicted a good later therapeutic alliance.

This point is underscored by a finding from Tang and DeRubeis's (1999a) investigation of sudden gains. They found that in the therapy session before the sudden gains, the therapeutic alliance was not significantly better than that observed in the control sessions. But, in the therapy session *after* the sudden gain, therapeutic alliance rose to a significantly higher level.

Taken together, these results raise serious questions concerning the interpretation of past findings on the positive correlation between alliance and psychotherapy outcome. Most such studies have used the average score of alliance from several or all treatment sessions, and have shown a relation between this average score and symptom change. Thus it is possible that the correlations reported from these studies reflect the impact of good outcome on the alliance, rather than any causal effect of the alliance on symptom improvement.

FUTURE DIRECTIONS

Although an impressive set of findings has been published attesting to the benefits of cognitive therapy, there is much more to be learned about the extent of those benefits; the scope and limits of the applicability of cognitive therapy; its ability to be learned by therapists and applied faithfully outside the context of carefully controlled, carefully monitored clinical trials; and its essential elements and processes. In the following, we call for research that will build on the knowledge that has accrued about cognitive therapy since the first research reports on it appeared in the 1970s.

The TDCRP findings, especially those that cast doubt on the potency of cognitive therapy for more severe forms of depression (Elkin et al., 1995), have had a substantial impact on how researchers and policy makers view the benefits of cognitive therapy—in part because of the TDCRP's relatively large sample size, and because of design features that were lack-

THE THERAPIES

ing in other comparison studies of cognitive therapy versus medication. However, recently completed large-scale efficacy studies (e.g., Jarrett et al., 1999) as well as others that are underway (e.g., studies by Thase and colleagues at the University of Pittsburgh, and by DeRubeis, Hollon, and their colleagues at the University of Pennsylvania and Vanderbilt University, respectively) have employed the design features that caused the field to give such credence to the TDCRP findings, such as inclusion of a control group. In the near future, then, there will be no longer be any good reason to grant the TDCRP findings the preeminent status they were accorded in the 1990s. Jarrett et al.'s findings—that cognitive therapy outperformed a pill placebo by the same margin as antidepressant medication among patients with atypical depression—have already had an impact. The aggregation of these findings with others that will become available in the next decade will allow for more precise estimates of the average benefit of cognitive therapy for depression, relative to antidepressant medications and to placebo controls. These data can then be used as a starting point in the calculation of the benefits that can be expected if mental health delivery systems hire well-trained cognitive therapists and allow them to conduct the intensive yet still relatively short-term treatments that have been conducted in outcome studies.

It could be argued that carefully conducted cognitive therapy efficacy studies, from the first one (Rush et al., 1977) to the Jarrett et al. (1999) study and those currently underway, tell us about the benefits of cognitive therapy under optimal conditions, so that they yield overestimates of the expected benefit patients can expect in mental health clinics and the like. We note that it has also been argued, to the contrary, that such efficacy studies may yield *underestimates* of the benefits that would generally be achieved by such treatment (see Seligman, 1995). The fact that it is not known whether outcome studies overestimate or underestimate the effects that cognitive therapy can achieve in private practices and mental health centers indicates that studies of the generalizability of cognitive therapy are sorely needed. This is very likely to happen in the next decade or two, as funding agencies such as the National Institute of Mental Health have made "effectiveness" research a clear priority. Characteristically, in cognitive therapy efficacy research, therapists (and patients) are carefully selected, and extensive resources are allocated to the training and monitoring of therapists, with the aim of testing the effects of high-quality therapy that adheres to the description of cognitive therapy provided in a cognitive therapy manual (e.g., Beck et al., 1979). One way to view findings from the efficacy studies conducted to date is that they tell us what could be achieved in the future, if typical therapist-training programs were to produce trainees who can provide high-quality therapy that adheres to the principles of cognitive therapy. But it is nonetheless vital that pragmatic answers be obtained to this question: How well does cognitive therapy, as it is currently delivered by mental health practitioners, reduce (and prevent) problems with depression?

Other questions that are relevant to the effectiveness of interventions should also be addressed in relation to cognitive therapy. In particular, the long-term benefits of cognitive therapy must be more carefully documented. Thus far, research has focused primarily on the ability of cognitive therapy to prevent relapse in the months following treatment termination, and studies have tended to include sample sizes too small to yield precise estimates of even this medium-term benefit. Larger studies with longer follow-ups will be needed to provide estimates of both the relapse prevention (medium-term) and recurrence prevention (longer-term) effects of cognitive therapy.

Policy makers, managed care companies, and insurers are becoming more interested in and sophisticated about pragmatic issues in the delivery of mental health care. Cognitive therapy, because it is a relatively short-term treatment with an impressive record of efficacy evidence behind it, has been considered to be well suited to the present climate of cost-consciousness. The field needs large-scale, sophisticated efforts to estimate the costs and benefits of cognitive therapy, as well as other treatments, such as the more widely used antidepressant medications. Even though cognitive therapy is somewhat more expensive than antidepressant medications in the short run, cost–benefit analyses may reveal that it pays for itself within a short time following treatment termination, considering its potential to confer resistance to relapse and recurrence (see Antonuccio, Thomas, & Danton, 1997).

Most therapy process/mechanism research is conducted via correlational analyses (but see Jacobson et al., 1996, for a notable exception). A variable (M) is suspected to be an important mechanism; M is then measured at time T, and its correlation with outcome (O) is calculated. This approach is subject to the two usual problems of correlational analysis: the ambiguity of the causal direction, and the possibility that a third variable caused both M and O.

There is a straightforward way to deal with the first problem, ambiguity of causal direction. If M is measured earlier than O, the possibility that O caused M can be ruled out. An example of this approach is the Feeley et al. (1999) study, in which four process variables were assessed in the second therapy session and then correlated with subsequent symptom improvement. The significant correlation these researchers obtained—that greater use by the therapist of Cognitive Therapy—Concrete techniques predicted better outcome—cannot be dismissed as resulting from the fact that good outcome leads to greater use of Cognitive Therapy—Concrete techniques.

It should be noted that outcome does not just occur at the end of treatment. Outcome begins to accumulate from relatively early in therapy (Ilardi & Craighead, 1994; Tang & DeRubeis, 1999b). Thus, to apply the above-described method, it is not enough just to measure variable M before the end of treatment. Rather, it appears to be necessary to measure suspected causal variables very early in treatment. However, this solution does not resolve the second problem with correlational analyses—the possibility that third variables affect both therapeutic processes and the outcomes of therapy. Indeed, this problem cannot be completely resolved without random assignment to experimental and control conditions, which is often difficult or impossible in research on therapeutic mechanisms. However, there are alternative ways to conduct correlation analyses that tackle the third-variable problem from different angles. If a diverse array of methods all point to the same causal relationship, our confidence in the relationship can be much higher, even if no single method is sufficient.

One promising approach is time course analysis. Most theories about how a mechanism produces therapy outcome contain implications about how the causal relation unfolds over time. If the observed time course of change is consistent with the time course implied in the theory, then it helps to validate the theory. If the observed time course is inconsistent with the expected time course, then the theory is called into question. A recent example of this is the debate between Ilardi and Craighead (1994) and Tang and DeRubeis (1999b). Ilardi and Craighead pioneered the use of this method in cognitive therapy mechanism research and charged that the observed time course of change is inconsistent with the time course of change implied by Beck's cognitive mediation hypothesis of cognitive therapy. Tang and DeRubeis countered that when correct assumptions about cognitive therapy are used, the observed time courses are in fact consistent with Beck's original hypothesis. (This debate is briefly summarized above, in the section "The Time Course of Change in Cognitive Therapy.")

Other potentially useful approaches, such as task analysis (Greenberg, 1986; Rice & Greenberg, 1984), have also been proposed and applied in investigations of cognitive therapy's mechanism. If researchers continue to look beyond correlation analyses and randomized experiments to explore a greater variety of methods, it would benefit our understanding of the mechanisms through which cognitive therapy exerts its short- and long-term benefits.

Aside from the weakness in inferring causality, the typical correlation analysis suffers from at least two other problems. First, variable M is often analyzed in isolation from other important process variables, and even if it is analyzed together with other process variables, often only linear interactions are considered. This leaves more complex interactions unexplored. For example, Tang and DeRubeis (2000) recently identified a complex interaction, "determination by the weakest link," among therapy process variables. In a preliminary investigation of cognitive therapy for depression, they found that therapy progress was best predicted by how good the worst aspect of the therapy was, which would vary from case to case. That is, in some cases the alliance was weak, and in other cases adherence to cognitive therapy was poor; in both types of cases, outcome tended to be relatively poor. However, in cases in which both the alliance and therapist adherence were acceptable, outcome was very good. This finding highlights the idea that the contribution of one process variable to outcome depends on the context formed by other process variables.

Another potential complexity that needs to be reflected in research is that important therapeutic changes may be concentrated in certain critical sessions, rather than spread evenly across the treatment process. As a consequence, the common research approach of analyzing correlation between variables in a random sample of sessions may overlook some of the most important events in therapy, because this approach will reveal what happens in typical sessions, but not necessarily what happens in the few sessions that matter most (Elliott, 1983, 1984; Lambert, DeJulio, & Stein, 1978). To overcome this problem, researchers need to investigate how to identify and analyze critical sessions. Using sudden gains as a marker for critical sessions, Tang and DeRubeis (1999a) identified what appeared to have been critical sessions in about 50% of cognitive therapy responders. Their findings suggested that the critical session is responsible for triggering substantial symptom improvements. Future explorations of critical events and critical sessions may provide insight into the mechanisms of cognitive therapy.

To some, research on therapeutic mechanisms might seem to be an abstract pursuit, unrelated to the welfare of patients. However, we believe that mechanism research is at least as important to cognitive therapy's future as efficacy research, if not more so. Whereas successful demonstrations of cognitive therapy's efficacy may help to give cognitive therapy the position it deserves in health delivery systems, a better understanding of the mechanisms of cognitive therapy will point toward the systematic improvement of the efficacy and efficiency of cognitive therapy in the future. It is sobering to note that even in successful cognitive therapy trials, such as that reported by Jarrett et al. (1999), only 58% of patients responded to cognitive therapy. This was the same response rate as was achieved by antidepressant medication, and it was significantly better than placebo (28%); however, with 42% of patients not responding to cognitive therapy, there remained considerable room for improvement.

However, since the initial tests of the efficacy of cognitive therapy, there have been few if any research-based or research-tested improvements of cognitive therapy. This stands in contrast to the research efforts in the pharmaceutical industry, on which vast resources are spent to improve the efficacy and side effect profiles of antidepressant medications. Eventually, a new generation of antidepressants may come along that is significantly more effective than today's cognitive therapy. In order to serve our patients better, and to assure that the progress of cognitive therapy keeps pace with that of alternative treatments, clinical researchers need to improve and refine cognitive therapy and the training of cognitive therapists, so that more patients can benefit from it. To do so, we need first to understand better how cognitive therapy achieves its effects.

REFERENCES

American Psychiatric Association. (1993) Practice guideline for major depressive disorder in adults. *American Journal of Psychiatry, 150*(Suppl. 4), 1–26.

Antonuccio, D. O., Thomas, M., & Danton, W. G. (1997). A cost-effectiveness analysis of cognitive behavior therapy and fluoxetine (Prozac) in the treatment of depression. *Behavior Therapy, 28,* 187–210.

Barber, J. P., & DeRubeis, R. J. (1989). On second thought: Where the action is in cognitive therapy for depression. *Cognitive Therapy and Research, 13,* 441–457.

Barber, J. P., & DeRubeis, R. J. (1992). The Ways of Responding: A scale to assess compensatory skills taught in cognitive therapy. *Behavior Assessment, 14,* 93–115.

Barlow, D. H., Rapee, R. M., & Brown, T. A. (1992). Behavioral treatment of generalized anxiety disorder. *Behavior Therapy, 23,* 551–570.

Baron, R. M., & Kenny, D. A. (1986). The moderator–mediator variable distinction in social psychological research: Conceptual, strategic, and statistical considerations. *Journal of Personality and Social Psychology, 51,* 1173–1182.

Beck, A. T. (1961). A systematic investigation of depression. *Comprehensive Psychiatry, 2,* 305–312.

Beck, A. T. (1963). Thinking and depression. *Archives of General Psychiatry, 9,* 324–333.

Beck, A. T. (1964). Thinking and depression: 2. Theory and therapy. *Archives of General Psychiatry, 10,* 561–571.

Beck, A. T. (1972). *Depression: Causes and treatment.* Philadelphia: University of Pennsylvania Press.

Beck, A. T., & Beamesderfer, A. (1974). Assessment of depression: The depression inventory. In P. Pinchot (Ed.), *Psychological measurements in psychopharmacology, modern problems in pharmacopsychiatry* (Vol. 7, pp. 151–169). Basel: Karger.

Beck, A. T., Brown, G., Steer, R. A., & Weissman, A. N. (1991). Factor analysis of the Dysfunctional Attitude Scale in a clinical population. *Psychological Assessment, 3,* 478–483.

Beck, A. T., Emery, G., & Greenberg, R. L. (1985). *Anxiety disorders and phobias.* New York: Basic Books.

Beck, A. T., & Greenberg, R. L. (1974). *Coping with depression*. New York: Institute for Rational Living.

Beck, A. T., & Hurvich, M. (1959). Psychological correlates of depression. *Psychosomatic Medicine, 21,* 50–55.

Beck, A. T., Rush, A. J., Shaw, B. F., & Emery, G. (1979). *Cognitive therapy of depression*. New York: Guilford Press.

Beck, A. T., Steer, R. A., & Brown, G. K. (1996). *BDI-II manual*. San Antonio, TX: The Psychological Corporation.

Beck, A. T., & Ward, C. H. (1961). Dreams of depressed patients: Characteristic themes in manifest content. *Archives of General Psychiatry, 5,* 462–467.

Beck, A. T., Weissman, A., Lester, D., & Trexler, L. (1974). The measurement of pessimism: The Hopelessness Scale. *Journal of Consulting and Clinical Psychology, 42,* 861–865.

Beck, J. S. (1995). *Cognitive therapy: Basics and beyond*. New York: Guilford Press.

Beckham, E. E. (1989). Improvement after evaluation in psychotherapy of depression: Evidence of a placebo effect? *Journal of Clinical Psychology, 45,* 945–950.

Blackburn, I. N., Bishop, S., Glen, A. I. M., Whalley, L. J., & Christie, J. E. (1981). The efficacy of cognitive therapy in depression: A treatment trial using cognitive therapy and pharmacotherapy, each alone and in combination. *British Journal of Psychiatry, 139,* 181–189.

Blackburn, I. M., & Moore, R. G. (1997). Controlled acute and follow-up trial of cognitive therapy in out-patients with recurrent depression. *British Journal of Psychiatry, 171,* 328–334.

Chambless, D. L., & Gillis, M. M. (1993). Cognitive therapy of anxiety disorders. *Journal of Consulting and Clinical Psychology, 61,* 248–260.

Clark, D. M. (1996). Panic disorder: From theory to therapy. In P. M. Salkovskis (Ed.), *Frontiers of cognitive therapy* (pp. 318–344). New York: Guilford Press.

Clark, D. M., Salkovskis, P. M., & Chalkley, A. J. (1985). Respiratory control as a treatment for panic attacks. *Journal of Behavior Therapy and Experimental Psychiatry, 16,* 23–30.

Compas, B. E., Haaga, D. A. F., Keefe, F. J., & Leitenberg, H. (1998). Sampling of empirically supported psychological treatments from health psychology: Smoking, chronic pain, cancer, and bulimia nervosa. *Journal of Consulting and Clinical Psychology, 66,* 89–112.

Cooper, J. M. (Ed.). (1997). *Plato: Complete works*. Indianapolis, IN: Hackett.

DeLongis, A., Coyne, J. C., Dakof, G., Folkman, S., & Lazarus, R. S. (1982). Relationship of daily hassles, uplifts, and major life events to health status. *Health Psychology, 1,* 119–136.

DeRubeis, R. J., & Crits-Christoph, P. (1998). Empirically supported individual and group psychological treatments for adult mental disorders. *Journal of Consulting and Clinical Psychology, 66,* 37–52.

DeRubeis, R. J., & Feeley, M. (1990). Determinants of change in cognitive therapy for depression. *Cognitive Therapy and Research, 14,* 469–482.

DeRubeis, R. J., Gelfand, L. A., Tang, T. Z., & Simons, A. (1999). Medications versus cognitive behavioral therapy for severely depressed outpatients: Mega-analysis of four randomized comparisons. *American Journal of Psychiatry,* *156,* 1007–1013.

DeRubeis, R. J., & Hollon, S. D. (1999). *Mediation of the relapse prevention effect* *of cognitive therapy for depression.* Unpublished manuscript, University of Pennsylvania.

DeRubeis, R. J., Hollon, S. D., Evans, M. D., Garvey, M. J., Grove, W. M., & Tuason, V. B. (1990). How does cognitive therapy work? Cognitive change and symptom change in cognitive therapy and pharmacotherapy for depression. *Journal of Consulting and Clinical Psychology, 58,* 862–869.

Dobson, K. S. (1989). A meta-analysis of the efficacy of cognitive therapy for depression. *Journal of Consulting and Clinical Psychology, 57,* 414–419.

Durham, R. C., Murphy, T., Allan, T., Richard, K., Treliving, L. R., & Fenton, G. W. (1994). Cognitive therapy, analytic psychotherapy, and anxiety management training for generalized anxiety disorder. *British Journal of Psychiatry, 165,* 315–323.

Elkin, I., Shea, M. T., Watkins, J. T., Imber, S. D., Sotsky, S. M., Collins, J. F., Glass, D. R., Pilkonis, P. A., Leber, W. R., Docherty, J. P., Fiester, S. J., & Parloff, M. B. (1989). National Institute of Mental Health Treatment of Depression Collaborative Research Program: General effectiveness of treatments. *Archives of General Psychiatry, 46,* 971–982.

Elkin, I., Gibbons, R. D., Shea, M. T., & Sotsky, S. M. (1995). Initial severity and differential treatment outcome in the National Institute of Mental Health Treatment of Depression Collaborative Research Program. *Journal of Consulting and Clinical Psychology, 63,* 841–847.

Elkin, I., Gibbons, R. D., Shea, M. T., & Shaw, B. F. (1996). Science is not a trial (but it can sometimes be a tribulation). *Journal of Consulting and Clinical Psychology, 64,* 92–103.

Elliott, R. (1983). That in your hands . . . : A comprehensive process analysis of a significant event in psychotherapy. *Psychiatry, 46,* 113–129.

Elliott, R. (1984). A discovery-oriented approach to significant change events in psychotherapy: Interpersonal process recall and comprehensive process analysis. In L. N. Rice & L. S. Greenberg (Eds.), *Patterns of change* (pp. 249–286). New York: Guilford Press.

Ellis, A. (1984). Rational–emotive therapy. In R. J. Corsini (Ed.), *Current psychotherapies* (3rd ed., pp. 196–238). Itasca, IL: Peacock.

Ellis, A., & Harper, R. A. (1975). *A new guide to rational living.* North Hollywood, CA: Wilshire Books.

Evans, M. D., Hollon, S. D., DeRubeis, R. J., Piasecki, J., Grove, W. B., & Tuason, V. B. (1992). Differential relapse following therapy and pharmacotherapy for depression. *Archives of General Psychiatry, 49,* 802–808.

Fava, G. A., Grandi, S., Zielezny, M., Rafanelli, C., Canestrari, R., & Morphy, M. A. (1994). Cognitive behavioral treatment of residual symptoms in primary major depressive disorder. *American Journal of Psychiatry, 151,* 1295–1299.

Fava, G. A., Grandi, S., Zielezny, M. C., & Canestrari, R. (1996). Four-year outcome for cognitive behavioral treatment of residual symptoms in major depression. *American Journal of Psychiatry, 153,* 945–947.

Fava, G. A., Rafanelli, C., Grandi, S., Conti, S., & Belluardo, P. (1998). Prevention of recurrent depression with cognitive behavioral therapy. *Archives of General Psychiatry, 55,* 816–820.

Feeley, M., DeRubeis, R. J., & Gelfand, L. (1999). The temporal relation of adherence and alliance to symptom change in cognitive therapy for depression. *Journal of Consulting and Clinical Psychology, 67,* 578–582.

Folkman, S., & Lazarus, R. S. (1980). An analysis of coping in a middle-aged community sample. *Journal of Health and Social Behavior, 21,* 219–239.

Frank, J. D. (1973). *Persuasion and healing.* Baltimore: Johns Hopkins University Press.

Freud, S. (1957). Mourning and melancholia. In J. Strachey (Ed. and Trans.), *The standard edition of the complete psychological works of Sigmund Freud* (Vol. 14, pp. 237–260). London: Hogarth Press. (Original work published 1917)

Gaston, L., Marmar, C., Gallagher, D., & Thompson, L. (1991). Alliance prediction of outcome beyond in-treatment symptomatic change as psychotherapy processes. *Psychotherapy Research, 1,* 104–112.

Gemar, M., Segal, Z., & Sagrati, S. (1999, November). Contributions of effortful and implicit measures of cognition to a risk marker for depressive relapse/recurrence. In D. Kraft (Chair), *Improving the long-term well-being of depressed patients by predicting and preventing relapse.* Symposium conducted at the 33rd Annual Convention of the Association for Advancement of Behavior Therapy, Toronto.

Greenberg, L. S. (1986). Change process research. *Journal of Consulting and Clinical Psychology, 54,* 4–9.

Greenberg, L. S. (1984). *Research on the process of change.* New York: Guilford Press.

Greenwald, A. G., McGhee, D. E., & Schwartz, J. L. K. (1998). Measuring individual differences in implicit cognition: The implicit association test. *Journal of Personality and Social Psychology, 74,* 1464–1480.

Hamilton, M. (1960). A rating scale for depression. *Journal of Neurology, Neurosurgery and Psychiatry, 23,* 56–62.

Hollon, S. D. (1999). Rapid early response in cognitive behavior therapy: A commentary. *Clinical Psychology: Science and Practice, 6,* 305–309.

Hollon, S. D., & Beck, A. T. (1979). Cognitive therapy of depression. In P. E. Kendall & S. D. Hollon (Eds.), *Cognitive-behavioral interventions: Theory, research, procedures* (pp. 153–201). New York: Academic Press.

Hollon, S. D., DeRubeis, R. J., & Evans, M. D. (1996). Cognitive therapy in the treatment and prevention of depression. In P. M. Salkovskis (Ed.), *Frontiers of cognitive therapy* (pp. 293–317). New York: Guilford Press.

Hollon, S. D., DeRubeis, R. J., Evans, M. D., Wiemer, M. J., Garvey, M. J., Grove, W. M., & Tuason, V. B. (1992). Cognitive therapy and pharmacotherapy for depression: Singly and in combination. *Archives of General Psychiatry, 49,* 774–781.

Hollon, S. D., Emerson, M., & Mandell, M. (1982). *Psychometric properties of the Cognitive Therapy Scale.* Unpublished manuscript, University of Minnesota/ St. Paul–Ramsey Medical Center.

Hollon, S. D., Evans, M. D., Auerbach, A., DeRubeis, R. J., Elkin, I., Lowery, A.,

Tuason, V. B., Kriss, M., & Piasecki, J. (1985). *Development of a system for rating therapies for depression: Differentiating cognitive therapy, interpersonal psychotherapy, and clinical management pharmacotherapy.* Unpublished manuscript, University of Minnesota/St. Paul–Ramsey Medical Center.

Hollon, S. D., Evans, M. D., & DeRubeis, R. J. (1985). Preventing relapse following treatment for depression: The cognitive–pharmacotherapy project. In N. Schneiderman & T. Fields (Eds.), *Stress and coping* (Vol. 2, pp. 227–243). Hillsdale, NJ: Erlbaum.

Hollon, S. D., & Kriss, M. R. (1984). Cognitive factors in clinical research and practice. *Clinical Psychology Review, 4,* 35–76.

Ilardi, S. S., & Craighead, W. E. (1994). The role of nonspecific factors in cognitive-behavior therapy for depression. *Clinical Psychology: Science and Practice, 1,* 138–156.

Jacobson, N. S., Dobson, K. S., Truax, P. A., Addis, M. E., Koerner, K., Gollan, J. K., Gortner, E., & Prince, S. E. (1996). A component analysis of cognitive-behavioral treatment for depression. *Journal of Consulting and Clinical Psychology, 64,* 295–304.

Jacobson, N. S., & Gortner, E. T. (2000). Can depression be de-medicalized in the 21st century: Scientific revolutions, counter-revolutions and the magnetic field of normal science. *Behaviour Research and Therapy, 8,* 103–117.

Jacobson, N. S., & Hollon, S. D. (1996a). Cognitive-behavior therapy versus pharmacotherapy: Now that the jury's returned its verdict, it's time to present the rest of the evidence. *Journal of Consulting and Clinical Psychology, 64,* 74–80.

Jacobson, N. S., & Hollon, S. D. (1996b). Prospects for future comparisons between drugs and psychotherapy: Lessons from the CBT vs. pharmacotherapy exchange. *Journal of Consulting and Clinical Psychology, 64,* 104–108.

Jarrett, R. B., Basco, M. R., Risser, R., Ramanan, J., Marwill, M., Kraft, D., & Rush, A. J. (1998). Is there a role for continuation phase cognitive therapy for depressed outpatients? *Journal of Consulting and Clinical Psychology, 66,* 1036–1040.

Jarrett, R. B., Schaffer, M., McIntire, D., Witt-Browder, A., Kraft, D., & Risser, R. C. (1999). Treatment of atypical depression with cognitive therapy or phenelzine. *Archives of General Psychiatry, 56,* 431–437.

Klein, D. F. (1996). Preventing hung juries about therapy studies. *Journal of Consulting and Clinical Psychology, 64,* 81–87.

Kovacs, M., Rush, A. J., Beck, A. T., & Hollon, S. D. (1981). Depressed outpatients treated with cognitive therapy or pharmacotherapy: A one-year follow-up. *Archives of General Psychiatry, 38,* 33–39.

Lambert, M. J., DeJulio, S. J., & Stein, D. M. (1978). Therapist interpersonal skills: Process, outcome, methodological considerations, and recommendations for future research. *Psychological Bulletin, 85,* 467–489.

Lazarus, R. S., & Folkman, S. (1984). *Stress, appraisal, and coping.* New York: Springer.

Meichenbaum, D. (1977). *Cognitive-behavior modification.* New York: Plenum Press.

Miranda, J., & Persons, J. B. (1988). Dysfunctional attitudes are mood-state dependent. *Journal of Abnormal Psychology, 97,* 76–79.

Morgan, R., Luborsky, L., Crits-Christoph, P., Curtis, H., & Solomon, J. (1982). Predicting the outcomes of psychotherapy by the Penn Helping Alliance Rating Method. *Archives of General Psychiatry, 39,* 397–402.

Murphy, G. E., Simons, A. D., Wetzel, R. D., & Lustman, P. J. (1984). Cognitive therapy and pharmacotherapy: Singly and together in the treatment of depression. *Archives of General Psychiatry, 41,* 33–41.

Nisbett, R., & Ross, L. (1980). *Human inference: Strategies and shortcomings of social judgment.* Englewood Cliffs, NJ: Prentice-Hall.

Overholser, J. C. (1993a). Elements of the Socratic method: I. Systematic questioning. *Psychotherapy, 30,* 67–74.

Overholser, J. C. (1993b). Elements of the Socratic method: II. Inductive reasoning. *Psychotherapy, 30,* 75–85.

Pearlin, L. I., & Schooler, C. (1979). The structure of coping. *Journal of Health and Social Behavior, 19,* 337–356.

Persons, J. B. (1989). *Cognitive therapy in practice: A case formulation approach.* New York: Norton.

Rice, L. N., & Greenberg, L. G. (Eds.). (1984). *Patterns of change.* New York: Guilford Press.

Rush, A. J., Beck, A. T., Kovacs, J. M., & Hollon, S. D. (1977). Comparative efficacy of cognitive therapy and pharmacotherapy in the treatment of depressed outpatients. *Cognitive Therapy and Research, 1,* 17–37.

Salkovskis, P. M. (1985). Obsessional–compulsive problems: A cognitive behavioural analysis. *Behaviour Research and Therapy, 23,* 571–583.

Salkovskis, P. M. (1996). The cognitive approach to anxiety: Threat beliefs, safety-seeking behavior, and the special case of health anxiety and obsession. In P. M. Salkovskis (Ed.), *Frontiers of cognitive therapy* (pp. 48–74). New York: Guilford Press.

Segal, Z. V., Gemar, M., & Williams, S. (1999). Differential cognitive response to a mood challenge following successful cognitive therapy or pharmacotherapy for unipolar depression. *Journal of Abnormal Psychology, 108,* 3–10.

Seligman, M. E. P. (1995). The effectiveness of psychotherapy: The *Consumer Reports* study. *American Psychologist, 50,* 965–974.

Seligman, M. E. P., Abramson, L. Y., Semmel, A., & von Baeyer, C. (1979). Depressive attributional style. *Journal of Abnormal Psychology, 88,* 242–247.

Shea, M. T., Elkin, I., Imber, S. D., Sotsky, S. M., Watkins, J. T., Collins, J. F., Pilkonis, P. A., Beckham, E., Glass, D. R., Dolan, R. T., & Parloff, M. B. (1992). Course of depressive symptoms over follow-up: Findings from the National Institute of Mental Health Treatment of Depression Collaborative Research Program. *Archives of General Psychiatry, 49,* 782–787.

Simons, A. D., Murphy, G. E., Levine, J. L., & Wetzel, R. D. (1986). Cognitive therapy and pharmacotherapy for depression: Sustained improvement over one year. *Archives of General Psychiatry, 43,* 43–48.

Tang, T. Z., & DeRubeis, R. J. (1999a). Sudden gains and critical sessions in cognitive behavioral therapy for depression. *Journal of Consulting and Clinical Psychology, 67,* 894–904.

Tang, T. Z., & DeRubeis, R. J. (1999b). Reconsidering rapid early response in cognitive behavioral therapy for depression. *Clinical Psychology: Science and Practice, 6,* 283–288.

Tang, T. Z., & DeRubeis, R. J. (2000). *Determination by the weakest link: Predicting critical sessions and sudden gains with therapy mechanism variables.* Manuscript in preparation.

Tang, T. Z., DeRubeis, R. J., & Beberman, R. (1999). *Cognitive changes in the critical sessions and sudden gains: A replication study with an improved measure of in-session cognitive changes.* Manuscript in preparation.

Van Oppen, P., de Haan, E., Van Balkom, A. J. L. M., Spinhoven, P., Hoogduin, K., & Van Dyck, R. (1995). Cognitive therapy and exposure in vivo in the treatment of obsessive compulsive disorder. *Behaviour Research and Therapy, 33,* 379–390.

Weissman, A. N., & Beck, A. T. (1978, November). *Development and validation of the Dysfunctional Attitude Scale: A preliminary investigation.* Paper presented at the meeting of the American Educational Research Association, Toronto.

Young, J., & Beck, A. T. (1980). *The development of the Cognitive Therapy Scale.* Unpublished manuscript, Center for Cognitive Therapy, Philadelphia.

11

Varieties of Constructivism in Psychotherapy

ROBERT A. NEIMEYER
JONATHAN D. RASKIN

The universe is not an idea of mine;
My idea of the universe is an idea of mine.
Night doesn't fall before my eyes;
My idea of night falls before my eyes.
Apart from my thinking and my having thoughts
The night concretely falls,
And the stars' shimmering exists like a weighable thing.
—FERNANDO PESSOA (1998, p. 80)

As the broad scope of this volume demonstrates, cognitive therapy and cognitive-behavioral therapy (CBT) have experienced impressive growth over the last 20 years. Developing from their early "home base" in the treatment of depression (Beck, Rush, Shaw, & Emery, 1979), cognitively oriented psychotherapies now address a vast range of disorders and human problems, from impulse control difficulties in childhood to relational dissatisfaction in adult life. Dobson and Pusch (1993) have aptly characterized this growth as occurring mainly on a plane of *breadth*, pressing back the frontiers of application of CBT, while at the same time making only relatively modest modifications in the basic philosophy and methods of CBT itself. Thus the essential cognitive paradigm—with its focus on monitoring and correction of irrational, distorted, or maladaptive thoughts that mediate one's emotional and behavioral responses to problematic situations or persons—has proven remarkably elastic, being stretched to fit nearly every conceivable form of personal distress.

Accompanying this horizontal proliferation of CBT models has been another form of growth, which has occurred more on a dimension of *depth* rather than breadth (Dobson & Pusch, 1993). Viewed from this perspective, cognitively oriented therapies have "deepened" across time by refining their approaches to less easily accessed core features of personal knowledge, and by reaching toward models more adequate to the complexity of human meaning systems and their social embeddedness (R. A. Neimeyer, 1995b). It is to this second, depth dimension of development that constructivist, narrative, and social-constructionist theorists and therapists have made the greatest contribution. Our goals in this chapter are to review several prominent expressions of this broad constructivist trend,[1] to describe their common points of departure from traditional CBT, and to point toward research that is coherent with a constructivist perspective. Equally important, we try to give the reader a flavor of the therapeutic strategies associated with these perspectives by providing illustrative case vignettes derived from our own practice as constructivist therapists.

THE EPISTEMOLOGICAL SHIFT

Occasionally developments quite outside the discipline of psychology conspire to trigger far-reaching changes in the nature of psychological theory, and equally basic changes in the practice of psychotherapy. For example, a shift from continental, hermeneutic philosophies of science toward more logico-empirical forms (Radnitsky, 1973) in the 1920s helped foster a shift from the more elaborate, inferential theorizing preferred by psychoanalysts to a more spare, parsimonious form of research and therapy associated with behaviorism. More recently, the advent of computers in the 1950s triggered sweeping changes in models of mind, providing new currency for "mentalistic" concepts, and contributing directly and indirectly to the "cognitive revolution" whose echoes continue to reverberate in psychological research and therapy (Mahoney, 1995). Far from being illegitimate sources of influence on psychological theory, broad culture shifts like these often breathe new life and creative vision into psychology, prompting successive generations of scientists and practitioners to transcend the conceptual limitations of their predecessors.

Constructivism, too, is partly the offshoot of cultural developments in the late 20th century. Although its roots can be traced to the philosophies of Vico, Kant, Vaihinger, and Korzybski, with their emphases on the active, form-giving nature of human cognition (Mahoney, 1991; Neimeyer,

2000a), constructivism did not fully flower until "postmodernism" began to cultivate an intellectual landscape congenial to its growth. As a broad movement spanning developments in art and architecture as well as social theory, postmodernism reacts against the confining strictures of modernism, with its faith in an orderly, knowable reality, whose forms and functions can be mirrored by the human mind and its products (Appignanesi & Garratt, 1995). At a conceptual level, postmodern theorists specifically dispute traditional views of knowledge as having a firm foundation in either unquestioned authority or "immaculate perception." Likewise, they regard as subtly oppressive attempts to formulate a "grand unified theory" or "grand narrative" that expresses the full truth of the human condition (Botella, 1995). Instead, "posties" acknowledge and even celebrate the "foundationlessness," "fragmentariness," and "constructed" character of human knowing, which yields at best local (even personal), positional, and historically limited "truths" whose value is determined less by their validity than by their pragmatic utility (Polkinghorne, 1992). Stated succinctly, a postmodern sensibility shifts the central concern of epistemology, or the theory of knowledge, from the question "Is this belief true, rationally defensible, or empirically justified?" to "What are the consequences of holding this belief for the self and others, and what practices does it support (and suppress) in a social context?"

Transposed into the domain of psychotherapy, postmodernism has given impetus to constructivist, narrative, and social-constructionist approaches that depart from the realist epistemology underpinning traditional schools of counseling and psychotherapy. In the eyes of their critics, such postmodern therapies are suspiciously "antirealist," carrying the subversive implication that psychotherapy is something less than the rigorously "rule-governed," "systematic," and "replicable" enterprise to which scientific psychology aspires (Held, 1995). However, constructivists rarely deny the existence of a "real world" (Efran & Fauber, 1995); what they dispute is the long tradition of psychotherapy, from Freud to contemporary cognitive therapists, who construe psychotherapy as an authoritative procedure for improving a client's degree of "reality contact." Indeed, constructivist therapists are

> only vaguely interested in the ontological question of whether a real world exists in any meaningful sense beyond our construction of it. . . . [But they are] far more interested in what psychotherapy might look like if it were liberated from the quest to judge a client's personal reality by extraspective criteria of rationality or objectivity. (R. A. Neimeyer, 1995c, pp. 341–342)

Of course, if one abandons the goal of eliminating a client's "cognitive distortions" by means of authoritative interpretation, rational disputation, empirical testing, and psychoeducational instruction, then by what criteria does a therapist diagnose difficulties, and how might he or she intervene in them? Many constructivist therapists are beginning to answer this question (Neimeyer & Raskin, 2000a). As they do so, constructivists face the challenge of applying idiographic, meaning-oriented perspectives within a dominant professional framework that advocates global categories of client disorders, such as those found in the American Psychiatric Association's *Diagnostic and Statistical Manual of Mental Disorders,* fourth edition (DSM-IV). We see constructivist practitioners as part of the loyal opposition when it comes to employing DSM-IV diagnostic classifications (Neimeyer & Raskin, 2000b). On the one hand, constructivists, like other clinicians, sometimes pragmatically use terms like "major depression" or "posttraumatic stress disorder" when communicating with colleagues or insurers, or when conducting clinical research. On the other hand, they are sensitive to and critical of the potentially stigmatizing features of traditional diagnostic systems. In this regard, when constructivist clinicians choose to employ categorical labels, they do so from the perspective that such diagnoses, like all systems devised for conceptualizing people's problems in living, are constructions of disorder rather than categories that carve nature at its joints (Raskin & Lewandowski, 2000). As such, the primary problem with DSM-IV is its preemptive application to such an extent that alternative ways of construing clients are dismissed or subordinated, instead of placed on equal footing as thoroughly viable alternative models of psychological functioning (Raskin & Lewandowski, 2000).

The remainder of this chapter considers five distinguishable thematic emphases in constructivist psychotherapy, and the distinctive conceptual and practical features associated with each. In our view, these represent not so much unique *divisions* of constructivist therapy so much as *dimensions* along which different therapies and therapists vary.[2] However, in the sections to follow we orient our discussion around one prototypical expression of each theme for the sake of clarity, focusing on key features of its (1) theory and epistemology, (2) clinical theory of disorder, (3) psychotherapeutic strategies, and (4) supportive research. We begin with a discussion of those themes perhaps most familiar to CBT-oriented readers, and then progress to those that are more novel, or even radically divergent, from a traditional cognitive therapy perspective. Thus we briefly summarize, illustrate, and evaluate each of the following emphases: psychotherapy as "personal science," psychotherapy as "developmental reconstruction," psychotherapy as "radical questioning," psychotherapy as "narrative reauthoring," and psychotherapy as "discursive critique." We close the chapter with a few thoughts on the relationship between CBT and constructivist therapies, and the problems and prospects of psychotherapy integration.

PSYCHOTHERAPY AS PERSONAL SCIENCE

Theory

One implication of the postmodern shift in epistemology is that the warrant for belief systems is displaced from the world of objective facts to the realm of subjective meanings. This shift is nowhere more evident than in George Kelly's (1955/1991) personal construct psychology (PCP), whose personal science metaphor has since been elaborated by both contemporary construct theorists (Neimeyer & Neimeyer, 1990–2000) and kindred constructivist therapists (Mahoney, 1980). In this view, people function as incipient scientists, actively devising personal theories to permit them to anticipate future events and channel their relationships with others. Kelly (1955/1991) postulated that the dimensions of meaning that constitute this personal construct system are bipolar in nature. In other words, Kelly believed that people organize their social lives in terms of implicit contrasts, as when a woman who is a client in marital therapy construes herself as "moral," "honest," and "economically responsible," and places her husband on the contrast poles of each of these dimensions—as "degenerate," "lying," and "untrustworthy with money." Each person develops a hierarchical network of idiosyncratic bipolar personal construct dimensions, organized around a set of core role constructs that define the person's central identity commitments, which are typically highly resistant to change.

A key element in PCP theory involves people's quest for validation of the constructs they apply to events. Like scientists, people tend to test their constructs and to maintain those that prove most useful in predicting the outcomes of their ventures, although they may be reluctant to relinquish even inadequate constructions if no compelling alternatives are available. Adding to the complexity of revising the construct system is the inaccessibility of external reality in any direct form, insofar as it is inevitably filtered through one's personal interpretations. This, and the general viability of many alternative constructions of the same events (e.g., different constructions of the same family problem), frequently make straightforward rational or empirical disputation of a client's constructions a fruitless undertaking.

One easily misunderstood implication of the personal science metaphor is that it does not bestow privileged status upon forms of knowledge developed within the parameters of the scientific method. Systems of knowledge not devised through formal scientific means (such as law, art, philosophy, history, religion, and even "folk wisdom") remain products of personal science, insofar as they involve the active development of systems of meaning that people rely upon and refine as they navigate life (Botella, 1995). In this regard, the idea of personal science is broader than is commonly assumed within CBT, emphasizing the ongoing process of constructing increasingly complex hierarchical meaning systems, whose central features are passionately defended from invalidation across the course of living (Neimeyer, 1987).

Disorder

Constructivist interpretations of psychological disturbance drawing on the personal science metaphor differ substantially from traditional approaches to "psychopathology." Numerous PCP critiques of category-based diagnostic systems have been offered, all of which discourage reliance on nomothetic categories and encourage a focus on the idiographic meanings that structure a client's experience and action (Faidley & Leitner, 1993; Honos-Webb & Leitner, 1997; Raskin & Epting, 1993, 1995; Raskin & Lewandowski, 2000). Although PCP theorists have empirically evaluated models of numerous disorders (Winter, 1992), at root they see problems as originating in the continued use of personal constructs despite their repeated invalidation, as judged by their incongruity with more concrete outcomes assessed within a person's own system (Kelly, 1955/1991).

A distinctive feature of PCP theory is that it focuses less on disorders of construct *content* (e.g., having negative beliefs about the self, world, and future) than on disorders of construct system *processes* and *structures*. For example, Kelly (1955/1991) defined "dilation" as broadening one's perceptual field, leading to the application of constructs to a wide array of scenarios and experiences. When done to an extreme extent, dilation prevents one from making clear discriminations about whether one's constructions are usefully applied in any given instance. For example, the "manic" client's

> "perceptual field" is so broadened that almost everything is relevant. There is so much to do. There is no time to sleep. . . . Until such time as he is able to limit his perceptual field to something that is manageable, he cannot make the time to reconstrue. (Fransella, 1993, p. 123)

On the other hand, "constriction" involves narrowing one's perceptual field in order to avoid incompatibilities in one's construct system. Landfield and Leitner (1980) provide a nice example of constriction with the "therapy client who had dedicated himself to becoming the world's leading authority on buffaloes in western Nebraska. The entire area of interpersonal relationships was out of bounds" (p. 12). In the clinical domain, constriction is often associated with depression, in which the person's engagement with the world is reduced to a minimum to ward off the threat of further invalidation by events that could erode precarious core identity constructs.

"Loosening" and "tightening" are other forms of construing that, in exaggerated form, can lead to difficulties. Loose constructs are those that lead to varying predictions, whereas tight construing yields unvarying pre-dictions (Kelly, 1955/1991). All people fluctuate between looser and tighter construing, as the former allows them to entertain new but not fully devel-oped constructions, while the latter is necessary for them to apply con-structs effectively in designated circumstances. Unfortunately, excessively loose construing makes the very purpose of construing—prediction as a foundation for making life choices—all but impossible. On the other hand, overly tight construing prevents one from entertaining new and possibly liberating constructions of events. Excessively loose construing is analogous to the fragmented thinking associated with schizophrenia, whereas exces-sively tight construing resembles the rigid, inflexible thinking associated with the traditional diagnosis of obsessive–compulsive personality disorder (Johnson, Pfenninger, & Klion, 2000).

"Disorders of transition" focus on difficulties that arise when a person perceives imminent change within his or her construct system. For example, "guilt" occurs when one violates core constructions of self-identity. If you are experiencing guilt, "you may find yourself doing things which you would not have expected to find yourself doing, had you been the sort of person you thought you were" (Bannister, 1977, pp. 32–33). "Anxiety" occurs when a person realizes that his or her construct system is inadequate to account for a critical situation: "The person does not have sufficient structure to under-stand the events around him. The system fails!" (Landfield & Leitner, 1980, p. 13). As such, a certain level of anxiety is inevitable whenever one attempts to explore new experiences that are not comfortably accommodated by one's existing construct system. "Threat" occurs when one seems poised on the brink of comprehensive change in the construct system (Kelly, 1955/1991), as when an abused woman is paralyzed in leaving a destructive relationship by the threat of sweeping revisions in her view of herself and life without her partner. Finally, "hostility" is characterized by efforts to extort validational evidence to support constructions that are clearly failing (Kelly, 1955/1991), as when the abusive partner in the example above literally forces his resistant partner into his construction of her role. An intriguing implication of this view is that negative emotions are not "caused" by "maladaptive" ways of thinking, as in conventional CBT models, but are instead expressions of im-pending transitions in the fundamental constructions of meaning that regu-late our lives with others (Bannister, 1977; McCoy, 1977). It follows that the goal of therapy is not to "control" negative emotions, but instead to under-stand the sometimes subtle changes in one's basic framework for living to-ward which they point (Mahoney, 1991).

Psychotherapy

Theorists who work within a PCP paradigm are technically eclectic, en-couraging clinicians to employ the full range of therapeutic strategies available, but to do so within a consistent conceptual framework. However, one therapy technique unique to PCP theory is "fixed-role therapy" (Epting, 1984; Fransella, 1995; Kelly, 1955/1991). In this brief therapy format, clients are asked first to write character sketches of themselves, as if they were characters in a play, from the standpoint of someone who knows them intimately and sympathetically. A therapist reworks aspects of a client's sketch, introducing novel construct dimensions that structure different forms of interactions with others. The client is then given opportunities to practice the new role with the therapist, and is asked to enact the part in daily life, metaphorically sending his or her usual self on vacation and allowing the new identity to step in for a fixed period of time. The rationale for the fixed-role sketch is that it allows clients to experiment with new behaviors and self-constructions while wearing the protective mask of make-believe (G. J. Neimeyer, 1995), at the same time mitigating the guilt and threat that might accompany failure to remain true to a core role.

This same respectful and invitational stance characterizes other variations of PCP therapy, such as Leitner's (1995) focus on the ways in which clients struggle to establish intimate "role relationships" with other persons. Because of their potential to affirm and extend people's deepest sense of themselves, role relationships can be the most rewarding of human experiences if one's core constructions are validated by another, or they can be the most devastating when one's core constructions are invalidated. For this reason, engaging in role relationships is often terrifying and difficult, especially for people who have been hurt in the past when they allowed themselves to be vulnerable. Therapy revolves around helping clients to risk rather than retreat from role relationships, by first allowing themselves to be known deeply by the therapist and eventually by other people in their lives. A practical example combining features of Leitner's experiential PCP therapy with use of a fixed role can be seen in the case of Carla, a college student seeking therapy with one of us (J. D. R.—the "I" in what follows) because of anxiety about her future.

Carla reported feeling unsure of herself in a variety of personal and professional contexts, often unable to recognize or experience feelings that might help her ascertain her own point of view on any given topic. Carla connected much of this difficulty to her relationship with her parents, especially her father. She initially described her father as a loving figure, but as therapy progressed we found ourselves talking regularly about how he imposed his ideas upon her about what Carla should do, believe, and be. Although her father's intentions were to protect and assist Carla in the difficult process of growing up, the result had been that she had immense difficulty identifying her own desires and interests. She learned from her father to defer to others and not attend to her own feelings.

Fixed-role therapy entered the equation when I asked Carla to act out a role quite different from the passive one she saw as her true self. We conjured up "Ruth," an assertive, gregarious character who was not afraid to stand up for her beliefs. "Ruth" was still a loving and concerned daughter, but did not always abide by the wishes of family and friends. While remaining sensitive to those around her, "Ruth" would not hesitate to act upon her own needs and feelings as she struggled to develop into the person she wanted to become. I asked Carla to act out the role of "Ruth" in between sessions. Initially she found this quite difficult to do, and dejectedly returned to sessions worried that she had disappointed me. In this respect, the fixed-role work provided important grist for the therapeutic mill. Her initial failure to comply with my request that she act out the fixed role provided a basis on which we could explore the role relationship we were developing. Although it was difficult for her to elaborate, Carla eventually expressed a concern that if she did not act out the fixed role, she would disappoint me and I would reject her—a form of openness that itself was compatible with "Ruth's" role. However, Carla became noticeably upset upon talking about this concern, as it was one that loomed even larger in her relationship with her father. The role relationship I had with Carla became a focal point of therapy, as she was quite surprised by my reaction to her not acting out the fixed role; I told her that she knew what felt comfortable and that I respected her decision not to enact it. Not surprisingly, it took Carla some time to believe experientially that I would not reject her for failing to perform the fixed role. However, as we continued across several sessions to discuss the role relationship we had developed, Carla began choosing to act out aspects of the new role. She said that what made it easier was that she was doing so because *she* wanted to, not because she was trying to please me to avoid my rejecting her. As she began to perform the fixed role in self-selected areas of her daily life, she found herself incorporating many of "Ruth's" characteristics into her own sense of self. Her impression of herself as a passive, uncertain person incapable of making life decisions waned, and was replaced by an ever more assertive character who was even beginning to renegotiate her relationship with her father through a series of difficult but ultimately transforming interactions.

Like other constructivist change strategies, the playful form of fixed-role enactment of an alternative self, rather than focusing on the disputation of irrational beliefs or errors in logical thinking, instead targets the creation of both new personal realities and revised role relationships.

Research

PCP theory has generated a substantial empirical literature—numbering literally thousands of studies (Neimeyer & Martin, 1996)—that have explored not only topics of direct relevance to psychotherapy, but also a broad range of issues in social, personality, cognitive, and educational psychology (Neimeyer & Neimeyer, 1990–2000). The majority of these studies make use of adaptations of "repertory grid technique" to elicit the personal construct systems of individuals in their own terms, and to examine how these systems are used to organize perceptions of important people and events (Fransella & Bannister, 1977; G. J. Neimeyer, 1993). As such, grids have proven useful in predicting which clients are likely to respond to interpersonal versus behavioral interventions (Winter, 1990), and how people come to reconstrue themselves across the course of successful psychotherapy (Winter, 1992). Along with traditional clinical measures, grids have also been used to document the process and outcome of distinctive forms of PCP, such as nonthreatening group therapy formats for survivors of sexual abuse (Alexander, Neimeyer, & Follette, 1991; Alexander, Neimeyer, Follette, Moore, & Harter, 1989; Neimeyer, Harter, & Alexander, 1991).

In light of the common tendency to categorize constructivist approaches to personal science with more rationalist therapies like those of Beck (1993) or Ellis (1993), it is noteworthy that empirical research on the process of the two approaches suggests that they are quite different. For example, applying a number of reliable process scales to therapy transcripts with dozens of clients, Winter and Watson (1999) found that cognitive therapists showed a more negative attitude toward their clients, but also more direct expressions of approval, information, and guidance, than did PCP clinicians. For their part, clients in the constructivist condition showed greater participation and involvement in therapy, and the constructivist therapy on the whole was characterized by a greater frequency of more complex levels of differentiation with external and analytic focus, reevaluation, and integration. However, there were no significant differences in the extent to which clients in the two conditions saw their therapists as offering basic Rogerian facilitative conditions. Research such as this points to distinctive features in the two therapies that deserve further study in terms of their links to client outcome.

PSYCHOTHERAPY AS DEVELOPMENTAL RECONSTRUCTION

Theory

Several constructivist theories focus on the dialectics of self-construction, an ongoing effort that begins in the crucible of early attachment relationships and continues throughout life. Common to these approaches is an emphasis on the centrality of core ordering processes that regulate our sense of reality, identity, power, and emotion (Mahoney, 1991). The postrationalist cognitive therapy developed by Vittorio Guidano (Arciero & Guidano, 2000; Guidano, 1991) exemplifies this orientation, drawing heavily on research into cognitive psychology and human bonding patterns to conceptualize individual variations in how people construct personal theories of self and world. From this perspective, the form of one's relationships with primary caregivers in early life (e.g., anxious, ambivalent, or secure) influences the prototypical emotional schemata that one employs in subsequent relationships (e.g., by sensitizing one to the fearful anticipation of danger, failures in the self, or the threat of abandonment). Moreover, because the continuity of personal meaning processes rests on the interplay between the individual and his or her network of contemporary intimate relationships, the most disrupting emotions that can be experienced in life are those involved in establishing, maintaining, and breaking such bonds (Guidano, 1987).

At the heart of Guidano's theorizing are two levels of knowledge processes, which form a coalition between an explicit self-theory and a shifting array of tacit self-boundaries. Significantly, it is the tacit level of self-awareness, represented by images, feelings, and emotional schemata rather than by clear verbal labels, that organizes the flow of the person's experience and directs attention to particular themes in the world. For example, a woman raised with the threat of parental abandonment may come to have a delicate sensitivity to any nuance of withdrawal or distancing in subsequent relationships, even if she finds it difficult to "rationally defend" this intuition at a conscious level. This tacit awareness of potential abandonment may then activate a whole ensemble of emotional schemata (such as fear, anger, or self-protective rejection of the other), all of which pose challenges to her explicit sense of identity and her constructions of the relationship. In comparison to the highly articulated tacit level of processing, the person's explicit self-image consists of a more limited and conscious set of models of self and world (e.g., as self-reliant or resilient), whose verbalizability permits a measure of self-reflection and problem solving that is unique to human beings.[3] Thus, rather than representing a set of traits or a static achievement, personal identity is an ongoing process that seeks historical continuity through the coordination of tacit and explicit systems of self-knowledge.

Disorder

Problems arise in terms of this model when a person is confronted by a tacit awareness that cannot be adequately encoded in terms of an explicit self-image. In such a case, the person can move in the direction of a "progressive" shift in self-knowledge by extending his or her model of personal identity to accommodate the awareness, or toward a "regressive" reorganization that preserves the existing self-definition by "explaining away" the tacit emotional arousal. An example of the "personal cognitive organization" associated with agoraphobia illustrates this process.

Guidano hypothesized that persons prone to agoraphobia experience constraints on their autonomous exploration of the world during their childhood, which are indirectly imposed by overprotective parents who paint the world as dangerous or unsupportive, or who threaten desertion if the child ventures out on his or her own. Thus, in contrast to the healthy child, for whom exploration is encouraged by the "secure base" provided by attachment to the parent, the phobia-prone child comes to experience closeness and separation as antagonistic, mutually exclusive orientations. Under such a circumstance, normal impulses toward freedom and independence come to imply loneliness and the loss of protection of a powerful other, all of which are keenly felt rather than explicitly discussed. As a result, the child moves toward adulthood by walking a tightrope between perceived constraints imposed by others on the one hand, and desertion and loneliness on the other. This delicate balance involves excluding from explicit recognition all tacit experiences that activate needs for independence, and developing a growing set of somatic complaints to "explain" the troubling feelings, while at the same time ensuring proximity to a protective figure. The resulting adjustment is precarious, however, because the constant fluctuation between the need for freedom and the need for protection establishes fear as the most easily recognized feeling in the person's emotional range. As a consequence, the person with agoraphobia comes to structure an explicit model of self as "in control" not only of (potentially dangerous) interpersonal situations, but also of personal emotions, which come to be seen as shameful weaknesses. However, the carefully maintained exclusion of any feelings of dependence actually renders the maintenance of close relationships difficult, especially when a strong tacit need for independence or closeness upsets the balance and threatens the individual with loss of control. Guidano and his colleagues have devised similar models of several other prototypical cognitive organizations for such conditions as depression, obsessive–compulsive disorder, and eating disorders (Guidano, 1987, 1991; Guidano & Liotti, 1983).

Therapy

This conceptualization of disorder implies two primary goals for therapy. In an immediate sense, the therapist assists the client to attend to and "decode" problematic feelings that are "decentered" from the self, which then become data that can be used to progressively extend and restructure the client's explicit attitudes toward self and world. In the context of longer-term therapy the therapist can also direct the client in a "developmental review" that traces the origins of his or her explicit self-theories, and examines how these have precluded a more satisfying way of engaging the self and world. Detailed case studies illustrating such developmental reconstruction have been provided elsewhere (Arciero & Guidano, 2000; Guidano, 1991). Here we limit ourselves to an illustration of a "decoding" intervention in the context of a brief, eight-session treatment for a client presenting to one of us (R. A. N.—the "I" in what follows) with an anxiety disorder.

Karen was a 43-year-old, self-employed organizational consultant with a lucrative career, who had begun to experience pervasive anxiety that interfered with her work performance. A quick review of her past adjustment disclosed a long but infrequent history of panic attacks dating to her early 20s, which had nevertheless been untreated at the time. Although the seemingly inexplicable fear, heart palpitations, diffuse sweating, and lightheadedness that accompanied these episodes had been dismissed as "psychological" by Karen's general practitioner, she had gradually learned to minimize them through modifying her activities so as to avoid triggering such arousal. Recently, however, the panic was becoming more frequent and was accompanied by a growing baseline anxiety, which compounded her worries that something was seriously wrong with her. Pressed by her physician to consult a psychiatrist, Karen was subsequently referred to me for cognitive therapy when he became concerned about her potential addiction to the antianxiety medication he had prescribed.

Interpersonally, Karen came across as a somewhat driven, logical person, who described a relentless need to be "in control" of staff meetings, presentations, and business relationships in the corporate environment. Although she apparently related comfortably to others in such settings, she also hinted at the emotional barrenness of most of her adult life, which had been characterized by only superficial friendships and fleeting relationships with men. The clearest exception to this pattern was her current, apparently paradoxical relationship with her "underachieving" partner, Don, a part-time worker at an automotive supply store who idled away his time around the house, but who nonetheless had "been there" for her for the past 3 years. Now, however, their somewhat ambivalent but reliable relationship seemed jeopardized by forces outside their control, as Karen's company was changing its base of operations to a distant city, requiring them either to transplant the relationship, to abandon it, or to have Karen change her line of work. Although she complied willingly enough with a preliminary exploration of these issues, Karen was clear about her therapeutic goals: an elimination of the anxiety symptoms, beginning with the increasingly frequent breakthroughs of panic. Accepting this charge, I first established the contexts most likely to elicit the panic—being somewhere other than work, on her own, unprotected by Don. I then suggested a straightforward behavioral homework assignment: to take a walk by herself from her home in the direction of the local mall, and monitor both her level of anxiety and the accompanying "automatic thoughts" she experienced as she did so. Karen willingly accepted the assignment.

The next session, I was astonished by Karen's report that in keeping with the assignment, she had walked several miles, but without so much as a hint of anxiety. As we inquired more deeply into this unexpected outcome, an explanation gradually took shape: She could perform any such assignment *as (home)work*, although engaging in precisely the same exploratory behavior *of her own initiative* would immediately overwhelm her with paralyzing fear. The problem, therefore, was at the level of meaning, not overt behavior, necessitating a deeper inquiry into the significance of the disturbing feelings that began to surface during her anxiety attacks. As we focused more closely on these, Karen spontaneously flashed to an experience of similar terror in her early 20s, when she was "on the road" as a sales representative for a manufacturing firm. At that time, she recalled, she had felt a keen sense of loneliness, and had gone to the hotel bar to seek some human companionship. Karen became visibly anxious (requiring a structured relaxation intervention) as she recounted how she was subsequently followed back to her room by one of the men she met, who forced his way into her room and proceeded to rape her savagely.

In retrospect, we came to realize, Karen had assimilated this traumatic experience by developing a deep tacit rule that might be verbalized as follows: "I'm safe as long as I only do what I need to for my *work*, but I am vulnerable the moment I do something for *myself*." Karen's recent development of a nondemanding, "manageable" relationship with Don had permitted her to meet some of her needs for closeness within a personal cognitive organization centered on work and self-control. Now, however, the threat to this precarious arrangement posed by the impending relocation had led to a resurfacing of the old conflict between the "safety" of work-oriented loneliness and "threat" of seeking a more satisfying interpersonal life, perhaps without Don's protection. With these conflicting feelings made explicit rather than tacit, Karen noticed a drop in her baseline anxiety, and accepted my suggestion that she and Don come in together to work on the status of their relationship. Couple counseling further reduced Karen's propensity to panic, as both partners considered the meaning of a deeper commitment to each other, and ultimately decided to make the work-related move and seek further relational therapy in the new location.

Research

Guidano's developmental approach to therapy is anchored in several programs of basic research, such as Abelson's (1981) investigation of cognitive scripts and Bowlby's (1980) work on childhood attachment. Moreover, its extensive grounding in studies of childhood and adult psychopathology, primate behavior, and emotion give it a far broader base of scientific support than typifies most psychotherapies. On the other hand, specific interventions compatible with a developmental, reconstructive therapy (Guidano, 1995) are only beginning to be evaluated. The results of preliminary studies of various methods of enhancing clients' awareness of their tacit and explicit self-processing are encouraging, however (Mahoney, 1991). Moreover, the ongoing development of process coding manuals should permit future researchers to test presumed mechanisms of change in Guidano's "postrationalist" psychotherapy, such as the movement toward greater self-coherence resulting from a developmental review (Levitt & Angus, 1999). Finally, recent research on prospective users of psychotherapy suggests a general preference for developmental constructivist over cognitive/rational and behavioral interventions, suggesting the acceptability of such treatment to clients (Vincent & LeBow, 1995). More important, when clients' identification with the presenting problem was controlled for, this study found that individuals with an internal locus of control evaluated the constructivist therapy more favorably, whereas those with an external locus of control favored more traditional cognitive and behavioral interventions. Such findings suggest the complementarity of the two approaches and the possible utility of matching treatments to clients, rather than promoting a single form of therapy indiscriminately.

PSYCHOTHERAPY AS RADICAL QUESTIONING

Theory

One implication of constructivist epistemology is that because people have *constructed* what they take to be reality, they can quickly and efficiently *deconstruct* this same reality once they become vividly aware of their role in having created it in the first place. Difficulties arise when the higher-order constructions of self and world that make a particular symptomatic construction, action, or emotion necessary are unconsciously held, providing hidden coherence for the symptom in the person's overall ecology of meaning. In such cases, therapy appropriately takes the form of "radical questioning," whose goal is to bring to light (in an experientially compelling way) the tacit constructions that require the painful symptom, and to lay the groundwork for their transformation.

The depth-oriented brief therapy (DOBT) approach designed by Bruce Ecker and Laurel Hulley (1996, 2000) exemplifies the stance of radical questioning. DOBT maintains that brevity and depth in therapy need not be contradictions in terms, if the therapist assumes that significant change is possible in every session, from the very first contact. Clients typically bring to therapy a conscious "antisymptom position"—an earnest wish to be free of the anxiety, sadness, conflict, indecision, or other symptoms that cause distress not only for them, but often for their significant others as well. Where DOBT diverges from more traditional therapies is in resisting the temptation to contract immediately with a client to work toward elimination of the presenting problem. Instead, using an experiential rather than interpretive or didactic procedure, the therapist inquires into the hidden order in the client's apparent disorder, prompting the client to articulate and "inhabit" the more deeply embedded and unconscious "prosymptom position" that makes maintaining the symptom a vital priority. Once this is brought to light, resolution of the problem can occur rapidly and spontaneously, as the client consciously affirms the once problematic symptom (e.g., when a man recognizes the deeper rationality of procrastinating in pursuing training in a career that was not of his own choosing). Alternatively, the symptom may dissolve when the client recognizes that the previously hidden purpose of the symptom no longer has contemporary relevance (e.g., when an adult woman who was sexually abused as a child suddenly grasps that her lonely self-reliance serves a now-outdated protective function in a current relationship).

Disorder

The very concept of "disorder" is qualified in a DOBT framework, insofar as a construction, action, or emotional stance that is apparently dysfunctional or irrational in the conscious view of the therapist, significant others, and even the client is revealed as highly functional[4] and "rational" at higher-order, nonconscious levels. Thus DOBT can be seen in some sense as the antithesis of rationalistic cognitive therapies: Rather than instructing clients in specific methods of demonstrating the "cognitive errors" concealed in seemingly logical "automatic thoughts," DOBT provides a nondidactic means of revealing the hidden logic of apparently maladaptive client positions. Stated differently, DOBT presumes that the symptom is actually coherent with a deeper construction of reality held by the client, and can only be relinquished if and when a reconstruction of this higher-order meaning and purpose is possible.

Therapy

DOBT requires an empathic attunement on the part of the therapist to the client's very real distress (the antisymptom position), but also a detective-like persistence in inquiring into the deeply rooted purposes of this same presenting problem. In practice, this stance gives rise to a highly focused, but measured pursuit of the "emotional truth" of the symptom—the higher-order tacit meaning that makes it crucial to maintain, despite the genuine suffering it causes. The means by which this "radical inquiry" (from the Latin *radix*, meaning "root") proceeds are varied, but it typically includes the reflection of the client's predicament in deeply etched, metaphorically vivid language that engages the client at more than a "cognitive" level. Inquiry is furthered through a number of specialized techniques, such as the construction of carefully crafted incomplete sentences that provide a kind of magnet for unconscious meanings, and the use of various forms of visualization and direct statement that crystallize the prosymptom position in the client's awareness. Holding the prosymptom "reality module" in full view, while simultaneously inhabiting the contrasting antisymptom position, sets the stage for an "experiential shift" in the direction of resolution of the presenting problem.

An example of this process is provided by my (R. A. N.'s) work with Sara and Geoff, a couple in their early 40s who had recently divorced their estranged spouses to marry one another. In the course of their 3-year relationship and 3-month marriage, they had been through a good deal together, including a geographic relocation on both their parts and a career change on Geoff's. Though these transitions were stressful, others were closer to the heart, including the progressive death of Sara's beloved father approximately 9 months before, during which Geoff had been a major support. Now, just as they were consolidating their sense of being a couple, new and apparently more divisive problems were arising in connection with their children. In particular, Geoff's 15-year-old daughter, Kalen, was visibly remote and "pissy" around her father's new wife—despite Sara's initial efforts to befriend her, and despite Kalen's close and "special" relationship to Geoff. Although similar tensions had occurred between Sara's own daughter, Samantha, and Geoff, both spouses reported that he had handled the problem straightforwardly and with good humor, persisting in making overtures to her and at the same time requesting a modicum of respect. As a result, his relationship with Samantha had gradually warmed, while Sara's relationship with Kalen had clearly grown colder. Depressed, Sara admitted that her anxiety about Kalen's weekly visits had escalated to the point that she found herself "shutting down" and "backing off," finding excuses to be away from the house as much as possible at these times. Perhaps more significantly, Geoff added with a hint of anger, he felt "frozen out" of the relationship with Sara, who would withdraw from him as well as Kalen, only to moodily and uncharacteristically "pick fights" with him after the visit. Speaking clearly from the antisymptom position, both partners desperately sought a way out of this cycle, but an answer to the pernicious dynamic had eluded them to this point.

My radical inquiry into the systems of meaning that maintained the problem involved first asking Sara to recount a vivid recent circumstance in which she had strongly felt this relational problem. She quickly accessed a memory from Kalen's visit the previous week, in which Kalen had sat across the dinner table from her, her body positioned in an exaggerated orientation toward her father (and away from Sara), engaged in animated conversation with him that (intentionally) excluded her. Hurt and resentful, Sara had "swallowed her feelings" and left the table quietly, only to vent her anger indirectly at Geoff over the next 2 days. At that point in the story, I asked Sara to close her eyes and "reenter" the scene, pausing to let her reexperience some of the visceral sadness and anger she had begun to feel at that time. Using the method of "symptom deprivation" (Ecker & Hulley, 1996), I then requested that she continue to imagine the scene, but to stay in it without "backing off," instead engaging Kalen and Geoff in a normal, three-way after-dinner conversation. Within moments Sara opened her eyes and said abruptly, "I can't. I feel like I'm taking her father away from her." Moisture welled in her eyes as she began to access a previously unacknowledged sense of guilt about "stealing" the "wonderful father" whom Kalen loved and clearly still needed. With the emotional truth of Sara's symptomatic withdrawal in clearer view, I formulated it on an index card, which I then read slowly and evocatively back to Sara, as Geoff listened in rapt silence. Fresh tears flowed as she affirmed the phenomenological accuracy of the statement. I then handed her the card, and asked her to visualize speaking directly to Kalen as she read the words inscribed on it. Choking on the words "silence" and "guilt," Sara then read:

> Even though I am filled with sadness, and retreat from Geoff in icy silence, I would rather continue to live in fearful anticipation of your arrival than to suffer the stab of guilt that would come, if I were to take from you the sort of father who has been taken from me.

Only the sound of Sara's sobs broke the minute of silence that followed. Eventually, with Geoff now holding her hand to comfort her, Sara said, "That's really it, isn't it? That's why I can't be open and involved with her, like I am in other relationships. That's so *true*, but I'd never seen that before." With the session coming to a close, I asked her to keep the card and read it once each morning and evening, to help hold this new prosymptom position in a conscious rather than nonconscious fashion in the week that followed. The experiential shift introduced by this new awareness became evident the ensuing week, as both she and Geoff reported Sara's spontaneous invitation to Kalen to assist in making dinner for Geoff—an invitation that Kalen somewhat warily accepted. Equally important, Sara and Geoff had had a moving discussion of the death of Sara's father, and had decided together to ask her mother to visit them in their new home during the forthcoming holiday season. The icy distance and helplessness that each had earlier displayed were clearly melting, to an extent that neither felt the need for further sessions in the immediate future.

A view of radical inquiry as the "treatment of choice" for self-deception (in the sense of the unacknowledged tension between consciously and unconsciously held positions) characterizes some other forms of constructivist inquiry in addition to DOBT (Efran & Cook, 2000). Ecker and Hulley (1996) and Neimeyer (2000b) have provided other examples of depth-oriented brief interventions.

Research

In part because of its recency, DOBT has yet to be evaluated in controlled outcome studies, although substantial research on psychotherapeutic change processes suggests that it holds considerable promise. For example, Martin (1994) has conducted an extensive program of research on critical moments in psychotherapy, and discovered that those that were most memorable and important were those that enhanced clients' personal awareness and increased their depth of processing. Moreover, these significant interactions were characterized by the elaboration of client's meanings through the use of figuratively rich language, and especially the collaborative construction of metaphors that captured aspects of clients' positions in poignant terms. Quantitative reviews of psychotherapy outcome studies also have demonstrated the efficacy of emotionally evocative procedures like those featured in DOBT and kindred experiential approaches (Greenberg, Elliott, & Lietaer, 1994). Because of its brevity, its apparent impact, and its artful integration of dynamic and humanistic traditions, a therapy featuring radical questioning procedures deserves the attention of a wider circle of constructivist practitioners and researchers.

PSYCHOTHERAPY AS NARRATIVE REAUTHORING

Theory

As constructivist epistemology has shifted away from logical and computational metaphors of mind, it has increasingly embraced alternative models emphasizing "narrative knowing" (Bruner, 1990). In its clinical expression, this narrative impulse takes two general forms: the first aligned more closely with the models of personal science and developmental reconstruction outlined above, and the second with social-constructionist approaches predicated on rather different conceptions of language, reality, and selfhood (Neimeyer, 1998c). In this section we highlight the key features of both of these strands of narrative theory, and allude to the prospect of their integration in the practice of psychotherapy as "narrative reauthoring."

From a "cognitive-constructivist" standpoint, narration represents the prototypical form in which human beings organize experience, "emplotting" significant events by placing them in a temporal sequence that is projected toward a meaningful goal (Neimeyer & Stewart, 1998). Moreover, the stories we tell often speak at deeper thematic levels as well, revealing the "landscape of intentionality" as well as the "landscape of action" on which the story unfolds (Bruner, 1990). Thus, whether we are relating the events of our day to a friend, reading a novel or short story, watching a movie or TV program, or sorting through the significance of a lifetime of suffering with a psychotherapist, our lives are saturated in storytelling. From this perspective, narration serves an important intrapersonal function: namely, to establish continuity of meaning in our lived experience (R. A. Neimeyer, 1995a). In particular, confronted with a welter of life experiences that challenge our sense of consistency, we are motivated to construct a coherent self-narrative that makes our experience recognizable as our own (Hermans & Hermans-Jansen, 1995).

From a more social-constructionist perspective (Burr, 1995; Gergen, 1991), however, narratives are not so much the results of an internal process of structuring experience as they are the distillations of cultural discourses that configure and constrain the "identity scripts" that any given person can enact. One implication of this sociocentric stance is that the "culture tales" in which we are immersed in a sense "colonize" the self (Sass, 1992), providing the very concepts by which we define ourselves as male or female; young or old; or members of a given race, religion, or profession. This more social reading also sensitizes us to what people are doing or attempting to do as discourse users (Edwards & Potter, 1992), in terms of the implicit positions to which they are assigning self and others. For example, although there may be no transcendentally "true" account of the conflict between angry parents and a rebellious adolescent, this is not to say that each party will not push for acceptance of his or her self-serving version of events with any audience who will listen. Thus, from a social-constructionist viewpoint, narration is seen not as an intrapsychic process for representing personal reality, but as a political process for constructing a social reality (Neimeyer, 2000b).

A middle road between the extremes of cognitive constructivism and social constructionism is provided by a focus on the centrality of human relationships, the dialogical context in which storied accounts are actually related and identities enacted in our daily lives (Gergen, 1994; Tappan, 1999). Because we are all "heterogeneously distributed" across many different social groups with their own (often conflicting) expectations and rules, we operate not with a single self but with multiple selves, which vie for dominance in any given context (Wortham, 1999). Particularly when we find ourselves at the crossroads of intersecting relationships, we can experience the "tug" of competing roles and identities, as when we struggle over incompatible "position calls" voiced by our families, careers, or friends. Particular self-narratives (of ourselves as devoted parents or children, serious professionals, or loyal friends) therefore serve an important dialogical function, seeking validation for the plausibility of a particular identity script from a given relevant audience. Thus narration (temporarily) asserts the primacy of a particular version of the "self" of the storyteller, constructing an "as if" frame within which not only one's life, but also one's identity, achieves fictional coherence (Neimeyer, 2000b).[5]

Disorder

The complementary emphases of a cognitive-constructivist and a social constructionist view of narration give rise to similarly complementary views of disorder, situated largely in the self versus social network, respectively. In the first case, self-narratives disintegrate and become fragmented when a person can discern no meaningful way to bridge the past with the present, or when critical life experiences fall outside the intelligible master narrative of the person's life (Polkinghorne, 1991). This fragmentation frequently arises, for example, in cases of trauma, as combat veterans, victims of sexual assault, and even survivors of natural disasters find no adequate way to integrate their losses into their previous life stories (Wigren, 1994). As a consequence, they are often left with incoherent personal histories— ones one in which their objective losses are compounded by the loss of their sense of who they were (Neimeyer & Stewart, 1998).

In a more social-constructionist account, people experience problems when their identities are subjugated to the demands of a dominant narrative, as when a client comes to construe him- or herself preemptively as an "anorexic," "alcoholic," or "depressive" (Monk, Winslade, Crocket, & Epston, 1996). Of course, not all dominant discourses concern psychiatric diagnoses; as feminist therapists are quick to point out, the socially conferred identity statuses for whole genders and races can sharply delimit the permissible range of self-narratives for those who do not resist these requirements (Brown, 2000). In this sense, a person's identity can become *too* coherent—so subordinated to the social script that no deviations in the form of personal idiosyncrasies are tolerated.[6]

Therapy

In keeping with the more individualistic and social strains of narrative theory, narrative therapy encompasses two broad sets of procedures for developing a more coherent sense of self on the one hand, or a preferred identity on the other. At a general level, however, both of these can be viewed as forms of "narrative reauthoring," in which one constructs not only a more satisfying story of oneself as a protagonist, but also a more competent sense of oneself as author.

Constructivists concerned with the traumatic disruption of clients' identities through profound loss, assault, and victimization have frequently drawn on narrative conceptualizations to help clients reestablish a sense of personal continuity and find a "place" for the trauma in the stories of their lives. For example, Stewart (1995) has devised several novel group therapy procedures for assisting traumatized combat veterans in finding ways to "bridge" the naive youth who went off to war with the disillusioned veterans who returned. Likewise, Neimeyer (1998b) has drafted numerous biographical, metaphoric, and narrative exercises for promoting new perspectives on losses resulting from bereavement, job loss, geographical dislocation, and relationship dissolution. Because such experiences typically entail invalidation of the "assumptive world" that underpins one's sense of stability, worth, and meaning (Janoff-Bulman & Berg, 1998), this work is often intense, tacking back and forth between emotional reliving of the traumatic event and reflective writing or dialogue to promote its gradual integration.

Narrative therapists contending against dominating socially constructed identities tend to place the process of reauthoring in a more political than personal frame. For example, White and Epston (1990) specifically contend against the "individualizing discourses" in Western culture (and psychotherapy) that situate problems "inside" of people—a practice that not only pathologizes and shames clients, but also constructs a disordered identity that too often becomes a self-fulfilling prophecy. As an alternative, they characteristically "externalize" the problem, inviting persons subjugated to it to muster their personal and social resources to resist its influence. For example, a divorced man conflicted about his new relationship out of a sense of guilt about the dissolution of his marriage may be asked to consider the "real effects" of guilt on his life. Gradually elaborating on how guilt requires him to distance from his children, refuse to commit to his new partner, and treat himself in self-punishing ways, he may begin to consider ways to "push back" against the oppressive weight of the guilt, and thus to reclaim authorship of a preferred life story. As Freeman, Epston, and Lobovits (1997) note, "In the space between person and problem, responsibility, choice, and personal agency tend to expand" (p. 8). Narrative therapists have been especially creative in consolidating this sense of agency through carefully crafted and metaphorically evocative questions that unmask the influence of the problem on the person, and consolidate the influence of the person on the problem (Eron & Lund, 1996). These gains are often substantiated through narrative productions on the part of both therapist and client, such as therapist-drafted letters that vividly recapitulate client gains and point toward more hopeful futures.

An illustration of this arose in the course of therapy with Gerri, a 50-year-old woman diagnosed with bipolar disorder and treated with lithium for the past 30 years. Gerri had weathered many storms over this period of time (e.g., the stillbirth of a wished-for child, a devastating affair associated with her first manic episode, and her husband's long-standing combative relationship with a "good-for-nothing" brother who was nearly destroying their family business). Recently, however, she had been encouraged by her psychiatrist to seek therapy with me (R. A. N.) when it became necessary to change her medication because of increasing signs of lithium poisoning. The depression that ensued could be attributed to many factors, including pharmacological rebound; grief over her daughter's recent miscarriage; her own feeling of powerlessness regarding her deteriorating health; and marginalization in her husband's company, in which she worked as an underpaid secretary. Moreover, these setbacks were substantially compounded by her once supportive husband's increasing reliance on alcohol "to relieve the stress," leading to frequent angry outbursts and overall worsened family relations. "Burdened" by hopelessness and "eaten up" with suppressed anger, Gerri had begun tearfully to wonder aloud whether there was any point in going on living, as she anticipated deepening despair rather than joy in the approaching holiday season.

As Gerri told her story, I engaged in figuratively rich "curious questioning" (Monk et al., 1996) about how hopelessness and anger had wormed their way back into her life. Over 15 minutes of metaphorical discussion, we constructed an image of hopelessness as a creeping fog that made it difficult for her to see ahead, or even to see the people around her who might be reaching out to her in gestures of support. Anger was sneakier, coming in under the cover of the fog and carefully covering its tracks, while continuing to sabotage her relationship to her husband, William, and his with her. An avid fan of TV wrestling, Gerri had positioned herself by the end of the session in opposition to the pernicious influence of the "tag team" of hopelessness and anger, and even enjoyed a laugh or two at their expense.

In the next session 2 weeks later, Gerri looked like a transformed woman. Although still cautious about her improvement and concerned about her medication, she reported that William had actually accompanied her to her psychiatrist's office and had contributed several observations about side effects of the new medications they were trying, prompting a helpful change in her drug regimen. Even more impressively, although he had declined my earlier invitation to accompany Gerri to our session, William had reduced his drinking to a single beer per night, and spontaneously helped Gerri prepare a barbecue dinner for her daughter and son-in-law. For her part, Gerri found herself tackling and accomplishing a difficult record-keeping task at work she had been avoiding, earning the compliments of her husband and other employees in the process. My questions helped to "historicize" these developments ("What let you know that you had the strength to start wrestling with the fog that almost had you pinned?") and to recruit an audience for a preferred narrative ("Who in your life would benefit from knowing more about the way you and William are shaking off the stranglehold of the anger that nearly choked all the life out of your marriage?"). As we neared the end of the session, I asked Gerri for 10 minutes to draft a brief letter for her to deliver to her husband:

> Dear William,
>
> Talking to Gerri today was a true pleasure. As I'm sure you can tell, it is as if the aliveness is returning to her, after a long period of deadening. It is especially good to see her cutting through the fog of hopelessness that had clouded her view, and to witness her new optimism about the future.
>
> While I'm sure that sorting out her medication—in which you seem to have played a critical role—was a part of what made this new beginning possible, I also suspect that the efforts that each of you made to wrestle with these problems as a team played an even bigger part in these positive new developments. I am especially impressed at the kindness you each have shown the other, and the patience you two have displayed about the inevitable imperfections that we all share as human beings.
>
> As I head into Thanksgiving with my family, I find that I am also thankful for the hopeful changes in yours. Needless to say, I appreciate your efforts at home and at work to make a life possible for both you and Gerri that is truly worth living. I look forward to updates, and to hearing your thoughts about what seems to be a new chapter in the story of your relationship.

The following week I received a call from William, who asked whether he could accompany his wife to her next session. Their story was continuing to unfold in positive directions, and he said he was interested in talking about some new ideas as to how the momentum could be sustained.

Research

The narrative perspective receives empirical support from basic research in cognitive science, which suggests that people intrinsically tend to encode experiences in terms of "event structures" and "story schemata" (Barsalou,

1988; Mandler, 1984). This "storying" of experience in conscious declarative memory is compromised, however, by traumatic experiences that enter iconic memory as "unmetabolized" images and sensations, which resist incorporation into verbalizable accounts (van der Hart & Brown, 1992; van der Kolk & van der Hart, 1991). The result is a dissociated but affectively charged set of memories that are unintegrated into the master narrative of a person's life. Research on combat veterans and persons exposed to mass murder indicates that those survivors who fail to integrate the event into their constructions of their lives are at greatest risk for developing posttraumatic stress disorder (Sewell, 1996, 1997; Sewell et al., 1996).

Narrative research has also begun to make inroads from the laboratory into the clinic, inspiring taxonomies of narrative structure (Neimeyer, 2000b) and process (Angus, Levitt, & Hardke, 1999) that hold promise for the study of client processing in therapy. Likewise, specific narrative therapy procedures such as problem externalization are beginning to be evaluated in large-scale outcome studies (Rohrbaugh, Shoham, Spungen, & Steinglass, 1995), as are expressive procedures using narrative methods. One prominent example of the latter trend is the series of controlled studies by Pennebaker and his associates (Pennebaker, 1997), which has repeatedly replicated the efficacy of relatively unstructured, emotionally vivid written recounting of traumatic experiences in improving physical and mental health outcomes. The promise of such interventions is all the more intriguing, insofar as they depart fundamentally from the more directive, disputational, and didactic interventions that typify traditional cognitive therapy.

PSYCHOTHERAPY AS DISCURSIVE CRITIQUE

Theory

Although the epistemological orientations of the postmodern perspectives described above depart subtly or substantially from the realism underpinning most forms of CBT, the philosophy associated with radical-critical perspectives is the one that breaks most sharply with mainstream assumptions. Indeed, in its purest expressions this postmodern variation does not merely propose an alternative nonrealist epistemology, but rejects epistemology altogether. Calling for an "end of knowing," Newman and Holzman (1997) argue that the appropriate focus of psychology is not personal or social knowledge, language, or narrative, but "activity"—a focus that requires a new methodology. According to Holzman (2000), "activity" is distinguishable from both "behavior" as construed by behaviorists, and "agentic action" as understood by humanists. Instead, she uses the word in the Marxist sense to denote "revolutionary, practical-critical activity, [a form of] human practice that is fully self-reflexive, dialectical, transformative of the totality [and] continuously emergent." Psychological method, in this view, is inseparable from the object to be studied; central to both is our human capacity to create new patterns of living through "performances" that transform both ourselves and our environment (Newman & Holzman, 1999). As a critical practice, such a view is ultimately unconcerned with academic debates about what theory or therapy is right or wrong, but it is deeply concerned about the ways that such theories or therapies instantiate or help undermine oppressive social institutions.

Disorder

In a sense, radical-critical psychology goes a step beyond even social-constructionist and narrative models, arguing that dominant social discourses do not merely *engender* disorders in persons subjugated to them; they *are* the disorders that must be resisted in a politically informed practice. Organized psychology is of course responsible for much of this discourse, touting a picture of persons as "rational, unitary subjects"—an image that is "shot through with racist and sexist assumptions" (Burman, 2000). As Burman (2000) observes, "psychology makes us mad, in the sense of pathologizing irrationality as well as individualizing political resistance into personal distress." She and others are sharply critical of the *"psy complex . . .* [that] dense network of theories and practices inside and outside the academy and clinic, [which is] a dangerous and pernicious regulative apparatus [that nonetheless] fails" (Parker, 2000). The oppressiveness of mainstream psychology, in this view, is reflected in its endorsement of diagnostic systems that place disorders within persons rather than social systems, in its tendency to aggrandize power in the hands of a therapeutic elite, and in its scientistic quantification of human traits and presumed deviations. Because these "techniques of power" (Foucault, 1970) are deeply etched in Western cultural biases, criticism is necessarily directed against not only traditional psychology, but also the broader capitalist social system that it supports.

Therapy

Not surprisingly, this molar social critique animates equally radical forms of "therapy." Although criticism of the "psy complex" is itself a form of cultural intervention, more affirmative varieties of "social therapy" have also taken shape. As a group, these practices are a response to this question: "What does psychology need to be in order to reinitiate people's development given how oppressive and non-growthful societal conditions are?" (Holzman, 2000). One answer to this question would be that psychologists need to promote the development of whole communities rather than of isolated individuals in them. For example, the Castillo Theatre in New York builds performances relevant to the lives of its various marginalized constituencies, showcasing issues concerning African American, Latino, lesbian and gay, and women's cultures (Holzman, 2000). Likewise, the All Stars Talent Show Network promotes an antiviolence campaign with urban youth through the organization of talent shows that become community-wide productions. Significantly, young people not only sing, rap, dance, and perform plays in this program, but also negotiate with schools and churches for space, develop a publicity campaign, and mentor younger performers and organizers. It thereby gives youth who are typically overidentified with destructive behavior an opportunity to experience themselves as creative, as resourceful, and as having something to give (Fulani, 2000). Developing the assets of economically distressed communities in collaboration with neighborhood associations can serve similar empowerment goals (Saleebey, 1998). One advantage of such efforts is that they bring the same level of interest, complexity, and elegance to constructions of the community as are reserved for constructions of self and family within usual psychological discourse.

Despite the focus of much radical critical work on community development, there is no reason why a similar spirit of responsiveness (Shotter, 2000) and resistance cannot infuse the practice of an experiential constructivist psychotherapy.

An example of this arose in the course of my (R. A. N.'s) therapeutic conversation (Neimeyer, 1998a) with Alan, a young counselor who felt a "stab" of malaise when he said to a recent client at the end of a session, "It's been good visiting with you." Noticing a slight trembling in his jaw when he repeated this expression, I asked him to close his eyes, to attend to any "felt sense" in his body associated with this experience, and to describe it in an appropriate image. Alan offered a depiction of an "anxious, tight ball" in his chest, which, when I invited him to loosen it, brought a tearful recognition of the "guilt" contained in its tangled mass. Further processing this tacit meaning, Alan placed it in a larger narrative whose central theme was his lack of "genuineness" in relationships, and the way this was painfully accentuated by his initial attempts to conduct psychotherapy. As we "tacked" from this self-narrative to the social dynamics that sustained it, Alan linked his sense of insufficient genuineness to stern injunctions delivered during his early graduate training to maintain professional distance. Further discussion established that this message in turn replicated broader disciplinary and cultural discourses of psychotherapy as a scientific procedure delivered with a minimum of personal involvement. With our own emotionally intimate encounter as a salient counterexample, I then joined Alan in critiquing the dominant narrative of psychotherapy as an impersonal technical intervention, and in exploring the hopeful possibility that his experience as a counselor might actually become a setting in which he could deepen rather than constrain his engagement with others. Thus Alan's initially vague awareness of an anxious discrepancy between who he was and who he wanted to be had functioned as a "unique outcome," representing the first emergence of resistance against an oppressive disciplinary script of self-monitoring and restraint. Alan's case therefore serves as a reminder that a critical, emancipatory attitude can find expression in individual therapy as well as broad-scale social action.

Research

In keeping with its rejection of epistemology, radical-critical theorists are typically dismissive of empirical research, contending that the performance of their method requires no justification beyond itself. As Holzman (2000) argues, "we don't take objective criteria to be valid tools to evaluate us. We don't accept the terms of the debate. Objective distance is precisely what we are critiquing, in practical-critical fashion, by building environments that do not depend on or have a use for it." However, it might be acknowledged that not all radical theorists are fully consistent in their rejection of objective data, as when they cite reductions in crime statistics in those neighborhoods that most actively develop a culture around the All Stars Talent Show Network or similar initiatives (Fulani, 2000). But even from a conservative perspective, it is clear that the evaluation of "revolutionary" community-based development initiatives would require very different methods and criteria from those that typify an individualizing psychotherapy featuring the correction of cognitive distortions and training in appropriate cognitive and behavioral skills.

CONCLUSIONS

Like all disciplines, the field of psychotherapy is evolving, in response to conceptual developments both internal to psychology and in the broader culture. In this chapter, we have reviewed one influential outgrowth of the postmodern epistemological shift—one that gives the construction of human meaning and activity a more personal and social grounding. The constructivist, narrative, and discursive approaches cultivated by these changes have arguably deepened the theoretical roots of the cognitive therapies, and have begun to bear fruit in novel forms of psychotherapeutic practice.

How are these constructivist developments likely to be received by more traditional cognitive theorists and therapists? At one level, a number of cognitive therapists have already shifted visibly in a constructivist direction, emphasizing the narrative organization of experience (e.g., Meichenbaum, 1995) or the role of problematic self-schemata arising from early developmental relationships (e.g., Bricker, Young, & Flanagan, 1993). Even Ellis (1997, 1998), who is often portrayed as the prototypical rationalist, has in recent years protested that his theory is constructivist and even postmodern in orientation! Thus it seems to be a safe prediction that cognitive theorists will continue to build bridges to constructivist approaches, at least to those characterized by relatively more familiar emphases on personal science or developmental reconstruction. Moreover, it is probable that many practitioners of CBT will experiment with less familiar but intriguing change strategies associated with radical questioning, narrative reauthoring, or (perhaps) even discursive critique.[7] Of course, as cognitive therapists would recognize, familiarity is in the eye of the beholder, so that the degree to which a given constructivist model can be assimilated by a given therapist says at least as much about the therapist's schemata as it does about the model being construed! From this more personal perspective, we hope that an engagement with selected constructivist ideas will challenge the reader to consider fresh possibilities for the conceptualization and treatment of psychological distress.

From a more theoretical perspective, however, we suspect that the full integration of traditional cognitive and constructivist models advocated by some authors (Ramsay, 1998) will encounter conceptual obstacles. If models of therapy are viewed as being built around a core set of theoretical and metatheoretical commitments, which in turn cohere with a formal theory, a set of clinical heuristics, and finally a repertory of characteristic techniques, then deep-level epistemological incompatibility can impede a meaningful synthesis of the resulting models (R. A. Neimeyer, 1993; Neimeyer & Feixas, 1990). For example, the prevailing tendency to situate "problems" in the cognitive worlds of individuals would be viewed with suspicion by radical-critical theorists and many narrative therapists, and a rationalistic, disputative, and didactic style of therapy would be eschewed by most constructivist approaches. For their part, some CBT theorists are likely to be uncomfortable with the emotionally evocative developmental and experiential methods reviewed here, and others would no doubt resist the enthusiastic call for an "unscientific psychology" voiced by radical-performative therapists. Thus it remains to be seen whether a genuine theoretical hybrid of constructivist and cognitive therapies will prove viable, or whether eclectic practitioners will resort to simply grafting the techniques of one system onto the rootstock of the other. In our view, the most progressive synthesis in the two perspectives would require a liberalization of the traditional realist epistemology associated with more rationalistic cognitive therapies. Such a shift would invite wider use of interventions promoting greater coherence, complexity, and consensual validation of a client's constructed meanings, with a corresponding deemphasis on clients' avoiding a putative list of "cognitive errors" or squaring their beliefs with a presumed "objective reality" (R. A. Neimeyer, 1995b). Although there are signs that such a "paradigm shift" is under way, work in the philosophy of science suggests that changes in the "hard core" of a field's sustaining assumptions are not completed quickly or easily (Kuhn, 1972; Lakatos, 1974).

A related question concerns the viability of constructivist approaches in the current climate of managed care, with its emphasis on short-term interventions and therapist "accountability." In many respects, constructivist and narrative therapies seem well positioned to compete or even thrive in such an environment (Neimeyer & Raskin, 2000b). For example, Kelly's (1955/1991) fixed-role therapy, with its active emphasis on promoting significant change within a fixed interval of 2 to 4 weeks, represented the original form of brief therapy. The recent proliferation of DOBT and a range of broadly constructivist solution-focused therapies (Hoyt, 1998) has continued this trend, as such therapies have found widespread acceptance among practitioners in all of the helping professions. Managed care executives and treatment planners are not epistemologists, and are likely to embrace any responsible approach that proves expedient and efficacious in reducing client distress and enhancing client satisfaction in "real-world" settings, as assessed by straightforward outcome measures implemented ultimately by third-party payers. There is evidence that this orientation toward cost containment will "level the playing field" among practitioners of many orientations, as long as they adopt the "attitude and expectation—supported by various theories, methodologies, and findings—that significant and beneficial changes can be brought about relatively quickly . . . and that patients can then maintain and often expand the benefits on their own" (Hoyt, 1995, pp. 442–443).

How constructivist therapies will fare in the world of academic psychology is a separate question, but one that also seems to be yielding a cautiously optimistic answer. On the one hand, references to constructivism, social constructionism, and narrative approaches have burgeoned in the past decade, forming a vast if not wholly integrated professional literature in the form of journal articles, scholarly volumes, and practitioner sourcebooks. On the other hand, the theoretical emphasis of some of this work can prove daunting to students and researchers, both of whom show a preference for simple, parsimonious interventions that can be easily learned and operationalized. The general resistance of constructivists to this level of manualization of therapy methods, combined with their greater interest in studying basic psychotherapeutic change processes than outcomes of specific "name-brand" theories, may limit the growth of the perspective in more conservative academic departments. However, virtually every significant shift in psychological theory—from psychoanalysis through behavioristic, humanistic, systemic, and cognitive perspectives—has been ushered in by a passionate period of conceptual elaboration and defense, prior to the refinement of concrete interventions and empirical research. Viewed from the standpoint of the sociology of science, there is ample evidence that constructivism as a "theory group" is currently undergoing just such a shift toward more differentiation and widespread institutionalization, during which programs of research and application will diversify (Neimeyer, 1987; Neimeyer & Martin, 1996).

Does this imply that constructivist approaches will soon be "mainstreamed" to the point at which they will become the establishment position in academic psychology? Although such an outcome is not inconceivable—recall that only a generation ago, cognitive perspectives were considered quite radical—we believe this is unlikely to happen for several reasons. One of these is the consistent iconoclasm of postmodern approaches in general, which gain much of their impetus from a critique of established structures, whatever their theoretical persuasion. The succession of constructivist emphases reviewed in this chapter shows just this sort of increasingly radical tendency, suggesting that at least some versions of postmodern theory will continue to develop at the margins of institutionalized psychotherapy, while other variants are more likely to work within established institutions. In our view, both are essentially constructive (and ineluctable) trends in the development of any social-scientific specialty, and help sharpen debates about issues and methods that ultimately promote more adequate and useful theories of human existence.

Whether or not full integration of the cognitive and constructivist therapies is feasible or desirable, it is clear that the latter are already making novel contributions to psychotherapeutic theory, research, and practice. We hope that this chapter furthers this trend, and that the resulting extensions increase the richness as well as the scope of the cognitive therapies.

NOTES

1. For convenience, we use the term "constructivist" to encompass the broad panoply of perspectives that emphasize those processes by which meaning is constructed by human beings in personal, interpersonal, and social contexts. As in any "family," relations among the burgeoning set of approaches sharing this moniker

are marked by occasional dissent as well as agreement, as we note in the pages to follow.

2. Indeed, constructivism itself represents not so much a dividing line segregating some therapies from others, as a dimension along which therapies of all kinds can be arrayed. Thus constructivist and narrative themes have begun to permeate not only CBT, as argued here, but also psychodynamic, systemic, and humanistic therapies as well (Neimeyer & Feixas, 1990). This perspective helps account for the reduced enthusiasm constructivist researchers display for "horse race" comparisons of different therapies, and their greater interest in studies of constructive change processes in therapies of all persuasions (Angus & Hardke, 1994; Toukmanian & Rennie, 1992). However, several groups of constructivist researchers are indeed committed to evaluating the outcome of their approaches, as work cited in this chapter and described in greater length elsewhere demonstrates (R. A. Neimeyer, 1995b).

3. Elsewhere, Guidano (1991) described this two-level process in terms of the basic dialectic between "experiencing" (associated with the tacit level) and "explanation" (linked to the explicit level of processing). Prior to his death in August 1999, he had also begun to reformulate this model in narrative terms that aligned it more closely with the cognitively oriented narrative work summarized below (Arciero & Guidano, 2000).

4. Because of the brevity of coverage required in this chapter, our example and discussion focus on a simpler case of symptomatology that serves a function at higher-order levels of the person's system of meaning. However, symptoms may also be "functionless" by-products of a compellingly necessary unconscious construction and may still be resolved through the same process of radical questioning and experiential shift. For a detailed case example along these lines, see Ecker and Hulley (2000).

5. From a more humanistic or cognitive standpoint, the reader might raise the question of whether these various personas or self-images vary in their authenticity or validity. From the more social-constructivist position summarized here, however, the question is not whether one image is more *valid* than another, but whether one will be *validated* by relevant audiences in the social world. Thus the defining feature of the stories we tell or enact is that they seek validation through the response of others, imparting a provisional structure to the shifting fiction that constitutes the only sense of identity we can achieve. For a more thorough discussion of these themes, see Neimeyer (2000b).

6. Neimeyer and Levitt (2000) have construed disorder in terms of the "dialectics of coherence" in one's narrative of life transitions, yielding a matrix of problematic narratives that vary by context (intrapersonal, interpersonal, cultural) and by type of problem (disrupted narratives vs. dominating narratives). Disrupted narratives are further divided into two types (problems of chaos and conflict), as are dominating narratives (problems of consistency and conformity). However, an explication and illustration of the resulting 12 patterns of narrative disorder would carry us beyond the scope of this summary coverage.

7. The use of cognitive therapy in the discursive deconstruction of oppressive cultural narratives regarding homosexuality, for example, characterizes Christine Padesky's (1997) cognitive work with gay and lesbian clients.

REFERENCES

Abelson, R. P. (1981). Psychological status of the script concept. *American Psychologist, 36*, 715–729.

Alexander, P. C., Neimeyer, R. A., & Follette, V. M. (1991). Group therapy for women sexually abused as children: A controlled study and investigation of individual differences. *Journal of Interpersonal Violence, 6*, 219–231.

Alexander, P. C., Neimeyer, R. A., Follette, V. M., Moore, M. K., & Harter, S. L. (1989). A comparison of group treatments of women sexually abused as children. *Journal of Consulting and Clinical Psychology, 57*, 479–483.

Angus, L., & Hardke, K. (1994). Narrative processes in psychotherapy. *Canadian Psychology, 35*, 190–203.

Angus, L., Levitt, H., & Hardke, L. (1999). Narrative processes and psychotherapeutic change: An integrative approach to psychotherapy research and practice. *Journal of Clinical Psychology, 55*(10), 1255–1270.

Appignanesi, R., & Garratt, C. (1995). *Postmodernism for beginners.* Cambridge, England: Icon/Penguin.

Arciero, G., & Guidano, V. F. (2000). Experience, explanation, and the quest for coherence. In R. A. Neimeyer & J. D. Raskin (Eds.), *Constructions of disorder: Meaning-making frameworks for psychotherapy* (pp. 91–117). Washington, DC: American Psychological Association.

Bannister, D. (1977). The logic of passion. In D. Bannister (Ed.), *New perspectives in personal construct theory* (pp. 21–38). London: Academic Press.

Barsalou, L. W. (1988). The content and organization of autobiographical memories. In U. Neisser & E. Winograd (Eds.), *Remembering reconsidered* (pp. 193–243). Cambridge, England: Cambridge University Press.

Beck, A. T. (1993). Cognitive therapy: Past, present, and future. *Journal of Consulting and Clinical Psychology, 61*, 194–198.

Beck, A. T., Rush, J., Shaw, B., & Emery, G. (1979). *Cognitive therapy of depression.* New York: Guilford Press.

Botella, L. (1995). Personal construct theory, constructivism, and postmodern thought. In R. A. Neimeyer & G. J. Neimeyer (Eds.), *Advances in personal construct psychology* (Vol. 3, pp. 3–35). Greenwich, CT: JAI Press.

Bowlby, J. (1980). *Attachment and loss: Vol. 3. Sadness and depression.* London: Hogarth.

Bricker, D., Young, J. E., & Flanagan, C. M. (1993). Schema focused cognitive therapy. In K. T. Kuehlwein & H. Rosen (Eds.), *Cognitive therapies in action* (pp. 88–125). San Francisco: Jossey-Bass.

Brown, L. (2000). Discomforts of the powerless. In R. A. Neimeyer & J. D. Raskin (Eds.), *Constructions of disorder: Meaning-making frameworks for psychotherapy* (pp. 287–308). Washington, DC: American Psychological Association.

Bruner, J. (1990). *Acts of meaning.* Cambridge, MA: Harvard University Press.

Burman, E. (2000). Method, measurement and madness. In L. Holzman & J. Morss (Eds.), *Postmodern psychologies and societal practice.* New York: Routledge.

Burr, V. (1995). *An introduction to social constructionism.* London: Routledge.

Dobson, K., & Pusch, D. (1993). Towards a definition of the conceptual and empirical boundaries of cognitive therapy. *Australian Psychologist, 28*, 137–144.

Ecker, B., & Hulley, L. (1996). *Depth-oriented brief therapy*. San Francisco: Jossey-Bass.

Ecker, B., & Hulley, L. (2000). The order in clinical "disorder": Symptom coherence in depth-oriented brief therapy. In R. A. Neimeyer & J. D. Raskin (Eds.), *Constructions of disorder: Meaning-making frameworks for psychotherapy* (pp. 63–90). Washington, DC: American Psychological Association.

Edwards, D., & Potter, J. (1992). *Discursive psychology*. Newbury Park, CA: Sage.

Efran, J. S., & Cook, P. F. (2000). Linguistic ambiguity as a diagnostic tool. In R. A. Neimeyer & J. D. Raskin (Eds.), *Constructions of disorder: Meaning-making frameworks for psychotherapy* (pp. 121–143). Washington, DC: American Psychological Association.

Efran, J. S., & Fauber, R. L. (1995). Radical constructivism: Questions and answers. In R. A. Neimeyer & M. J. Mahoney (Eds.), *Constructivism in psychotherapy* (pp. 275–302). Washington, DC: American Psychological Association.

Ellis, A. (1993). Reflections on rational–emotive therapy. *Journal of Consulting and Clinical Psychology, 61*, 199–201.

Ellis, A. (1997). Postmodern ethics for active–directive counseling and psychotherapy. *Journal of Mental Health Counseling, 19*, 211–225.

Ellis, A. (1998). How rational emotive behavior therapy belongs in the constructivist camp. In M. F. Hoyt (Ed.), *The handbook of constructive therapies: Innovative techniques from leading practitioners* (pp. 83–99). San Francisco: Jossey-Bass.

Epting, F. R. (1984). *Personal construct counseling and psychotherapy*. New York: Wiley.

Eron, J. B., & Lund, T. W. (1996). *Narrative solutions in brief therapy*. New York: Guilford Press.

Faidley, A. J., & Leitner, L. M. (1993). *Assessing experience in psychotherapy: Personal construct alternatives*. Westport, CT: Praeger.

Foucault, M. (1970). *The order of things: An archaeology of the human sciences*. New York: Pantheon.

Fransella, F. (1993). The construct of resistance in psychotherapy. In L. Leitner & G. Dunnett (Eds.), *Critical issues in personal construct psychology* (pp. 117–134). Malabar, CA: Krieger.

Fransella, F. (1995). *George Kelly*. London: Sage.

Fransella, F., & Bannister, D. (1977). *A manual for repertory grid technique*. New York: Academic Press.

Freeman, J., Epston, D., & Lobovits, D. (1997). *Playful approaches to serious problems*. New York: Norton.

Fulani, L. (2000). Race, identity and epistemology. In L. Holzman & J. Morss (Eds.), *Postmodern psychologies and societal practice*. New York: Routledge.

Gergen, K. J. (1991). *The saturated self*. New York: Basic Books.

Gergen, K. J. (1994). *Realities and relationships*. Cambridge, MA: Harvard University Press.

Greenberg, L., Elliott, R., & Lietaer, G. (1994). Research on experiential therapies. In A. E. Bergin & S. L. Garfield (Eds.), *Handbook of psychotherapy and behavior change* (4th ed., pp. 509–539). New York: Wiley.

Guidano, V. F. (1987). *Complexity of the self*. New York: Guilford Press.

Guidano, V. F. (1991). *The self in process*. New York: Guilford Press.

Guidano, V. F. (1995). Self-observation in constructivist psychotherapy. In R. A. Neimeyer & M. J. Mahoney (Eds.), *Constructivism in psychotherapy* (pp. 155–168). Washington, DC: American Psychological Association.

Guidano, V. F., & Liotti, G. (1983). *Cognitive processes and emotional disorders.* New York: Guilford Press.

Held, B. S. (1995). *Back to reality.* New York: Norton.

Hermans, H. J. M., & Hermans-Jansen, E. (1995). *Self-narratives: The construction of meaning in psychotherapy.* New York: Guilford Press.

Holzman, L. (2000). Performance, criticism and postmodern psychology. In L. Holzman & J. Morss (Eds.), *Postmodern psychologies and societal practice.* New York: Routledge.

Honos-Webb, L., & Leitner, L. M. (1997, July). The *DSM* and the destruction of self-meanings: A client speaks. In T. Anderson (Chair), *Disruptions in the therapeutic relationship: Influences of morality, ecology, diagnosis, and other cutting edge issues.* Symposium conducted at the 12th International Congress on Personal Construct Psychology, Seattle, WA.

Hoyt, M. F. (1995). Brief psychotherapies. In A. Gurman & S. Messer (Eds.), *Essential psychotherapies* (pp. 441–486). New York: Guilford Press.

Hoyt, M. F. (Ed.). (1998). *The handbook of constructive therapies: Innovative techniques from leading practitioners.* San Francisco: Jossey-Bass.

Janoff-Bulman, R., & Berg, M. (1998). Disillusionment and the creation of values. In J. H. Harvey (Ed.), *Perspectives on loss: A sourcebook* (pp. 35–47). Philadelphia: Brunner/Mazel.

Johnson, T. J., Pfenninger, D. T., & Klion, R. E. (2000). Constructing and deconstructing transitive diagnosis. In R. A. Neimeyer & J. D. Raskin (Eds.), *Constructions of disorder: Meaning-making frameworks for psychotherapy* (pp. 145–174). Washington, DC: American Psychological Association.

Kelly, G. A. (1991). *The psychology of personal constructs* (Vols. 1–2). New York: Routledge. (Original work published 1955)

Kuhn, T. (1972). *The structure of scientific revolutions.* Chicago: University of Chicago Press.

Lakatos, I. (1974). Falsification and the methodology of scientific research programs. In I. Lakatos & A. Musgrave (Eds.), *Criticism and the growth of knowledge* (pp. 91–196). Cambridge, England: Cambridge University Press.

Landfield, A. W., & Leitner, L. M. (1980). Personal construct psychology. In A. W. Landfield & L. M. Leitner (Eds.), *Personal construct psychology: Psychotherapy and personality* (pp. 3–17). New York: Wiley.

Leitner, L. M. (1995). Optimal therapeutic distance. In R. A. Neimeyer & M. J. Mahoney (Eds.), *Constructivism in psychotherapy* (pp. 357–370). Washington, DC: American Psychological Association.

Mahoney, M. J. (1980). Psychotherapy and the structure of personal revolutions. In M. J. Mahoney (Ed.), *Psychotherapy process* (pp. 157–180). New York: Plenum Press.

Mahoney, M. J. (1991). *Human change processes.* New York: Basic Books.

Mahoney, M. J. (1995). The continuing evolution of the cognitive sciences and psychotherapies. In R. A. Neimeyer & M. J. Mahoney (Eds.), *Constructivism in psychotherapy* (pp. 39–65). Washington, DC: American Psychological Association.

Mandler, J. (1984). *Scripts, stories, and scenes: Aspects of schema theory*. Hillsdale, NJ: Erlbaum.

Martin, J. (1994). *The construction and understanding of psychotherapeutic change*. New York: Teachers College Press.

McCoy, M. (1977). A reconstruction of emotion. In D. Bannister (Ed.), *New perspectives in personal construct theory* (pp. 93–124). London: Academic Press.

Meichenbaum, D. (1995). Cognitive behavioral therapy in historical perspective. In B. Bongar & L. Beutler (Eds.), *Comprehensive textbook of psychotherapy* (pp. 141–158). New York: Oxford University Press.

Monk, G., Winslade, J., Crocket, K., & Epston, D. (1996). *Narrative therapy in practice*. San Francisco: Jossey-Bass.

Neimeyer, G. J. (1993). *Constructivist assessment: A casebook*. Newbury Park, CA: Sage.

Neimeyer, G. J. (1995). The challenge of change. In R. A. Neimeyer & M. J. Mahoney (Eds.), *Constructivism in psychotherapy* (pp. 111–126). Washington, DC: American Psychological Association.

Neimeyer, R. A. (1987). An orientation to personal construct therapy. In R. A. Neimeyer & G. J. Neimeyer (Eds.), *Personal construct therapy casebook* (pp. 3–19). New York: Springer.

Neimeyer, R. A. (1993). Constructivism and the problem of psychotherapy integration. *Journal of Psychotherapy Integration, 3*, 133–157.

Neimeyer, R. A. (1995a). Client-generated narratives in psychotherapy. In R. A. Neimeyer & M. J. Mahoney (Eds.), *Constructivism in psychotherapy* (pp. 231–246). Washington, DC: American Psychological Association.

Neimeyer, R. A. (1995b). Constructivist psychotherapies: Features, foundations, and future directions. In R. A. Neimeyer & M. J. Mahoney (Eds.), *Constructivism in psychotherapy* (pp. 11–38). Washington: American Psychological Association.

Neimeyer, R. A. (1995c). Limits and lessons of constructivism: Some critical reflections. *Journal of Constructivist Psychology, 8*, 339–361.

Neimeyer, R. A. (1998a). Cognitive therapy and the narrative trend: A bridge too far? *Journal of Cognitive Psychotherapy, 12*, 57–66.

Neimeyer, R. A. (1998b). *Lessons of loss: A guide to coping*. New York: McGraw-Hill. (Distributed by PsychoEducational Resources, P.O. Box 2196, Keystone Heights, FL 32656)

Neimeyer, R. A. (1998c). Social constructionism in the counselling context. *Counselling Psychology Quarterly, 11*, 135–149.

Neimeyer, R. A. (2000a). Constructivist psychotherapies. In *Encyclopedia of psychology*. Washington, DC: American Psychological Association.

Neimeyer, R. A. (2000b). Narrative disruptions in the construction of self. In R. A. Neimeyer & J. D. Raskin (Eds.), *Constructions of disorder: Meaning making frameworks for psychotherapy* (pp. 207–241). Washington, DC: American Psychological Association.

Neimeyer, R. A., & Feixas, G. (1990). Constructivist contributions to psychotherapy integration. *Journal of Integrative and Eclectic Psychotherapy, 9*, 4–20.

Neimeyer, R. A., Harter, S., & Alexander, P. C. (1991). Group perceptions as predictors of outcome in the treatment of incest survivors. *Psychotherapy Research, 1*, 149–158.

Neimeyer, R. A., & Levitt, H. (2000). What's narrative got to do with it?: Construction and coherence in accounts of loss. In J. H. Harvey & E. D. Miller (Eds.), *Loss and trauma*. Philadelphia: Brunner Mazel.

Neimeyer, R. A., & Martin, J. M. (1996). Looking back, looking forward: Personal construct therapy in sociohistorical perspective. In W. Dryden (Ed.), *Developments in psychotherapy* (pp. 140–166). London: Sage.

Neimeyer, R. A., & Neimeyer, G. J. (Eds.). (1990–2000). *Advances in personal construct psychology* (Vols. 1–5). Greenwich, CT: JAI Press/Elsevier.

Neimeyer, R. A., & Raskin, J. D. (Eds.). (2000a). *Constructions of disorder: Meaning-making frameworks for psychotherapy*. Washington, DC: American Psychological Association.

Neimeyer, R. A., & Raskin, J. D. (2000b). On practicing postmodern therapy in modern times. In R. A. Neimeyer & J. D. Raskin (Eds.), *Constructions of disorder: Meaning-making frameworks for psychotherapy* (pp. 1–14). Washington, DC: American Psychological Association.

Neimeyer, R. A., & Stewart, A. E. (1998). Trauma, healing, and the narrative employment of loss. In C. Franklin & P. S. Nurius (Eds.), *Constructivism in practice* (pp. 165–184). Milwaukee, WI: Families International.

Newman, F., & Holzman, L. (1997). *The end of knowing*. New York: Routledge.

Newman, F., & Holzman, L. (1999). Beyond narrative to performed conversation. *Journal of Constructivist Psychology, 12*, 23–40.

Padesky, D. (1997). *Psychotherapy with gay and lesbian clients: Coming out* (Videotape). Philadelphia: Taylor & Francis.

Parker, I. (2000). Four story theories about and against postmodernism in psychology. In L. Holzman & J. Morss (Eds.), *Postmodern psychologies and societal practice*. New York: Routledge.

Pennebaker, J. (1997). *Opening up*. New York: Guilford Press.

Pessoa, F. (1998). *Fernando Pessoa & Co.* New York: Grove Press.

Polkinghorne, D. E. (1991). Narrative and self-concept. *Journal of Narrative and Life History, 1*, 135–153.

Polkinghorne, D. E. (1992). Postmodern epistemology of practice. In S. Kvale (Ed.), *Psychology and postmodernism* (pp. 146–165). Newbury Park, CA: Sage.

Radnitsky, G. (1973). *Contemporary schools of metascience*. Chicago: Regnery.

Ramsay, J. R. (1998). Postmodern cognitive therapy: Cognitions, narratives, and personal meaning-making. *Journal of Cognitive Psychotherapy, 12*, 39–55.

Raskin, J. D., & Epting, F. R. (1993). Personal construct theory and the argument against mental illness. *International Journal of Personal Construct Psychology, 6*, 351–369.

Raskin, J. D., & Epting, F. R. (1995). Constructivism and psychotherapeutic method: Transitive diagnosis as humanistic assessment [Annual Edition]. *Methods: A Journal for Human Science*, 3–27.

Raskin, J. D., & Lewandowski, A. M. (2000). The construction of disorder as human enterprise. In R. A. Neimeyer & J. D. Raskin (Eds.), *Constructions of disorder: Meaning-making frameworks for psychotherapy* (pp. 15–40). Washington, DC: American Psychological Association.

Rohrbaugh, M., Shoham, V., Spungen, C., & Steinglass, P. (1995). Family systems therapy in practice: A systemic couples therapy for problem drinking. In B.

Bongar & L. Beutler (Eds.), *Comprehensive textbook of psychotherapy* (pp. 228–253). New York: Oxford University Press.

Saleebey, D. (1998). Constructing the community: Emergent uses of social constructionism in economically distressed communities. In C. Franklin & P. S. Nurius (Eds.), *Constructivism in practice* (pp. 291–310). Milwaukee, WI: Families International.

Sass, L. A. (1992). The epic of disbelief: The postmodern turn in contemporary psychoanalysis. In S. Kvale (Ed.), *Psychology and postmodernism* (pp. 166–182). Newbury Park, CA: Sage.

Sewell, K. W. (1996). Constructional risk factors for a post-traumatic stress response following a mass murder. *Journal of Constructivist Psychology, 9,* 97–108.

Sewell, K. W. (1997). Posttraumatic stress: Towards a constructivist model of psychotherapy. In G. J. Neimeyer & R. A. Neimeyer (Eds.), *Advances in personal construct psychology* (Vol. 4, pp. 207–235). Greenwich, CT: JAI Press.

Sewell, K. W., Cromwell, R. L., Farrell-Higgins, J., Palmer, R., Ohlde, C., & Patterson, T. W. (1996). Hierarchical elaboration in the conceptual structure of Vietnam combat veterans. *Journal of Constructivist Psychology, 9,* 79–96.

Shotter, J. (2000). From within our lives together. In L. Holzman & J. Morss (Eds.), *Postmodern psychologies and societal practice.* New York: Routledge.

Stewart, J. (1995). Reconstruction of the self: Life-span oriented group psychotherapy. *Journal of Constructivist Psychology, 8,* 129–148.

Tappan, M. B. (1999). Authoring a moral self: A dialogical perspective. *Journal of Constructivist Psychology, 12,* 117–132.

Toukmanian, S. G., & Rennie, D. L. (1992). *Psychotherapy process research: Paradigmatic and narrative approaches.* Newbury Park, CA: Sage.

van der Hart, O., & Brown, P. (1992). Abreaction re-evaluated. *Dissociation, 5,* 127–138.

van der Kolk, B. A., & van der Hart, O. (1991). The intrusive past: The flexibility of memory and the engraving of trauma. *American Imago, 48,* 425–454.

Vincent, N., & LeBow, M. (1995). Treatment preference and acceptability: Epistemology and locus of control. *Journal of Constructivist Psychotherapy, 8,* 81–96.

White, M., & Epston, D. (1990). *Narrative means to therapeutic ends.* New York: Norton.

Wigren, J. (1994). Narrative completion in the treatment of trauma. *Psychotherapy, 31,* 415–423.

Winter, D. A. (1990). Therapeutic alternatives for psychological disorder. In G. J. Neimeyer & R. A. Neimeyer (Eds.), *Advances in personal construct psychology* (Vol. 1, pp 89–116). Greenwich, CT: JAI Press.

Winter, D. A. (1992). *Personal construct psychology in clinical practice.* London: Routledge.

Winter, D. A., & Watson, S. (1999). Personal construct theory and the cognitive therapies: Different in theory but can they be differentiated in practice? *Journal of Constructivist Psychology, 12,* 1–22.

Wortham, S. (1999). The heterogeneously distributed self. *Journal of Constructivist Psychology, 12,* 153–171.

Index

"ABC" model
  applications of, 339
  assessment and, 318, 322–323
  description of, 13, 299
  philosophical change and, 311–312
  research on, 338
Absolutistic cognitions, 301, 303,
    307–310
"Acceptance" (Ellis), 306
Acceptance of client by therapist, 314,
    315–317
"Activating Situations," 95–96, 97
Activity record, 355–356
Activity schedule, 160–161, 356–357
ADHD (attention-deficit/hyperactivity
    disorder)
  CBT and, 275–277
  parents of children with, 257–258
  reward conditions and, 264–265
  self-evaluation training and, 266
Adler, Alfred, 297
Adolescents. See ADHD; Conduct
    disorder; Youth, CBT with
Affective arousal techniques, 154
Affective education, 259–260
Affective states
  developmental level and, 250
  efficacy expectations and, 177
  evaluative judgment and, 182

Aggression in children
  CBT and, 266–268
  problem-solving and, 254
  social-cognitive factors in, 248–249
Agoraphobia
  assessment of, 52–53
  constructivism and, 404
  CT and, 366–369
Agoraphobic Cognitions Questionnaire
    (ACQ), 52–53
All-or-nothing thinking, 353
All Stars Talent Show Network, 419,
    420
Amygdala, 119
"Antiawfulizing" (Ellis), 305–306
Antidepressants. See Pharmacotherapy
Antiprocrastination exercise, 329
Antisymptom position, 408–409
Anxiety
  cognitive assessment of, 49–58
  cognitive therapy and, 16
  constructivism and, 399, 405–406
  depression compared to, 55
  depression with, 58
  perceived danger or risk in, 55, 57–
    58, 184
  REBT and, 331–333
  self-management therapy and, 184–
    187

Anxiety *(cont.)*
  sensitivity to, 50
  social type, 51–52, 57, 270
  in youth, treatment of, 268–271
  See also Agoraphobia; Panic
    disorder
Anxiety management training (AMT),
    19–20
Anxiety Sensitivity Index (ASI), 50
Anxious Self-Statement Questionnaire,
    54
Anxious Thoughts Inventory, 51
Approach-retreat method, 159
Articulated thought in simulated
    situations (ATSS), 42–43, 46, 48–
    49
Artificial intelligence (AI)
  computer-based therapy, 125–126
  field of, 117
  models of disorders and, 123–125
Assertiveness, self-report measures for,
    52
Assertive Self-Statement Test (ASST), 52
Assessment
  continuum of procedures, 41, 42
  CT and, 364
  of efficacy, 200–201
  Frequency of Self-Reinforcement
    Questionnaire, 199
  Learned Resourcefulness Scale, 199
  REBT and, 318, 322–323, 334–337
  relational/problem-solving model
    and, 221
  Self-Control Questionnaire, 198–
    199
  self-monitoring and, 196–198
  SIT and, 201–202
  See also Cognitive assessment
Assumption of patient control, 28
ATSS. *See* Articulated thought in
    simulated situations (ATSS)
Attachment theory, 148, 402–403, 404
Attentional paradigms in anxiety, 57–
    58
Attention-deficit/hyperactivity disorder.
    See ADHD (attention-deficit/
    hyperactivity disorder)

Attributional Style Questionnaire
    (ASQ)
  CT and, 376–378, 379
  description of, 60–61
  priming and, 69–70
Attribution retraining, 255–256
Attributions
  in depression, 190
  efficacy expectations and, 176
  measurement of, 60–61
  of parents, 257–258
  in problem solving, 214
  in self-management, 183–184
  in youth, 249
Automatic thoughts, 130, 352
Automatic Thoughts Questionnaire
    (ATQ)
  description of, 59, 68, 70
  self-management and, 202
Autonomy, 162–163
"Awfulizing" (Ellis), 303

B

Bandura, Albert
  motivation theory of, 256
  self-efficacy model of, 6, 175–178,
    184–185, 187–188, 190, 200–
    201
  social learning theory and, 8, 115
Beck, Aaron
  automatic thoughts and, 130
  as cognitive-behavioral researcher,
    10, 115
  cognitive theory of depression of,
    87, 88, 93–98, 105
  cognitive therapy and, 12, 14–16
  on depression, 62–63, 66–67, 74,
    349
  philosophy and, 118
  on psychopathology, 86
  See also Cognitive therapy (CT,
    Beck)
Beck Depression Inventory (BDI), 61,
    68, 364
Beck Self-Concept Test (BST), 62–63
Behavioral analysis, 98
Behavioral contingencies, 264–266

Behavioral therapy
  CBT compared to, 7, 8, 9
  CT compared to, 150
  REBT and, 297
  scope of, 146
Behaviorism
  clinical psychology and, 114–115
  criticisms of cognitive approach
    from, 112
  decline of, 117
Bibliotherapy, 326, 364
Bipolar disorder, constructivist therapy
    and, 398, 415–416
Blaming, inappropriate, 353
Body Sensations Questionnaire (BSQ),
    52–53
Booster sessions, 365–366
Borderline personality disorder, 88,
    91–92
Brainstorming, 215, 230–231

C

Case formulation
  components overview, 89
  Diagnosis, 93–94
  evidence-based psychotherapy and,
    105–108
  form for, 90–91
  levels of, 87–89
  overview of, 86–87
  Problem List, 89, 91–93, 100, 102–
    103, 106
  Strengths and Assets, 99
  in treatment, 102–105
  Treatment Plan and, 99–102
  Working Hypothesis, 94–99, 103,
    106, 107
Castillo Theatre (New York), 419
Catastrophic Cognitions Questionnaire
    (CCQ), 53
Cathartic models of therapy, 8, 330
CBT. See Cognitive-behavioral therapy
    (CBT)
Change in cognitive therapy, 375–379
Children
  self-control and, 248, 258–259
  SIT and, 180

See also ADHD; Aggression in
    children; Conduct disorder;
    Youth, CBT with
Chronicity and treatment efficacy,
    153–154
"Chunking," 357
Client obstacles, 325
Clinical interview as retrospective
    cognitive assessment tool, 45
Clinical psychology
  behaviorism and, 114–115
  cognitive perspective and, 115–116
Coaching analogy in working with
    youth, 247, 260
Cognition
  clinical science and, 113
  conceptual models of, 116
  developmental level in youth, 250
  errors in, 352–353, 362
  role of, 111–112
  See also Cognitive science
Cognition Checklist (CCL), 54
Cognitive appraisal processes, 5, 6,
    219
Cognitive assessment
  of anxiety, 49–58
  contextual cues associated with, 48–
    49
  of depression, 58–72
  future directions for, 72–74
  information-processing model and,
    40–41
  methods of, 41–45
  of patients in remission, 68–69
  of processes, 40–41, 54–56, 64–66,
    170
  of products or content, 41, 49–54,
    59–64
  self-report methods for, 43–46
  structured measures for, 45–46
  of structures, 40, 56–58, 66–72
  validity of, 46–49
Cognitive-behavioral therapy (CBT)
  classes of, 6–8, 12
  definition of, 4, 247
  diversity of, 11–12, 29–31
  efficacy of, 10–11, 149–154

Cognitive-behavioral therapy *(cont.)*
    growth in, 393–394
    history of, 3, 8–11, 114–116
    as integrationist, 147–148
    propositions of, 4–6
    similarities in types of, 27–29
Cognitive-behavior modification
    CT compared to, 354
    description of, 4
Cognitive Bias Questionnaire (CBQ),
    63, 68, 70
Cognitive distortions, 303–304
Cognitive Intrusions Questionnaire
    (CIQ), 54
Cognitive Response Test (CRT), 63–
    64
Cognitive restructuring
    description of, 12
    PST and, 226
    with youth, 254–258
Cognitive revolution, history of, 112–
    113
Cognitive science
    artificial intelligence, 123–126
    change processes and, 130–131
    connectionism and, 126–128
    history of, 116–117
    integration of cognition and affect,
        129
    linguistics and cultural
        anthropology, 128–129
    neuroscience and, 119–123
    overview of, 117–118
    philosophy and, 118
    usefulness of, 131–132
Cognitive therapy
    CBT compared to, 7–8
    overview of, 14–16
    structural psychotherapy compared
        to, 25, 26
Cognitive Therapy and Research
    (journal), 10
Cognitive therapy (CT, Beck)
    adaptation of techniques of, 155,
        158–159, 162, 164
    behavioral methods of, 355–357
    beliefs and, 350–351

cognitive behavior modification
    compared to, 354
cognitive errors, 352–353, 362
cognitive methods of, 358–363
collaborative relationship in, 156–
    157
constructivist therapy compared to,
    402
Daily Record of Dysfunctional
    Thoughts, 358–360, 365
depression and, 364–366, 370–373
downward arrow technique, 361
eclectic principles and, 145–146
efficacy of, 150, 375–379
expectations of, 350–351
future of, 381–386
history of, 146–148, 349
nonoptimal type, 363
panic disorder, agoraphobia, and,
    366–369, 373
REBT compared to, 353–354
relapse prevention and, 365–366,
    372–373
research on, 373–374
scheduling activities in, 356–357
schema work, 352, 362–363, 365
self-monitoring in, 196, 197, 355–
    356
SIT compared to, 354
Socratic questioning, 363
theory of, 350
therapeutic interaction, 353–355,
    374–375, 380–381
three questions of, 360–361
time course of change in, 379–380
with youth, 256–257
Cognitive Therapy Package, 369, 373
Cognitive Therapy Scale (CTS), 374
"Cognitive triad," 350
Collaboration with patient, 103–104,
    353–355, 380–381
Collaborative Study Psychotherapy
    Rating Scale (CSPRS), 374–375
Commitment
    problem solving and, 214–215
    self-management and, 183
Common factors eclecticism, 142

Community, development of, 419, 420
Comorbidity
  aggression and, 266
  of depression and anxiety, 58
  treatment efficacy and, 153
Comparative research, need for, 30–31
Compensatory skills, 376, 378–379
Compliance with treatment and self-monitoring, 196
Conduct disorder, 266, 268
Constriction, 398
Constructivism
  overview of, 118, 394–395
  REBT and, 301
  therapies and, 424n. 2
Constructivist, definition of, 423–424n. 1
Constructivist therapy
  cognitive compared to social perspective, 412–413
  CT and REBT compared to, 402
  developmental reconstruction and, 402–407
  dimensions of, 396
  discursive critique and, 417–420
  epistemological shift, 394–396
  future of, 420–423
  integration with cognitive therapy, 421–422
  narrative reauthoring and, 411–417
  overview of, 26–27
  personal science and, 397–402
  radical questioning and, 407–411
  viability of, 422–423
Control
  assumption patient has, 28
  locus of and preference for therapy, 407
  perception of, 187–188, 214
Convergent-operations approach to cognitive assessment, 46
Coping
  definition and types of, 219–220
  measures of, 378
  modeling of, 262
Coping skills, CT and, 364–365

Coping skills therapies
  description of, 12
  uses of, 7
  See also Stress inoculation training
Coping style
  efficacy of treatment and, 152–153
  externalization versus internalization, 159–161
Coping with Depression (Beck & Greenberg), 364
Core beliefs. See Schema
Correlational analysis, 383–385
Cross-cultural research, 131
CT. See Cognitive therapy (CT, Beck)
Cultural anthropology and cognitive science, 128–129

D

Daily Record of Dysfunctional Thoughts (DRDT), 358–360, 365
Daily thought record (DTR), 160–161
Decision making, 215–216, 232
Decoding intervention, 405–406
Deep muscle relaxation, 261
Defensive processes, 148, 309
"Depreciation" (Ellis), 303
Depression
  anxiety compared to, 55
  anxiety with, 58
  brain activation and, 120
  cognitive assessment of, 58–59
  cognitive assessment of processes, 64–66
  cognitive assessment of products, 59–64
  cognitive assessment of structures, 66–72
  cognitive theory of, 87, 88, 93–98, 349
  cognitive therapy and, 15
  constriction and, 398
  CT and, 364–366, 370–373
  efficacy of treatment for, 149–150, 151
  irrational thinking in, 63
  manic depression, 398, 415–416
  negative self-schemata in, 66–68, 71

Depression *(cont.)*
  personality style and, 73–74
  PST and, 235–240
  REBT and, 333–334
  self-control therapy and, 23
  self-management therapy and, 190–196
  stress and, 73
  time course of CT in, 379–380
  in youth, 254, 271–275
"Depth" approaches, 365
Depth-oriented brief therapy (DOBT), 407–411, 422
Desensitization techniques and REBT, 315, 331
Desiring, philosophy of, 305–306
"Determination by the weakest link," 384–385
Developmental approach, 118, 406–407
Developmental level
  behavioral contingencies and, 264
  CBT and, 250
  cognitive restructuring and, 250
  integration of findings and, 280–281
Developmental reconstruction
  disorder in, 403–404
  research and, 406–407
  theory of, 402–403
  therapy and, 404–406
Diagnosis in case formulation, 93–94
Diagnostic and Statistical Manual of Mental Disorders (DSM-IV, APA), 396
Differentiated assessment of current thought, 51–52
Dilation, 398
Directive interventions, 159
Discomfort anxiety, definition of, 313–314
Discounting positives, 353
Discursive critique
  disorder in, 418
  research and, 420
  theory of, 417–418
  therapy and, 418–420

Disorders of transition, 399
Disputing irrational beliefs, 324, 326, 329
Distancing, 351
Downward arrow technique, 161–162, 361
DSM-IV (*Diagnostic and Statistical Manual of Mental Disorders,* APA), 396
Dysfunctional Attitude Scale (DAS)
  cognitive therapy and, 362–363, 376–378, 379
  description of, 67–68, 73
  self-management therapy and, 202
D'Zurilla, Thomas
  problem-solving therapy and, 21–22, 211, 213
  training manual of, 224

E

EASQ (extended Attributional Style Questionnaire), 61, 202
Eclectic psychotherapy, 140–146
Educative nature of cognitive-behavioral therapy, 28–29
Efficacy of cognitive-behavioral therapy
  disorders and, 149–154
  matching treatment to patient, 154–163, 164
  research on, 10–11
Efficacy of cognitive therapy
  for depression, 370–373
  for other disorders, 373
  research on, 375–379, 381–386
Ellis, Albert
  belief change and, 4
  as cognitive-behavioral researcher, 10, 115
  constructivism and, 421
  philosophy and, 118
  See also Rational emotive behavior therapy (REBT)
Emotional reasoning, 353
Emotional stress, 220–221

Endorsement methods of cognitive assessment, 44–46, 47–48, 49
Epictetus, 295
Epistemology
  description of, 118
  postmodernism and, 395, 397
  radical-critical perspective and, 417–418
Errors in thinking, 352–353, 362
Ethical humanism, 296, 313
Event-related potentials (ERPs), 120–121
Evidence-based psychotherapy, 105–108
Existentialism, 296, 313
Expectancy theory, 50
Expected-utility theory, 215
Experimental psychology, 114–115
Externalization, 159–161

F

Fear of Negative Evaluation (FNE) Scale, 50
Feedback loop model of self-management, 181–184
Fixed-role therapy, 330, 400–401, 422
Formulation of case. See Case formulation
Fortunetelling error, 353
Free-association method, 42
Frequency of Self-Reinforcement Questionnaire, 199
Functional-analytic approach to case formulation, 98–99
Functional MRI (fMRI), 119–120
Furman, W., 264

G

Gate control theory of pain, 188–189
Generalized anxiety disorder (GAD)
  assessment of, 56
  CT and, 366, 373
Goals
  of CT, 364
  setting in PST, 229–230
  of treatment, 100, 101, 102–103

Goldfried, Marvin
  background of, 12
  problem-solving therapy and, 21–22, 211, 213
  systematic rational restructuring and, 18–19
"Graded tasks," 357
Group therapy
  constructivist therapy and, 414
  for youth with depression, 272–274
Guidano, Vittorio
  postrationalist cognitive therapy of, 403, 404, 406–407, 424n. 3
  structural model of cognitive dysfunction of, 24–25
Guided discovery, 363
Guided imagery, 261

H

Hamilton Rating Scale for Depression (HRSD), 238
Haphazard eclecticism, 141–142, 163
Hedonism, 298–299, 325–326
"High frustration tolerance" (Ellis), 306
Homework, resistant patients and, 158–159
Hopelessness
  assessment of, 61–62
  CT and, 364
Hopelessness Scale (HS), 61–62, 202, 376–377
Humor as technique, 313, 317, 328
Hypothesis
  framing belief as, 351
  testing of, 357
  See also Working Hypothesis in case formulation

I

Imagery techniques, 327–328
Implicit Associations Test (IAT), 368, 379
Impulsive behavior and CBT, 275–276
Inference of cognitive activity, 6
Information-processing model, 9, 40–41, 117
Informed consent, 107

Integration, meanings of, 143
Integrationist movement, 141–142
Internalization, 159–161
Interpersonal cognitive problem-solving (ICPS) model
  alternative solution generation, 230–231
  decision making, 232
  overview of, 22, 216–217
  problem definition and formulation, 228–230
  problem orientation, 225–228
  solution implementation, 233–235
Interpersonal therapy, cognitive therapy compared to, 150
Interview as retrospective cognitive assessment tool, 45
Irrational, definition of, 299
Irrational beliefs
  biological basis of, 299–300
  disputing, 324, 326, 329
  emotional disturbance and, 303–305, 313
  maintenance of problems and, 309
  measures of, 63–64
  research on, 337
  See also Rational emotive behavior therapy (REBT); Schema

J

Jumping to conclusions error, 353

K

Kanfer, Frederick, 23, 181–184, 191
Kant, Immanuel, 295, 395

L

Labeling
  as error in thinking, 353
  of problems and situations, 226
Language
  development of and self-regulation, 16, 178, 248
  linguistics and cognitive science, 128–129
  semanticists, 296
  semantic techniques, 326–327

Learned helplessness model
  assessment based on, 60–61
  depression and, 190
Learned Resourcefulness Scale, 199
Level of impairment, 162
"Levels-of-processing" model of memory, 70
Linehan, M., 88, 91–92
Linguistics and cognitive science, 128–129
Locus of control and preference for therapy, 407
Long-term efficacy of treatment, 153–154, 383
Loose construct, 389–399
"Low frustration tolerance" (LFT, Ellis), 303, 308, 331
Luria, A.
  developmental sequence of, 17
  theory of, 16, 178, 248

M

Magnetic resonance spectroscopy (MRS), 121–122
Magnifying/minimizing error, 353
Mahoney, Michael
  on cognitive approach, 112
  as cognitive-behavioral researcher, 10, 12, 115
  on philosophical foundations, 118
Mania, 398
Mastery modeling, 262
"Match game," 265–266
Meaning
  narration and, 412
  in panic attack, 366, 367
  personal construct psychology and, 397–398
  techniques for uncovering, 360–361
  See also Constructivist therapy; Schema
Measurement
  of assertiveness, 52
  of attributions, 60–61
  of cognition, 5, 45–46
  of coping, 378
  of irrational beliefs, 63–64

of self-efficacy, 200–201
of social problem solving, 217–218
See also Outcome measures; Questionnaire measures of cognition
Mediational model
CBT and, 4–6
CT and, 377
description of, 27
research on, 9–10
Medication. *See* Pharmacotherapy
Meichenbaum, Donald
as cognitive-behavioral researcher, 10, 12, 115
constructivism and, 421
SIT and, 16–17, 178–181, 190–191, 201–202
stress inoculation training and, 20–21, 185–187, 188–190
Memory
"levels-of-processing" model of, 70
trauma and, 417
in youth, 250
Meta-Cognitions Questionnaire (MCQ), 51
Metacognitive beliefs, 51
Metaproblem, 323
Mind reading error, 353
Mischel, W., 8, 115, 248
Modeling
REBT and, 316, 317, 328
with youth, 262–263
Mood disorder
brain structure and, 119
perpetuation of, 307–310
personality and, 73–74
severity of and efficacy of treatment, 153–154
See also Anxiety; Depression
Mood record, 355
Multidimensional scaling, 57
Multimodal therapy, 145
"Musturbation" (Ellis), 303, 305

N

Narrative reauthoring
disorder in, 413
research and, 416–417
theory of, 411–413
therapy and, 414–416
Negative Affect Self-Statement Questionnaire, 54
Negative emotions, healthy vs. unhealthy, 306, 314
Neural network models, 126–128
Neuroscience
brain activation, 119–121
cognitive and pharmacological therapy comparisons, 122
neurochemistry, 121–122
pharmacological mood primes and, 122–123
Nondirective interventions, 159

O

Observational learning, 262–263
Obsessive and intrusive thought, assessment of, 53–54
Obsessive–compulsive disorder (OCD)
brain activation and, 120
CT and, 373
tight construing and, 399
in youth, 270–271
Obsessive Compulsive Thoughts Checklist (OCTC), 53–54
Obstacles
to client progress, 324–325
to scheduled activity, 357
to treatment, 100–101, 102, 104
Orbito-frontal complex, 120
Origins section of Working Hypothesis, 96, 97
Outcome measures
correlational analysis and, 383–384
goals and, 100
indices for, 7
questionnaires as, 48
in social problem solving, 217–218
Overgeneralizing, 353, 362

P

Padua Inventory—Washington State University Revision, 51
Pain and self-management therapy, 187–190, 197–198

Panic Appraisal Inventory (PAI), 53
Panic disorder
  assessment of, 52–53
  CT and, 368–369, 373
  description of, 367–368
  panic attack, description of, 366–367
  safety behaviors in, 368
  self-monitoring of thoughts in, 43
  See also Agoraphobia
Paradoxical interventions, 157–158
Parallel-distributed-processing
    framework, 126
Parents
  behavioral contingencies and, 265
  cognitive processing and, 257–258
  efficacy of CBT and, 274
  modeling and, 263
  problem-solving with youth, 253
  role of with youth, 250–251, 278–
    279
  treatment termination and, 271
Patient Cognitive Change Scale
    (PCCS), 379
Penalties in REBT, 315, 329–330
Penn State Worry Questionnaire
    (PSWQ), 50–51
Perception of control, 187–188, 214
Perfectionism Cognitions Inventory
    (PCI), 59–60
Performance
  efficacy expectations and, 176, 177–
    178
  self-evaluation of, 181–182
Perpetuation of psychological
    disturbance, 307–310
Persistence, problems of, 174–175,
    176
Personal construct psychology (PCP),
    397–398, 399–400, 401–402
Personality
  emotional disorder and, 73–74
  REBT and, 302
Personality Data Form, 319–321
Personal science
  disorder in, 398–399
  research and, 401–402

theory of, 397–398
  therapy and, 399–401
Pharmacotherapy
  ADHD and, 277
  cognitive therapy compared to, 150,
    151, 194
  CT compared to, 370–372, 376–
    377, 381–382, 385–386
  CT following, 372–373
  neuroscience and, 122–123
  PST compared to, 239–240
Philosophical change, effecting, 310–
    312
Philosophy
  cognitive science and, 118
  REBT and, 295–296
Physiological arousal and efficacy
    expectations, 177
Platte, J.
  interpersonal cognitive problem-
    solving model, 216–217, 252
  problem-solving therapy and, 211,
    225
Play methods, 250
Positive Automatic Thoughts
    Questionnaire (ATQ-P), 59
Positron emission tomography (PET),
    119–120
Postmodernism
  constructivist therapy and, 417–418,
    423
  epistemology and, 395, 397
Postrationalist philosophy, 25, 26
Posttraumatic stress disorder (PTSD)
  constructivism and, 413, 414, 417
  Meichenbaum and, 17
  neural network model of, 127
"Precipitants," 95–96, 97
Prescriptive matching or therapy, 145
Prescriptive model of social problem
    solving
  overview of, 213–214
  problem orientation, 214–215
  skills for, 215–216
Prevention of relapse, 365–366, 372–
    373, 383

Priming
    cognitive assessment and, 48–49, 69–70
    neuroscience and, 122–123
    Stroop Color-Naming Task and, 71–72, 73
Problem
    constructivist view of, 421
    definition of, 212–213, 219
Problem-focused nature of cognitive-behavioral therapy, 27–28
Problem-focused therapy compared to PST, 237–238
Problem-level case formulation, 87–88
Problem List in case formulation
    benefits of, 106
    development of, 89, 91–93
    goals of treatment and, 102–103
    obstacles to treatment and, 100
Problem solving
    definition of, 212, 220
    solution implementation compared to, 213
Problem-Solving Approach to Adjustment, The (Spivack, Platte, and Shure), 211, 216–217, 225
Problem-solving therapy (PST)
    concept definition for, 212–213
    depression and, 235–240
    description of, 12, 21–22
    innovations in, 240–241
    interpersonal cognitive problem-solving model, 216–217, 225–235
    measures of, 217–218
    open-ended clinical applications of, 222–223
    overview of, 211–212, 236
    prescriptive model of, 213–216
    stress model for, 219–222
    time-limited clinical applications of, 223–224
    with youth, 252–254
Process measures in social problem solving, 217–218
Process research, need for, 30
Prosymptom position, 409, 410

PST. *See* Problem-solving therapy (PST)
Psychodynamic model, 9, 138
Psychological disturbance
    acquisition and perpetuation of, 307–310
    personality and, 73–74
    severity of and efficacy of treatment, 153–154
Psychometric issues in cognitive assessment, 49
Psychotherapy
    eclectic and integrationist views in, 140–146
    evidence-based practice and, 138–140
PTSD. *See* Posttraumatic stress disorder (PTSD)

Q

Questionnaire measures of cognition
    anxiety and, 49–51
    assessment and, 44–45, 47–48, 49
    as primes, 69–70
    social problem solving and, 217
Questions, three in CT, 360–361

R

Radical-critical psychology, 417–418, 419, 420
Radical questioning
    disorder in, 408
    research and, 411
    theory of, 407–408
    therapy and, 408–411
Randomized controlled trials (RCTs), 105–106, 107–108
Random sampling of thinking, 43, 56, 66, 73
Rational, definition of, 298–299
Rational emotive behavior therapy (REBT)
    acquisition and perpetuation of disturbance and, 307–310
    anxiety case example, 331–333
    assessment stage of, 318, 322–323

Rational emotive behavior therapy
  (cont.)
  assessment technology of, 334–337
  behavioral techniques of, 329–330
  CBT compared to, 312–315
  cognitive techniques of, 326–328
  as constructivistic approach, 301
  constructivist therapy compared to,
    402
  CT compared to, 353–354
  depression case example, 333–334
  disputing phase, 324, 326, 329
  efficacy of, 337–339
  emotive techniques of, 328–329
  evolution of name of, 297
  future of, 339–340
  image of person and, 298–301
  induction procedures, 317–318
  influences on, 118, 295–297, 313
  irrational beliefs, research on, 337
  nature of disturbance and health
    and, 301, 303–307
  optimism of, 300, 310
  overview of, 12–14
  personality dimensions and, 302
  Self-Help Form, 327
  specialized vs. general, 315, 340n. 2
  technique overview, 325–326
  techniques avoided in, 330–331
  termination of, 325
  theory of, 310–312, 325–326
  therapeutic process of, 317–318,
    322–325
  therapist role in, 314, 315–317
  working-through phase, 324–325
  See also "ABC" model
Rationalism, 118
Reactance, potential for, 156
Reason and Emotion in Psychotherapy
  (Ellis), 14
Recordings of spontaneous speech, 41–
  42, 66
Recursive model, 108
Referenting techniques, 327
Referral for treatment, 250–251, 266
Reframing, 226
Rehm, Lynn, 23–24, 191–195, 197

Reiss, S., 50
Relapse, prevention of, 365–366, 372–
  373, 383
Relationship obstacles, 324
Relationship-oriented therapy, 142
Relationship therapy from con-
    structivist perspective, 409–411
Relaxation training
  overview of, 260–261
  panic disorder and, 368
Remission, cognitive assessment of,
  68–69
Repertory grid technique, 402
Repetition compulsion, 128
Research
  on "ABC" model, 338
  comparative, need for, 30–31
  on constructivist therapy, 401–402,
    406–407, 411, 416–417, 420
  cross-cultural, 131
  on CT, 373–374
  on irrational beliefs, 337
  on mediational model, 9–10
  on personal construct psychology,
    401–402
  process type, need for, 30
  on psychotherapy, 138–140
  randomized controlled trials, 105–
    106, 107–108
  theory and, 138–140
  on therapeutic mechanisms, 385
  Treatment of Depression
    Collaborative Research Program,
    370–372, 381–382
  validation efforts in, 280–281
  See also Efficacy of cognitive-
    behavioral therapy; Efficacy of
    cognitive therapy
Resistance
  potential for, 155–159, 163
  REBT and, 325
Response Styles Questionnaire (RSQ),
  65–66
Reverse-advocacy role-play strategy,
  225–226
Revised obsessional Intrusions
  Inventory (ROII), 54

Risk-taking exercise, 329
"Robot-ragdoll game," 261
Rochester Social Comparison Record (RSCR), 66
Role playing, 225–226, 263–264
Role relationships, 400
Rumination, 127–128

S

Safety behaviors in panic disorder, 368
Scheduling activities, 356–357
Schema
    AI and, 124–125
    CT and, 352, 365, 376
    defensive processes and, 148
    definition of, 15, 30
    identifying, 362–363
    Implicit Associations Test and, 368
    interpersonal type, 130–131
    problem orientation and problem perception, 214–215
    Working Hypothesis and, 95, 97, 104
Schizophrenia, 399
School-based intervention
    for aggression, 267
    for depression, 272, 274
School phobia treatment program, 268–270
Self-Consciousness Scale (SCS), 65
Self-control
    children and, 248, 258–259
    definition of, 173
Self-control model
    development of, 10
    of Kanfer, 181–184, 191, 258–259
    of Rehm, 191–195, 197
Self-Control Questionnaire (SCQ), 198–199
Self-control therapy, 23–24
Self-disclosure, 316, 328
Self-efficacy model (Bandura)
    anxiety and, 184–185
    depression and, 190
    fear and, 6

measurement in, 200–201
    overview of, 175–178
    pain and, 187–188
Self-evaluation
    assessment of, 62–63
    definition of, 259
    of performance, 181–182
    youth and, 265–266
Self-Focus Sentence Completion (SFSC), 64–65
Self-fulfilling prophecy phenomenon, 309–310
Self-image, explicit, 403–406
Self-instructional training (SIT)
    for adults, 180–181
    assessment and, 201–202
    for children, 180
    CT compared to, 354
    depression and, 190–191
    information gathering phase, 179
    overview of, 16–17, 178–179
    promoting change phase, 180
    trying on phase, 179–180
Self-management therapy
    anxiety and, 184–187
    assessment techniques and, 196–202
    Bandura model of, 175–178, 184–185, 187–188, 190, 200–201
    depression and, 190–196
    Kanfer model of, 181–184, 191
    manuals for, 194–195
    Meichenbaum model of, 178–181, 185–187, 188–191
    overview of, 173–175
    pain and, 187–190
    Rehm model of, 191–195
Self-monitoring
    as assessment technique, 196–198
    of behavior, 181
    CT and, 355–356
    definition of, 259
    goals of treatment and, 100
    PST and, 234–235
    of thoughts, 43
Self-recording, 259
Self-Referent Encoding Task (SRET), 70–72

Self-regulation
definition of, 173
depression and, 64–66
youth and, 258–259
Self-reinforcement
definition of, 259
PST and, 235
self-control and, 182, 192
youth and, 265
Self-report methods of assessment
agoraphobia and, 52–53
anxiety and, 50–52, 54
assertiveness and, 52
cognitive assessment and, 43–46,
47–48
future directions for, 73
obsessive and intrusive thoughts
and, 53–54
Seligman, M. E. P., 190
Semanticists, 296
Semantic techniques, 326–327
Severity of disorder and efficacy of
treatment, 153–154
Shame-attacking exercise, 329, 332
"Should" statements, 353
Shure, M.
interpersonal cognitive problem-
solving model, 216–217, 252
problem-solving therapy, 211,
225
SIT. *See* Self-instructional training
(SIT)
Situation-level case formulation, 88
Social anxiety
assessment of, 51–52, 57
in youth, 270
Social Avoidance and Distress (SAD)
Scale, 50
Social cognition, definition of, 248–
249
Social comparison and efficacy
expectations, 176–177
Social-constructionist perspective, 412,
413, 414–415, 424n. 5
Social Interaction Self-Statement Test
(SISST), 51–52

Social learning theory
in current behavior therapy, 146
development of, 115
self-management models and, 175
Social problem solving
definition of, 212
prescriptive model of, 213–216
See also Problem-solving therapy
(PST)
Social reinforcement (SR), PST
compared to, 235–237
Sociotropy, 162–163
Sociotropy-Autonomy Scale (SAS),
162–163
Socratic questioning, 363
Solution, definition of, 213
Solution implementation
clinical example of, 233–235
problem solving compared to, 213
steps for, 215–216
Spivack, G.
interpersonal cognitive problem-
solving model, 216–217, 252
problem-solving therapy, 211, 225
"Stay in there" activity, 329
Stimulus-response model, 7, 8
Strategic eclecticism, 142–143, 144–
145, 163
Strengths and Assets in case
formulation, 99
Stress
in parents, 278–279
relational/problem-solving model of,
219–222
Stressful life event, 220
Stress inoculation training
with anxiety, 185–187
overview of, 20–21
with pain, 188–190
Stroop Color-Naming Task, 71–72,
73
Structural psychotherapy, 24–26
Subjective level of distress, 161–162
Subjective Probability of Consequences
Inventory (SPCI), 52
Substance abuse assessment, 91

"Success therapy," 357
Sudden gains, 380, 381, 385
Symptom deprivation method, 410
Systematic desensitization, 18
Systematic rational restructuring, 18–19

T

Task analysis, 384
Technical eclecticism, 142–143, 144–145
Terminology, problems with, 29–30
Test anxiety, 44
Theoretical integrationism, 142–144, 163
Theory, overview of, 138–140
Therapeutic bond in REBT, 315–317
Therapeutic interaction in CT, 353–355, 374–375, 380–381
Therapist
  acceptance of client by, 314, 315–316
  CBT with youth and, 247
  collaboration with patient, 103–104, 353–355, 380–381
  obstacles of, 324–325
  REBT and, 314. 315–317
  self-disclosure by, 316, 328
Think-aloud procedures, 42, 46, 56, 58
"Thought bubbles" in cartoons, 255
Thought listing, 42, 44, 56, 58
Thought Record, 88, 103
Thought sampling. *See* Random sampling of thinking
Tight construct, 389–399
Time course analysis, 384
Time-limited nature of cognitive-behavioral therapy, 27–28
Training methods, 224
Trauma. *See* Posttraumatic stress disorder (PTSD)
Treatment
  compliance with, 196
  critical sessions in, 385, 411
  evidence-based practice, 138–140

history of development of strategies for, 115–116
long-term efficacy of, 153–154, 383
obstacles to, 100–101, 102, 104
referral for, 250–251, 266
school-based, 267, 272, 274
sudden gains in, 380, 381, 385
termination of, 271, 325, 365
Treatment of Depression Collaborative Research Program (TDCRP), 370–372, 381–382
Treatment Plan
  case formulation and, 99, 101–102
  goals, 100, 101, 102–103
  obstacles to, 100–101, 102, 104
"Turtle technique," 267

V

Validity
  of cognitive assessment, 46–49
  content versus construct, 47
Verbal persuasion and efficacy expectations, 177
Videotape thought reconstruction, 42–44, 46
Vygotsky, L., 16, 17, 248

W

Ways of Responding (WOR), 378–379
Working Hypothesis in case formulation
  cognitive-behavioral theory and, 98–99
  cognitive theory and, 94–98, 103
  individual treatment plan and, 106, 107
Worry, assessment of, 56
"W" questions, 228–229

Y

Youth, CBT with
  ADHD and, 275–277
  affective education, 259–260
  aggressive behavior and, 266–268
  anxiety disorders and, 268–271
  behavioral contingencies, 264–266

Youth, CBT with *(cont.)*
  CBT with adults compared to, 249–251
  cognitive restructuring, 254–258
  depression and, 271–275
  integration of findings, 280–281
  modeling, 262–263
  overview of, 246–247
  parental involvement and, 278–279
  problem-solving orientation and training, 252–254
  programmatic vs. prescriptive intervention, 279–280
  relaxation training, 260–261
  role playing, 263–264
  self-control and self-regulation techniques, 258–259
  theoretical influences on, 248–249
  therapist role in, 247
  transportability and, 280
  treatment termination, 271